DIGITAL EEG IN CLINICAL PRACTICE

DIGITAL EEG IN CLINICAL PRACTICE

Peter K.H. Wong, M.D., FRCP(C)

Professor, Division of Neurology
Department of Pediatrics
University of British Columbia
Director, Department of Diagnostic Neurophysiology
Children's Hospital
Vancouver, British Columbia

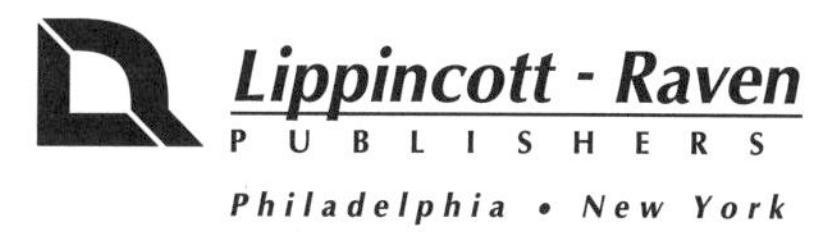
Lippincott - Raven
PUBLISHERS
Philadelphia • New York

**Lippincott - Raven Publishers, 227 East Washington Square,
Philadelphia, Pennsylvania 19106-3780**

Made in the United States of America

Library of Congress Cataloging-in-Publication Data

Wong, Peter K. H.
Digital EEG in clinical practice / Peter K.H. Wong
p. cm.
Includes bibliographical references and index.
ISBN 0-397-51635-5
1. Electroencephalography. I. Title.
[DNLM: 1. Electroencephalography. 2. Diagnosis, Computer-Assisted.
WL 150 W872d 1995]
RC386.6.E43W66 1995
616.8′047547—dc20
DNLM/DLC
for Library of Congress

95-32100
CIP

The material contained in this volume was submitted as previously unpublished material, except in the instances in which credit has been given to the source from which some of the illustrative material was derived.

Great care has been taken to maintain the accuracy of the information contained in the volume. However, neither Lippincott - Raven Publishers nor the author can be held responsible for errors or for any consequences arising from the use of the information contained herein.

9 8 7 6 5 4 3 2 1

To Elke, Carla, and Kelly

ERRATUM

a multiplication symbol (×) erroneously printed as a ˇ on:

page 9, lines 6, 8
page 13, lines 5, 6, 7
page 21, line 4

Digital EEG in Clinical Practice by Peter K. H. Wong
Lippincott-Raven Publishers, Philadelphia © 1996

CONTENTS

PREFACE

This book is written for the EEG practitioner who is familiar with traditional paper EEG technology who wishes to increase his/her skill in digital EEG methodology and technology. It assumes a basic knowledge of clinical EEG.

The novice reader is advised to start at the beginning of this book. The expert reader who already has some familiarity with digital techniques may skip the first two chapters. The last two chapters are for those readers who are interested in possibilities beyond routine digital EEG, but the material is by no means exhaustive, as this is an introductory text. The interested readers will be able to seek out the latest developments from the various laboratories which are in the forefront of the field.

Throughout the book, actual clinical examples are obtained from a specific manufacturer's instrument by direct screen print-out (the CEEGRAPH unit from Bio-Logic Systems Corporation, Mundelein, Illinois). The discussion is of general applicability however, and involves available features from other instruments, as well as from the author's own experience and imagination. This field of digital EEG is rapidly changing. Instruments that are in use today will be obsolete within a matter of years, or will have evolved to more sophisticated forms. Hopefully, by stressing the fundamental aspects of the technique, this book will retain its educational value and remain relevant for a longer while.

It is hoped that readers will notify me of any errors, omissions, or other items of interest that they feel should have been included. There are tentative plans for an interactive digital companion to this book for use with a standard computer, which can mimic a digital EEG machine. As your feedback will significantly influence publication plans, I urge you to send any comments to:

Peter K.H. Wong, M.D.
EEG Department, 1D43
B.C.'s Children's Hospital
4480 Oak Street
Vancouver, British Columbia
Canada V6H 3V4
E-mail: Peter_Wong@mtsg.ubc.ca

ACKNOWLEDGMENTS

The EEG technologists at the B.C. Children's Hospital worked hard at collecting consistently high quality data which form the basis for this book. The EEG department secretaries contributed in the design and implementation of the CMS clinical management software, as well as keeping the department running smoothly: without their help the EEG department would not function properly. Particular thanks to Yasmin Alibhai for her role in helping with EEG data selection, and to my friend Dr. John Ebersole for contributing his data as illustration.

FOREWORD

It has been nearly 70 years since Hans Berger demonstrated that human brains, like animal brains, generate electrical signals that can be recorded from the scalp, and named this phenomenon the electroencephalogram. Although the EEG did not gain immediate general acceptance among neurophysiologists, this first technique capable of measuring dynamic changes in human brain function was ultimately hailed as a revolutionary development in neurodiagnosis. In North America, the original, and for many years the only, neuroscience society was named the American EEG Society, recognizing that the EEG symbolized a new era in the exploration of brain and behavior. Within short order, EEG laboratories appeared in hospitals throughout the world and have remained an important part of clinical diagnosis in neurology ever since.

In recent years, neurology has witnessed a second diagnostic revolution, as a result of extraordinary developments in neuroimaging. Magnetic resonance imaging (MRI) quickly and easily displays multiple sections of human brain structure with a degree of spatial resolution barely dreamed of only a few years ago. Positron emission tomography (PET), single photon emission computed tomography (SPECT) and most recently, functional MRI, create three-dimensional images of various aspects of human brain function, which alone, or when coregistered with structural MRI, provide extraordinary localizing capability. MRI has become a diagnostic mainstay of neurologic practice, and many hospitals now also offer SPECT and even PET as routine clinical diagnostic procedures. As a result, clinical EEG has lost its utility in most situations where there are obvious structural abnormalities in the brain, and electrophysiology is no longer regarded as the most exciting discipline for investigating the substrates of human brain function.

Nevertheless, EEG retains supremacy in a number of diagnostic areas by virtue of its unparalleled temporal resolution, relative ease of application, and ability to monitor functional changes over long periods of time. Consequently, EEG remains an essential clinical diagnostic tool, particularly for neurologic disorders associated with brief transient cerebral disturbances, such as epilepsy, or subtle diffuse perturbations of cerebral function, as occur with metabolic disturbances, and for recording in the operating theater, in intensive care wards and on long-term monitoring units.

At first glance, it would appear that much of the excitement initially associated with EEG has now been transposed to neuroimaging; however, in the shadow of the diagnostic revolution engendered by the development of these techniques for actually seeing structure and function within the human brain, a second quiet revolution has been taking place in clinical neurophysiology. Just as computer applications have been necessary for generating images of MRI, PET and SPECT, computer applications have been used in association with EEG to facilitate data acquisition, storage, analysis, and display. Within the past decade, digital EEG has made it possible to manipulate EEG recordings, after the fact, in a number of ways that permit extraction of otherwise inaccessible information. With digital EEG available for routine clinical use, physicians or technologists can change filter settings, alter montages, count spikes, carry out frequency analysis or averaging, and even perform three-dimensional source localization after a routine study, with a flip of the switch, display the data in any way they wish, and write their report all at the same computer terminal.

Furthermore, coregistration of electrophysiological information with MRI, PET and SPECT, made possible by computer manipulation of digital data, will permit multimodality imaging capable of revealing more than any individual modality alone.

Digital EEG is cost-effective and time-saving, in addition to offering capabilities for clinical diagnosis and research far beyond those currently possible with analog equipment. As more practicing physicians have access to digital technology, novel observations will be made to extend our understanding of the diseased and normal human brain, and greatly expand the diagnostic application of EEG. It is likely that crucial diagnostic procedures that can only be performed by computer-assisted EEG will become routine, just as computer-assisted neuroimaging has become routine. Thus, digital EEG will come to be regarded not just as a convenient option, but as the accepted standard of practice. Consequently, all clinical neurophysiologists will eventually be required to understand and apply the principles of digital EEG.

This book is an excellent introduction to the field, written specifically to bring clinical practitioners up to date, and to prepare them for the future. It may not be hyperbole to suggest that mastery of the material included in this text could become essential for their professional survival.

Jerome Engel, Jr., M.D., Ph.D.
Professor
Director, Seizure Disorder Center
Reed Neurological Research Center
UCLA School of Medicine

DIGITAL EEG
IN
CLINICAL PRACTICE

1
Background

EVOLUTION OF THE DIGITAL ELECTROENCEPHALOGRAPH

Ever since the first digital unit hit the display stand in the late 1980's, it was evident that a revolution was underway. The basic electroencephalograph (EEG) instrument had not changed fundamentally since its inception. Transistorized circuit modules had replaced vacuum tubes, making the instruments at once more sophisticated and reliable. Miniaturization of the traditional electroencephalograph made it trim and portable, as well as decreasing power requirements; modern electronics further improved amplifier performance. But pens filled with ink still danced over paper folds. Unfortunately, once the waveforms were written out onto paper, the chart was not amenable to any subsequent manipulation or computation. If the wrong montage or sensitivity had been used to display a particular waveform, it was impossible to redisplay it using a different gain/filter settings or montage.

The first digital instruments were used for acquiring evoked potentials (EP) readings. In this case, the price and flexibility proved superior to the hard-wired averager. An analog to digital converter (ADC), or digitizer card, added to an inexpensive personal computer (PC), became a programmable multipurpose tool for all kinds of EP readings. The waveforms could be printed out on inexpensive dot-matrix printers, or displayed on the same computer's monitor. As these instruments became accepted and popular, manufacturers turned their attention to clinical EEG applications.

The acquisition of EEG readings in a clinical setting makes unique demands for copious annotations and for flexible and rapidly changeable filter/gain settings, which required a very particular design for the machine. The interaction between the technician and the machine became the subject of intense study, as this human-machine interface influenced how the instrument was viewed or accepted. The electronics available with digital technology greatly improved amplifier functioning. Now, amplifier parameters could be changed under software control, and automatic annotation of amplifier settings are stored into computer memory together with the EEG data: no longer is it necessary to constantly annotate gain and filter settings as these are displayed with the data.

Calibration now can be done once, and amplifier gain that is not exactly perfect can be automatically corrected by software to give the same gain across all channels. The EEG tracings therefore show the true voltages, as if painstaking calibration had been done on each channel. At the same time, during such autocalibration procedures, amplifier self-testing diagnostic tests can be run to ensure proper operations, thus reducing the chances of malfunction. Diagnostic tests may look for shorted-input noise level, linearity, gain error, and frequency response errors, among others, and can be quite comprehensive. Such internal testing facility greatly reduces the frequency of preventative maintenance servicing, thereby improving reliability. Amplifiers and pen mechanisms are the common culprits for malfunctions in analog systems. In a digital system, the only components that (rarely) break down are the mechanical components: disk drives and cables. Mechanical shock, dust, and static electricity are the main things to be avoided for trouble-free operation.

Calibration at different frequencies can be a built-in function, thus eliminating the need for biocalibration. By the same token, impedance testing can be done by software control. In fact, this is so quick that several impedance measurements can be done throughout a prolonged EEG recording automatically or at user-selectable intervals.

All of these software-controlled measurements can be stored onto a log, along with the EEG data. This information then is available for reference upon later playback (analysis), which can be helpful in sorting out unusual signals or artifacts.

COMPARISON WITH ANALOG MACHINES

There are certain features which we take for granted in the traditional analog instrument, but which will require a mental adjustment if a digital instrument is used. These include:

1. Display Height-Width Ratio (Aspect Ratio)

   At a paper speed of 30 mm/s, a 10 s page is 300 mm wide. At 20 mm per channel, a 20 channel print-out will be 400 mm high. For individual channels, a 10 μV/mm pen deflection for a 200 μV peak to peak signal is 20 mm high by 300 mm wide.

   As an example, a large (19") high-resolution computer display monitor has a viewing area 15" wide by 11" high, or 380 mm wide by 280 mm high, and is used to display 20 channels. Typical 21 channel paper is 300 mm wide by 400 mm high. At a 30 mm/s standard paper speed, the digitally displayed tracing is stretched out horizontally by approximately 40%, and so appears "flatter."

   Of course, to effect the same aspect ratio, it is only necessary to raise the gain. However, what most people object to is the apparent crowding of 20 channels onto the screen, which is aggravated by the smaller monitors used (15" or even 14").

2. Looking Back at Tracings From a Previous Time

   With paper recordings, it is easy to flip several pages back to the item of interest, and to fold the paper to compare waveforms. Digitally, this is not as convenient, but is possible with some equipment.

3. Annotation

   It is more cumbersome to "mark" or "draw" onto the digitized tracing. Any such interaction must be performed by a keyboard, mouse, light-pen, or touch-screen. In reality, for simple annotations there is nothing more natural than a pen. However, it is our experience that one quickly adjusts to the keyboard and mouse interface, and with familiarity comes increased ease of operation and improved annotation.

4. Pen Noise

   Rather than being a nuisance, technologists use the pen noise as a clue to synchronized discharges (e.g., large spikes, 3/s spike-waves, or other seizures) when they are intensely observing the patient and not the machine. This allows accurate synchronized observation of clinical details. At all other times the absence of pen noise is preferred, especially with pediatric, agitated, or uncooperative patients.

5. Matched Gains

Two significant advantages of digital units are auto-correction of amplifier gains and self-diagnostic tests of amplifier functions. Because of these characteristics, all EEG signals are then preconditioned to be perfectly matched across channels, for all signal frequencies. Such features are taken for granted in analog machines, although in reality the degree of precision is approximately 5% if one is scrupulously careful about the biocalibration; with digital units the gains of all the amplifiers can be matched to within 1 bit of accuracy.

ACCURACY AND PRECISION OF RECORDINGS

Let us assume an EEG voltage swing to be over 256 μV (i.e., from −128 to +128 μV). At 8 bits there are 256 digital values to represent this dynamic range (chosen to be also 256 μV for convenience). Successive digital values then reflect a 1 μV difference (this is also called the ADC resolution, or the digitization error). At 12 bits, the same dynamic range is represented by 4096 values, giving a much finer resolution of 0.0625 μV. Thus:

signal μV	8 bit digital	signal μV	12 bit digital
+128	255	+128	4095
		+127.9375	4094
		+127.875	4093
		+127.8125	4092
		+127.75	4091
+127	254	+127	4079
+126	253	+126	4063
.			.
.			.
0	127	0	2047
.		..	
.		..	
−126	2	−126	31
−127	1	−127	15
−128	0	−128	0

It is obvious that the 12 bit representation is far more precise, and can reflect much smaller changes in the signal amplitude. In effect, this yields greater details in wave shape that may not be seen with the 8 bit representation, so the digital result is a "high fidelity" rendition of the original signal. An 8 bit waveform may appear jagged on closer inspection, whereas the 12 bit waveform will appear smooth.

With 12 or more bits of analog to digital conversion precision, there is less concern for amplifier saturation: the amplifiers can be set at a much lower sensitivity of 70 or 100 μV/mm equivalent, thus allowing even high voltage signals (e.g., electrocorticography) to be recorded without clipping. This is done by selecting the greatest signal dynamic range before saturation, while still keeping the digitization noise small (the digitization noise is the voltage step represented by a 1 bit change, the so-called quantal or step noise). If 12 bits are available, we have ±2048 μV range with a resolution of 1 μV. As most amplifiers have an input short-circuit noise of approximately 1 μV, it would not be beneficial to have an ADC resolution much below this. As it turns out, this set of ADC parameters can be used with almost all EEG signals encountered in clinical practice, including artifacts.

At review or playback, the computer software can retrieve the digital signal, then condition and display it at the selected amplitude gain, so as to make it appear as though it had been recorded at 20 μV/mm, for example. The least precision in common use is 8 bits, but usually 11 or 12 bits are preferred.

The equivalent precision of paper EEG tracings is about 6 bits. This is arrived at by dividing the paper width for one channel by the pen thickness, arriving at an approximate value of 60 or 70 units. This is the maximal number of different voltage values which can be represented by that pen within the width of paper available, again similar to the ADC digital representation. As it happens, 6 bits allow 64 voltage levels to be represented within the peak to peak voltage swing (or dynamic range). On the monitor, the limiting consideration is the number of pixels available for the total number of channels. If the vertical resolution is 768, and allowing for overlap between tracings, a display precision of 6 bits or more can easily be achieved.

A paper speed of 30 mm/s with standard pen thickness can realize a time resolution of perhaps 10 to 20 ms. However, one has to remove some precision due to pen curvature and pen alignment errors, This can be improved upon by the use of an ink-jet writing mechanism instead of a pen. In practice, pen misalignment is an ever-present evil and cannot be entirely avoided. In the digital domain, 1024 horizontal dots on the screen (pixels) is used to display 10 s of data, yielding 100 or approximately 6.5 bits of precision at a resolution of 10 ms. Therefore, it can be seen that the achievable resolution of digital data is at least as good as paper. Ultimately, because of the absence of pen misalignment and because individual data segments can be "zoomed-in" and displayed using the entire screen, the maximum resolution available is limited only by the ADC rate, usually 200 Hz, giving an achievable resolution of 5 ms.

Thus it can be concluded that at standard display gain and "paper" speed, the resulting amplitude and time resolutions are quite similar. Digital display allows the entire screen to be used for displaying shorter segments of data, so that if 5 s is selected, then the time resolution can be doubled, allowing more details to be displayed. Such distortion-free display amplification can be done up to the original digitizing frequency and maximum raw data amplitude, which of course cannot be exceeded.

NEW CAPABILITIES

Customizability and Adaptability

One of the advantages of software-based instruments is that the operator interface can be customized to suit the particular operator's desires and idiosyncrasies, as well as the task at hand. Examples include: default selection (duration of hyperventilation [HV], protocol for photic stimulation [PS], choice of amplifier parameters from a "menu" to fit the given operator and task), specific comments (e.g., eyes open/eyes closed, movements, artifacts, awake, asleep, HV, PS, etc.), rapid execution of certain instructions which may require multiple key strokes (replacement by a single "hot key"), etc.

Connectivity

Inherent in their digital mode of data storage and computer-based operation (the "platform") is the fact that digital EEG machines can be connected together for communication of data (transfer of data files).

The communication details are handled by a local area network or LAN, which requires a interface card in each computer, as well as a network server (main dispatch and storage unit). Examples of network systems include the Novell, IBM, and Microsoft systems.

Once networked together, individual machines can transfer data files to each other, allowing separate EEG recording and reading stations. The EEG might have been recorded moments ago from the intensive care unit (ICU), but is available in the EEG department for immediate interpretation. There are many similar situations that would benefit from such connectivity. Letting our imagination soar, machines can monitor what is actually being recorded on another machine at that very moment (i.e., in real time), allowing no delay in diagnosis and intervention in acute situations like electrocorticography (ECoG) in the operating room (OR).

Growth Capability

With the above capabilities, complex recording protocols can be extended to monitoring patients under many difficult or demanding clinical environments, such as in the OR or ICU, using EEG or evoked potential recordings. This greatly enhanced flexibility and efficiency mean fewer personnel are required to achieve the same diagnostic results. On-line (real-time) or off-line spectral display (analysis of previously recorded data), as might be used in trend analysis, is another possibility now available to monitor long term EEG changes in the ICU patient.

Other analytical techniques available which can be applied to recorded digital EEG data are:

Topographic Analysis: studying the topographic distribution of certain waveforms (e.g., epileptiform discharges) in order to better understand their characteristics, or to allow discrimination across different clinical entities.

Source Localization: the mathematical deduction of the location, direction, and amplitude of a theoretical generator within the brain to account for the EEG.

Deblurring: the removal of the confounding effects of the skull in order to estimate the cortical EEG signal, based on the Laplacian technique. This is based on structural information from magnetic resonance imaging (MRI) slices.

Cortical Imaging: similar to deblurring, but using a different mathematical approach.

CLINICAL LABORATORY EXPERIENCE

At the Children's Hospital in Vancouver, B.C., Canada, the implementation of digital EEG technology in our busy pediatric neurophysiology laboratory was planned and executed in careful steps. We share our experience in the hope that those laboratories which are contemplating "plunging" into digital technology may be aware of our experience, so as to better prepare themselves for the change by taking the appropriate path.

1. Taking Stock of Our Existing Procedures

   An exhaustive documentation of the protocols for each of our diagnostic procedures was carried out. This allowed us to clearly state our needs and priorities when comparing different machines.
2. Thinking Ahead

We identified what our needs may be in the future, for example ICU/OR monitoring, epilepsy surgery work-up, ambulatory monitoring, EP, etc. This allowed us to assess the possibilities for future expansion, and to select the vendor based on stability and longevity in the digital EEG business.

3. Machine Trials

A small group of our technologists formed the working committee for hardware screening. They were sent to attend trade exhibitions with the specific mission of viewing each vendor's products. They arranged a demonstration of each digital EEG machine, as well as a question period with the most knowledgeable representative. A score sheet was used to keep track of each feature, listed in order of priority as previously determined. The top one or more machines were requested to be demonstrated at our laboratory on real patients. All decisions were made as a group.

4. Comparison of Instruments

Based on the score sheet and the performance of each machine, the group and the medical director met and discussed each instrument in turn. Major categories considered in detail were: ease of use, completeness of functions, compatibility with existing technology, connectivity with existing instruments, expandability, attractiveness of the vendor, pricing, etc. A consensus was arrived at for the best instrument.

5. Purchase and Installation

The installation of the instruments should be done with the help of the local biomedical engineer, as this person will be responsible for maintenance and emergency repairs. It is imperative for the unit to be thoroughly tested, including all test types.

6. Training

Prior to the installation, all technologists were encouraged to take training courses, including an introduction to microcomputers, disk operating system (DOS), and word processor skills. This imparted a familiarity with the keyboard and disk operations that are necessary for the successful operation of digital EEG machines.

Physicians were given a different introduction, by way of one-on-one teaching of the data analysis portion of the instrument. First, simple command keys were introduced (changing display gain and montage, paging backward and forward, reading a patient's data file from disk). Then more key commands were introduced (turning on/off the computer, starting the program from DOS, changing disk directories, automatic paging, half paging). The objective was to avoid intimidating the novice who may be computer-shy, and to gradually build confidence. A negative first impression will be difficult to overcome, and invariably cause resistance to learning all the steps necessary for smooth operation.

Once all are initiated into the daily operation of the systems, someone must be responsible for ensuring that proper procedures are followed. This requires the establishment of protocols for the handling of data files, their storage while awaiting interpretation, permanent archival storage, and system backup procedures. In Chapter 4 there will be a detailed discussion of the procedures in daily use in our own laboratory.

7. Precautions

Digital computers are subject to interference from external agents. A spark of static electricity to the keyboard can cause a computer to halt or "crash" (total cessation of computer function). This could be catastrophic in the midst of recording important data. Good software design allows for such incidents by automatically saving data to the hard disk (a less vulnerable form of permanent storage) as soon as it is acquired, so that at worst only the last few seconds of data may be lost.

Mechanical vibration should be avoided during operation: this may lead to damage to the hard disk, which may result in a "disk crash" where the disk unit is damaged permanently. Usually this does not happen with the minor amounts of movement an EEG machine is normally exposed to. An inactive computer (power off) is not vulnerable, except to mechanical vibrations that can cause loosening of electrical cable connections, which may occasionally be difficult to identify.

Dust build-up within and around the computer equipment will cause floppy disk errors and overheating. Problems arising in this manner are notoriously difficult to trace. It is a good practice to have regular scheduled preventative maintenance that includes cleaning and vacuuming.

2

Technology

DATA ACQUISITION PROCESS

After amplification and ADC, the EEG is now in the form of a long series of numeric values expressed as digital characters called “bytes.” This digital string forms a “time series,” where the position of each number is important, as their values reflect signal amplitude changes over time. For an EEG segment that may cover as much as 30 min of recording, the orderly collection of digital characters is called a “file.” This file of EEG signal information is digitally no different from a manuscript file produced by a word processor, except that it is longer.

Physically speaking, as the EEG is acquired in digital form, it is stored temporarily in the high-speed computer RAM or random access memory. As the RAM holding area (or “buffer”) is filled up, the data is relocated to the hard disk drive unit, which is a permanent storage device. When power is turned off, data residing in disk drives are safe, whereas data in RAM are lost. Typically, RAM capacities are in the millions of bytes (or megabytes, MB), while hard disk drives may be in the hundreds of megabytes, or even a gigabyte (a thousand million bytes, GB).

Routine EEG files covering 30 min of recording can be very large: for a frequency response of 0.1 to 100 Hz, ADC sampling has to be at least double the highest signal frequency (i.e., 200 Hz) in order to capture the signal with fidelity. If 12 bit ADC is used, each converted value occupies 2 bytes of space. Thus the data flow rate for a single channel is 200 conversions/s ˘ 2 bytes/conversion, or 400 bytes/s, or 0.4 KB/s (1 KB = 1000 bytes). For 20 channels, this is 8 KB/s. For 30 min of recording, this becomes 8 ˘ 60 ˘ 30 or 14.4 MB. By comparison, a 3.5” floppy diskette can hold 1.44 MB. A 1 GB drive can hold 60 to 80 such 30 min EEG files. For 8 bit ADC precision, this capacity is doubled to 120 to 160 files.

When the EEG recording is completed, this file then resides in the hard disk, and is available for review and interpretation by the electroencephalographer. Once a report has been generated, this file should be placed in archival storage, which in practice means drive units using removable optical disk cartridges, or digital tape cartridges. The former is convenient and fast for accessing, while the latter is slow but inexpensive. Archived files can then be removed from the working hard disk, thereby freeing up space for newer files. See Fig. 1 for an overview.

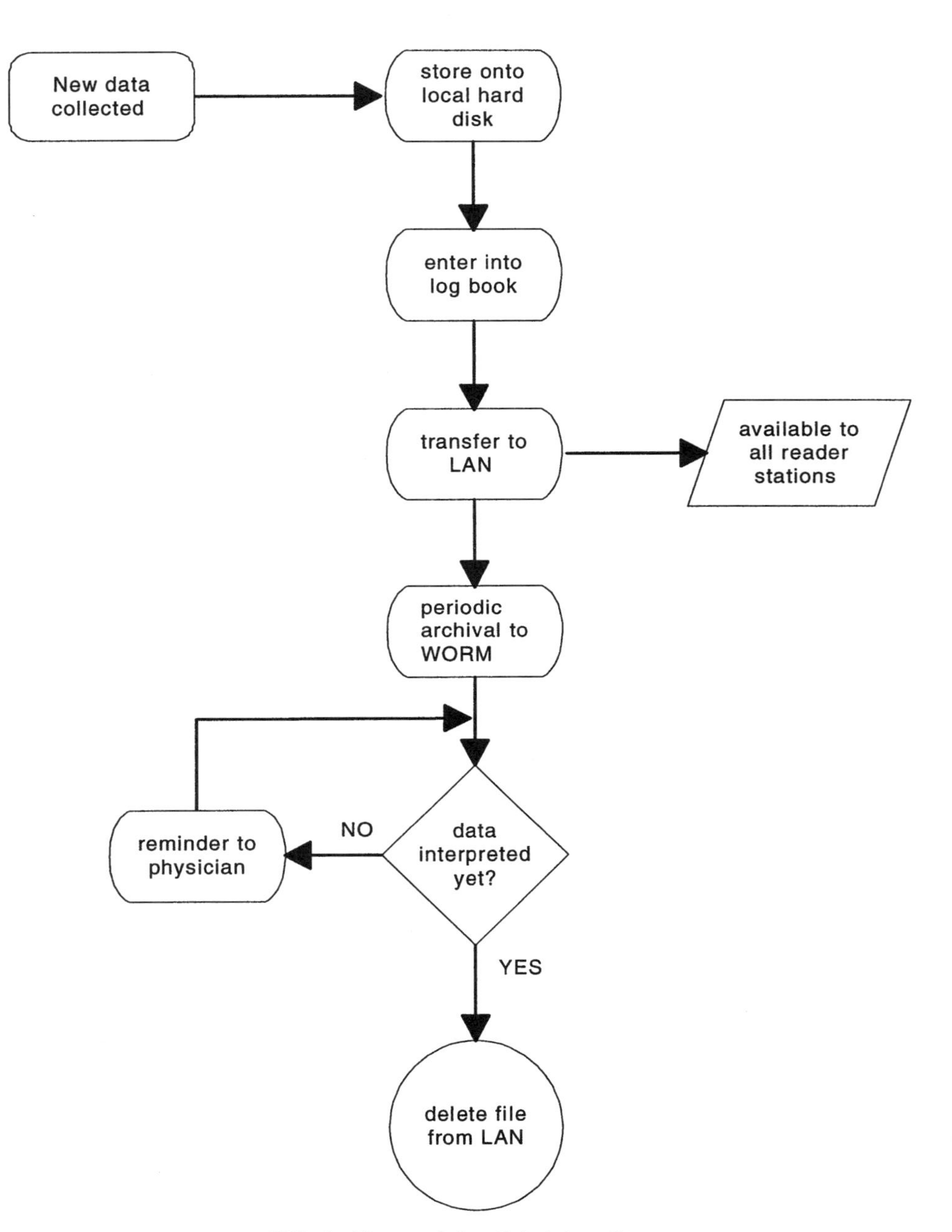

FIG. 1. Flow path for digital data files.

Factors to be considered for archival storage devices are reliability, cost, speed, capacity, and convenience. As it is often the sole means of storage, the digital EEG file is a legal document and must be safeguarded. Therefore reliability is paramount. An inconvenient archival procedure will encourage poor compliance, leading to errors and omissions, as well as higher labor costs. The best compromise in our experience is the optical disk. One cartridge holds 1 GB, or 60 to 100 routine EEG recordings. Storage cost for the cartridge itself is minimal, as 1,000 routine recordings can fit in 10 or 15 cartridges of 5” ˘ 5” ˘ 0.6” size, each weighing 200 or 300 g, all fitting in less than a foot of shelf space. Gone are the charges for microfilming, paper storage, accessioning, and handling etc., and the waiting periods to retrieve stored records.

Finally, digital data do not degrade: the tracings from last year’s file appear on the computer display screen exactly as when freshly acquired. True copies can be made, with 100% assurance of accuracy. Digital storage is, of course, still susceptible to risks like fire and water damage, mechanical trauma, theft, and human errors. These also prey on paper recordings. It would not be practical to require digital technology to be foolproof, as even traditional paper EEG technology is not.

CHANNEL REFORMATTING

From the electrodes on the scalp, each lead is connected to a single channel of the amplifier module. As the latter is under computer control, the switching of montages is digitally accomplished, as long as the amplifier input has a common reference (i.e., all recording leads referred to a common electrode). This enables the computer to calculate any desired montage (monopolar or bipolar, including common average reference and Hjorth’s source derivation) from the acquired data. At a given instant, the real signal voltage at an electrode lead is:

X_i = input signal for lead *i* (raw EEG of channel *i*, recorded with an ideal reference at infinity)

X_{ref} = voltage at the reference electrode (e.g., ear lobe), again referred to infinity

As the ideal reference is inaccessible, X_i and X_{ref} are of course unmeasurable. When a differential amplifier is connected, input one is connected to electrode *i*, and input two is connected to the reference electrode. In this case

$$V_i = X_i - X_{ref}$$

is the actual amplifier output of lead *i*, referred to the reference lead. To create a bipolar derivation, consider two channels, *i* and *j*. Then

$$\begin{aligned} V_{i-j} &= V_i - V_j \\ &= (X_i - X_{ref}) - (X_j - X_{ref}) \\ &= X_i - X_j \end{aligned}$$

The bipolar derivation of lead *i* referred to lead *j* can be simply calculated once the monopolar values of the individual leads are known. Generalizing, any derivation of leads can be calculated using a combination of recorded monopolar leads, as the only required steps involve subtraction of recorded real signal values. Examples are monopolar derivations referenced to another lead (e.g., referred to C_z with original reference being linked ears), common average reference with or without removal of leads with large signals (e.g., removal of frontal polar leads due to eye movement), etc. These different derivations need only to be programmed once into the computer, and then are available at any time thereafter.

There is a price for this convenience, though, and there are pitfalls unique to such a digital remontaging procedure. Certain precautions are necessary to ensure that the calculated EEG signals are accurate. Firstly, the same reference electrode must be used. This generally precludes the use of ipsilateral ears (A_1 for the left hemisphere, A_2 for the right), unless of course the individual A_1 and A_2 leads are also recorded referred to each other, in which case all references used are available for any montage.

It is unimportant where such a system reference is located, although common sense dictates that it should be in an electrically quiet location (away from muscle electromyogram, movement artifacts, etc.). Such contaminants to the reference electrode serve to introduce a large error into each scalp lead, and commonly cause problems by saturating the amplifier channels, causing clipping. Amplifiers which have a high dynamic range (i.e., the amplifier is capable of faithfully following large swings of input voltage, typically in the range of plus or minus several hundred microvolts) are necessary to avoid this problem. Additionally, the amplifier calibration, as well as the digital precision (i.e., number of bits), must be accurate enough so that sampling errors do not contaminate the calculated results. The following example is used to illustrate this point.

In the situation where a known calibrating signal is applied to each channel (100 μV), and assuming ± 5% error for each channel, we may have the following digital output values:

$$\text{Let } V_1 = \text{the output of channel 1} = 105\ \mu\text{V}\ (+5\%)$$
$$V_2 = \text{the output of channel 2} = 95\ \mu\text{V}\ (-5\%)$$

The errors are ± 5% for each channel. Displayed in a referential fashion, these calibration errors will not appear large. However, if a bipolar derivation of channels 1 and 2 is made, the output becomes:

$$\begin{aligned} V_{1\text{-}2} &= V_1 - V_2 \\ &= 105 - 95\ \mu\text{V} \\ &= 10\ \mu\text{V} \end{aligned}$$

In fact the correct value is 100 − 100 = 0 μV. Therefore the calculated derivation has an error which is very large, resulting from magnification of the individual 5% errors. This kind of error is, of course, unacceptable, as it grossly distorts the calculated bipolar derivation signals from their true values (as might have been obtained from actual error-free amplifier montaging). These errors are additive, thus they increase if more subtraction or computation steps are necessary to arrive at a certain derivation (e.g., Hjorth, common average reference, etc.).

Other errors also accumulate to produce distortions to the calculated bipolar derivations. Internal amplifier noise (input short circuit) errors due to random electronic signals from the silicon chip play a small role. ADC truncation errors are important if the conversion is based on 8 bits instead of 12 bits. For 8 bits, the input signal is represented by 256 different digital output values, arbitrarily called 0 to 255. For 12 bits, there are 4096 possible output values. The precision is therefore 1/256 (0.4%) and 1/4096 (0.02%) for 8 and 12 bit ADC respectively.

Ideally then, there should be high ADC precision (11 bits or more), good amplifier calibration, and automatic correction, in addition to the usual elements of good EEG amplifier design: high common mode rejection, high input impedance, low cross-talk between channels, high linearity, high stability (or low drift), high dynamic range, etc.

In summary, as long as the EEG was recorded using a single common reference electrode, any derivation can be recreated at will from the digital data. This is probably the single most important advantage of digital EEG. We have all had the experience of being in the wrong montage, seemingly whenever an interesting waveform is present. With digital reformatting capability, one merely selects the optimal montage to redisplay the data, showing the waveform to best advantage.

DISPLAY GRAPHICS

Computer Oriented

The current standard for PC graphics is the VGA (video graphics array) graphical interface, with resolutions of 640 dots ("pixels") horizontally and 480 lines vertically (referred to as 640 ˘ 480). There are enhanced Super VGA (or SVGA) versions, with resolutions of 800 ˘ 600, 1024 ˘ 768, and 1280 ˘ 1024. There are also nonstandard proprietary interfaces with resolutions up to 1600 ˘ 1200. The appropriate video monitors must be used with each standard. As well, there are both interlaced and noninterlaced monitors. The former are cheaper, but the display tracings may flicker or look jumpy. This situation is not present with the latter, which is more expensive, but will give a picture that is rock-steady.

Therefore, the ideal choice should be a large (19" or greater) noninterlaced monitor (regardless of the resolution), with a flat display tube and good color capability.

In Chapter 1, we stated that paper EEG has an equivalent resolution of 6 bits or 64 pixels in the vertical dimension. In the horizontal dimension (the time axis), there should be 100 pixels/inch or better. A 10 s page requires 1000 pixels. Therefore, a 1024 pixel time (horizontal) resolution would be the minimum requirement, with 1280 or higher being preferred.

Tracing Oriented

Like paper movement, computer displays of EEG tracings can be made to scroll in any direction. In addition, the scrolling speed can be varied to slower or faster "paper speeds": the slower the paper speed, the less high frequency resolution will be available for viewing. Of course, all the original EEG data is there, as the computer merely chooses every other point (or every 4th) of each channel for display.

More conveniently, data can be paged manually or automatically in adjustable steps (10 s, 20 s, 5 s, etc.). An extension of this idea allows half-page movements. Treating the screen as a window allows the idea of separate display units, each under separate control (e.g., showing different time points, display gains, or montages) that can be adjusted in size (zooming) and position within the computer screen.

Such split-screen capability can facilitate interpretation of EEG tracings, particularly as it allows simultaneous viewing of different segments of an EEG tracing for comparison purposes.

LINKAGE OF VIDEO AND EEG

There are advantages to recording the routine ambulatory EEG simultaneously with a video camera: any interesting clinical spell or EEG burst can be analyzed in detail retrospectively. Such electroclinical correlation can provide important information for the correct diagnosis of suspicious behavioral or electrical episodes. For this strategy to work, the effort involved must be minimal so as not to create an onerous task for the technologist. If nothing of interest occurred during the recording, then the video tape is recycled. It is retained for review otherwise.

Both EEG and video tape recording must be synchronized so as to display data recorded at the same time. This can be achieved by time codes embedded into the data streams, so that the data is always synchronized. Reliance upon the video recorder's timing display is not good enough, as an accuracy of better than half a second is required.

Various useful displays can be devised with such simultaneous video/EEG data, either for improved diagnostic interpretation, or for presentation to groups. The usual method is to run the EEG and video in real time, and to place the two monitors (for EEG and video separately) side by side. The operator can stop the playback at any item of interest, and either control the EEG display second by second or page by page (with the video slaved to follow in synchrony), or control the video display frame by frame, or in slow motion (with the EEG slaved to follow correctly, by way of a cursor pointing to the exact synchronized time of occurrence of the video frame under review). Either method (the EEG master, or the video master) should be natural, and the tedious intricacies of maintaining time synchrony should be entirely transparent to the operator.

For presentation at rounds, it is convenient to edit the video clip to include the EEG tracings of interest, by using the split-screen format. Video tape segments can be inexpensively copied for circulation or archival purposes. A variant of this analog video technology is to digitize the video and audio signals, and perform such editing entirely within the digital domain. There are many advantages: no reduction of display clarity with copying or editing, precise control of individual frames, digital visual effects (windows, picture in picture, pan/zoom), convenience (the material to be edited resides on hard disk, and can be retrieved much faster than from tape; manipulations are also more precise, as there are no mechanical tape/head movements to account for).

Such a procedure takes advantage of the multimedia revolution in the consumer electronics market, and it is conceivable that other new devices will be available soon that will facilitate and enhance the capabilities of such EEG/video systems.

It must be noted that video standards vary for different places, with the NTSC (National Television Standards Committee) standard for North America and the PAL (Phase Alternating Line) standard for Asia. Their equivalent vertical resolutions (number of distinct horizontal lines displayable) are 240 and 288 respectively. These standards define the video signals which are fed to the monitor. The format for video tape recording also varies. The common standards include VHS (Video Home System) and Super VHS for standard size video cassette recorders (VCR), and 8 mm and high 8 mm for the miniature 8 mm video camcorders. Generally, the Super VHS and High 8 mm formats have a vertical equivalent of 400 lines. When high definition television (HDTV) is available, the available resolution will again increase greatly.

3

B.C. Children's Hospital's Department of Diagnostic Neurophysiology Procedures

The following is an overview of the procedures and patient/data handling protocols in daily use at the Department of Diagnostic Neurophysiology at B.C. Children's Hospital.

PATIENT PROTOCOL OVERVIEW AND FLOWSHEETS

Since the objective of our department is to provide for clinical service, education, and research, it was decided at a very early stage that patient and EEG related information must be computerized and accessible. This would facilitate inquiries seeking clinical or administrative information, and would be particularly useful for research. A computerized patient database was initiated in our department in 1982.

Since then, this has been expanded to include many aspects of our service. Every referral to our department is entered into a specially designed computer software package called CMS (Clinical Management System), the specifications of which were designed as a group by the members of the department, with an outside software consultant contracted to write the software. See Fig. 2 for an overview of how it is integrated into patient flow. There are three main software components: scheduling, databasing, and reporting. The starting point for CMS is when a new request is received for an EEG test. The sequence of events is as follows:

(a) Scheduler. The scheduler displays sequentially the next available appointment openings for that given test type. When an acceptable date and time is found, it is reserved. Patient information is then immediately obtained.

(b) Patient Information Database. The patient information is entered into the database. Notification letters can be generated to the referring physician as well as the patient as reminders. At any time, the departmental staff can review any given day's appointments for room/technologist assignments. A EEG worksheet is generated on the day of the test. When the patient arrives, the worksheet is used by the

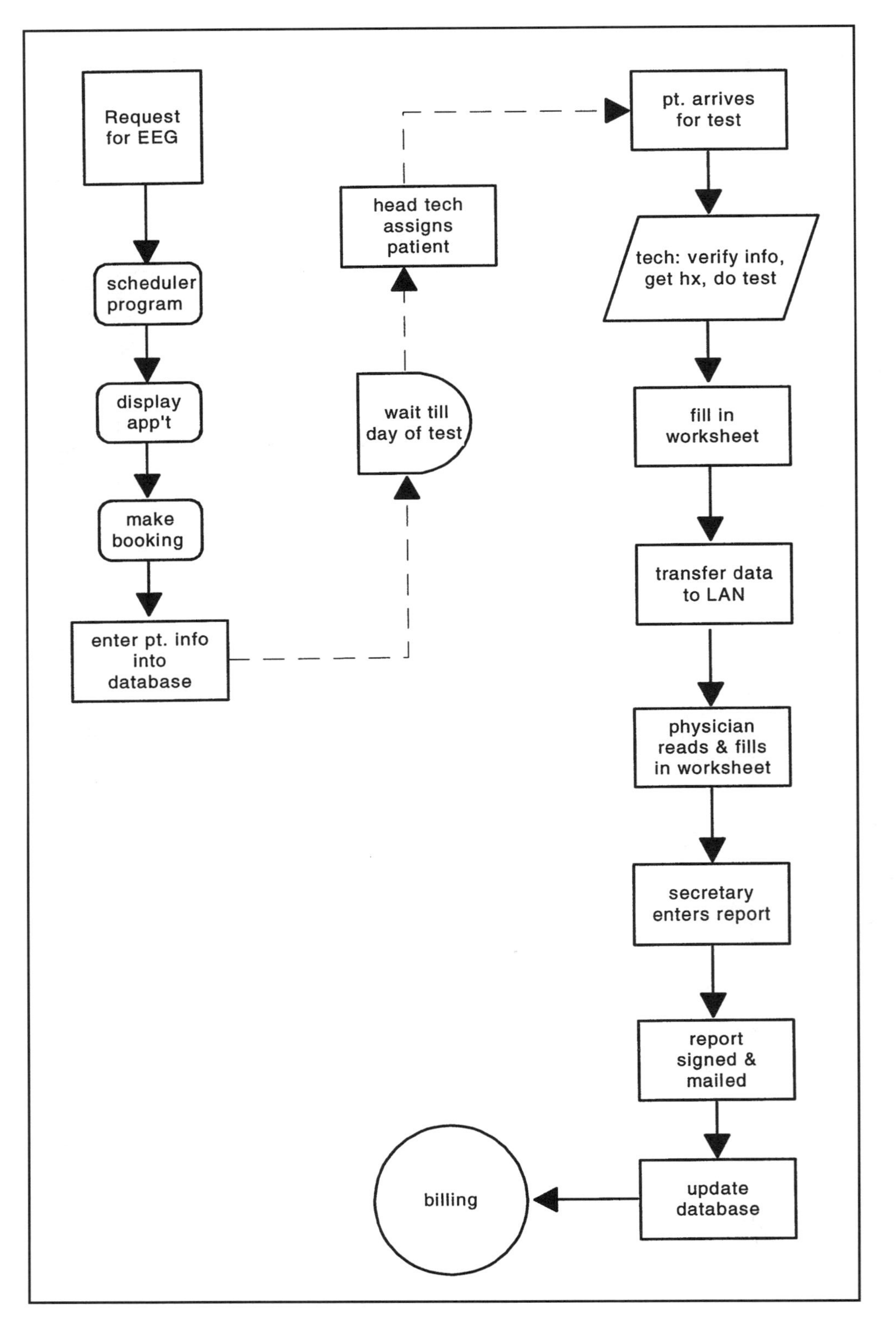

FIG. 2. Clinical Management System (CMS) overview.

technologist to obtain history relevant to the EEG. This is entered directly onto the worksheet. After the EEG is done, the recorded EEG data is transferred to the network, while the worksheet is left for the physician to fill in upon interpretation of the EEG.

(c) Report Generation. The worksheet is designed for rapid filling-in and transcription. An example is given for illustration (see Appendix A). Copies and addressing are automatically generated for distribution.

For completeness' sake, it was also necessary to devise an EEG classification and coding system that allows precise and succinct description of all EEG findings, both normal variants and abnormal findings. For such a system to be useful, it must be able to give descriptive information of waveforms and easily distinguish subtle differences between abnormalities (e.g., 3/s spike and wave versus atypical spike and wave). This is covered in a later section (and Appendix B).

CLINICAL MANAGEMENT SYSTEM (CMS) SOFTWARE DETAILS

The following information are included as "fields" in the database where manual entry is made (by the secretary or the technologist); a collection of fields are grouped into a "record." The analogy is a questionnaire form, each item constitutes a field, while the entire form constitutes a record.

Patient Database Structure

Multiple independent but linked databases are used to store information that is logically distinguishable:

(a) Patient Demographics (single record)

first name, surname, nickname, date of birth, address, telephone numbers, names of parents, hospital number, health insurance number

(b) History (multiple records)

birth weight, gestational age, delivery information, neonatal history; development, school, past medical and family history; seizure information (type, description, frequency, onset date); neurological findings; relevant laboratory findings (computed tomography [CT], MRI, single photon emission CT [SPECT], etc.)

(c) Clinical Profile (single record; this may be combined with the History database)

last visit date, family history, diagnoses, physicians involved, treatment

(d) Visit (multiple records)

EEG dates (same as visit dates), test type, names of technologist and interpreter, test protocol used (e.g., sedation, sleep deprivation), EEG findings (using the EEG classification system), technologist's comments.

Scheduling

An appointment booking system was devised which took into account our style of practice, number of technologists and test rooms, equipment resources, and appointment times. Various features were incorporated and automated so as to facilitate the booking process and minimize the time required. Following a phone request for a given service, a mutually acceptable date and time for the test are found, the necessary patient information is taken, and the customized paper forms for the technologist to use during the appointment are printed (this is usually done on the day prior to the appointment). The CMS system has to keep track of resources (test rooms, technologists, equipment, time), and reconcile discrepancies on an on-going basis.

The most important design attributes are user-friendliness, speed, and linkage to the database. Other useful features are automatic seeking of the next available opening for the desired test type, easy cancellation/rebooking (i.e., soft cancellation: a canceled patient is relegated to a cancellation list, so that the same patient can be later rebooked to another opening without having to reenter all the information), wait-list (automatic reminder whenever a cancellation occurs), rescheduling new time (i.e., simultaneous cancel/rebook), and editing of patient information.

Report Generation

The Visit database contains the entire EEG report, in a coded format. The purpose is to allow on-line printing of the final EEG report on the monitor on demand, instead of having to search through the filing system. This allows immediate display of the report in response to a telephone query, and an immediate printout for mailing purposes. All this can be done immediately as the single response to a telephone query.

To achieve a computerized report generation system, a procedure likened to "word and phrase salad" mixing is used. It is based on the premise that EEG reports routinely contain a small number of sentences with fixed format. There are relatively few variations, mostly involving the adjectives, nouns, and adverbs. By careful design of a few key sentences, and allowing for the appropriate selection of words and phrases, a collection of customized sentences can be built-up to adequately describe the EEG findings. To cover the requirement for free-form prose, anything can be directly grafted verbatim onto the report. Appendix A details the process for coding EEG findings onto the worksheet. The report subsequently generated is also listed. This computerized system is used in approximately 95% of our EEG reports. The time taken by the interpreter to manually enter the findings (by marking desired words and phrases) is under 1 min, and the time for the secretary to enter the database information and produce the final report is about 2 min. In addition to time savings, the code for the report becomes part of the Visit database record for that given date, and is available on-line.

EEG CLASSIFICATION SYSTEM

Appendix B gives a detailed description of the classification system, which was developed within our department from 1981 onwards. The original format was based in part on the Mayo Clinic system, but with many additional enhancements and provisions to adequately cover our needs.

Briefly, an EEG is broken down by states (Waking, Drowsiness, Sleep, Coma, sTupor—the upper case letter is the short-hand representation of the word), with the findings in each described separately. Such a description of findings consist of: class (normal variant, epileptiform, delta, background, etc.), location on scalp, and type of finding (spike, 3/s spike and wave, atypical spike and wave, polyspike, ctenoids, delta, beta, theta, complexes, etc.). This grouping allows for different findings of the same class, and can be repeated for different classes of findings. There are additional add-on codes for other descriptors: findings that are paroxysmal, rare, rhythmic waveforms, etc.

In our experience, this system can adequately account for over 90% of our EEG recordings in a manner that satisfactorily conveys the feel of the EEG. This system is also particularly useful when comparing sequential EEG reports. Its main strength is to greatly simplify retrieval of specific EEG findings of interest for retrospective studies. For example, it is easy to select all the EEGs based on the following criteria:

(a) any epileptiform discharges; optionally for a given period, gender, age, physician, occurrence in a given state (e.g., spikes only during waking),
(b) as in (a) but in association with other findings (delta, ctenoids, clinical manifestations),
(c) as in (a) but also requiring that the epileptiform discharge be in a given scalp location (frontal, central, parietal, temporal, occipital, midline, or combinations thereof),
(d) seizures within the first year of life,
(e) electrographic ictal patterns with or without simultaneous clinical manifestations,
(f) rhythmic spike discharges, optionally with restraints on location, state, companion findings,
(g) neonatal positive sharp waves, or
(h) paroxysmal delta activity, optionally in a given state.

The selected cases can be sorted, tabulated, and counted by various fields.

DIGITAL DATA HANDLING PROTOCOL

The main guiding principle in the design of our digital data handling procedures is that of data safety, followed by convenience and simplicity. A large stack of paper tracings is quite difficult to lose. In comparison, one can wipe out the digital EEG files from a dozen patients, by an inadvertent stroke at the keyboard. Therefore, a defined protocol needs to be scrupulously adhered to by all involved.

Fig. 3 gives an overview of the departmental network structure. Each EEG workstation is connected to the network through the fileserver, which is the central storage device and the network unit. Network cabling within the department connects all the workstations and reader stations. Cabling outside of the department connects to other areas of the hospital, allowing data collection from the ICU, OR, wards, etc. The fileserver is equipped with a hard disk drive capacity of 2 GB (either as a single drive, or spread over two drives), and a optical disk drive (for 1 GB rewritable and write-once removable optical cartridges). The hard disk unit is for dynamic storage of program software, as well as for temporarily holding data generated by the digital workstations. The optical media are for long-term (archival) storage. Once a file has been interpreted, it is off-loaded from the hard disk to an optical cartridge, and then deleted from the hard disk.

There are two kinds of optical cartridges. The rewritable ones can be reused by simply deleting the existing files. The deleted files are then permanently destroyed by this deletion and its space is available for new files. On the other hand, a file stored onto write-once cartridges is permanent. The space cannot be freed up to be reused again, and a deletion procedure merely removes the name of the deleted file from the cartridge's directory, but the actual file is not physically touched. It truly has been permanently etched onto the disk, and can be retrieved by rebuilding its entry in the directory. These write-once read-many times (WORM) cartridges are ideally suited for permanent EEG storage. There has been no upper limit determined for the maximum time which optical cartridges can be safely stored; certainly 10 years is not problematic.

Referring back to Fig. 1, Chapter 2, for the EEG data flow and handling procedure, the essential (human) feature is a log book that contains the following information: name, file number, WORM cartridge number, and interpreter. It serves as a daily reference of the workload and the archival status of the EEGs.

An EEG is recorded by the individual workstation (collection storage). The acquired data can be stored onto the local hard disk, in which

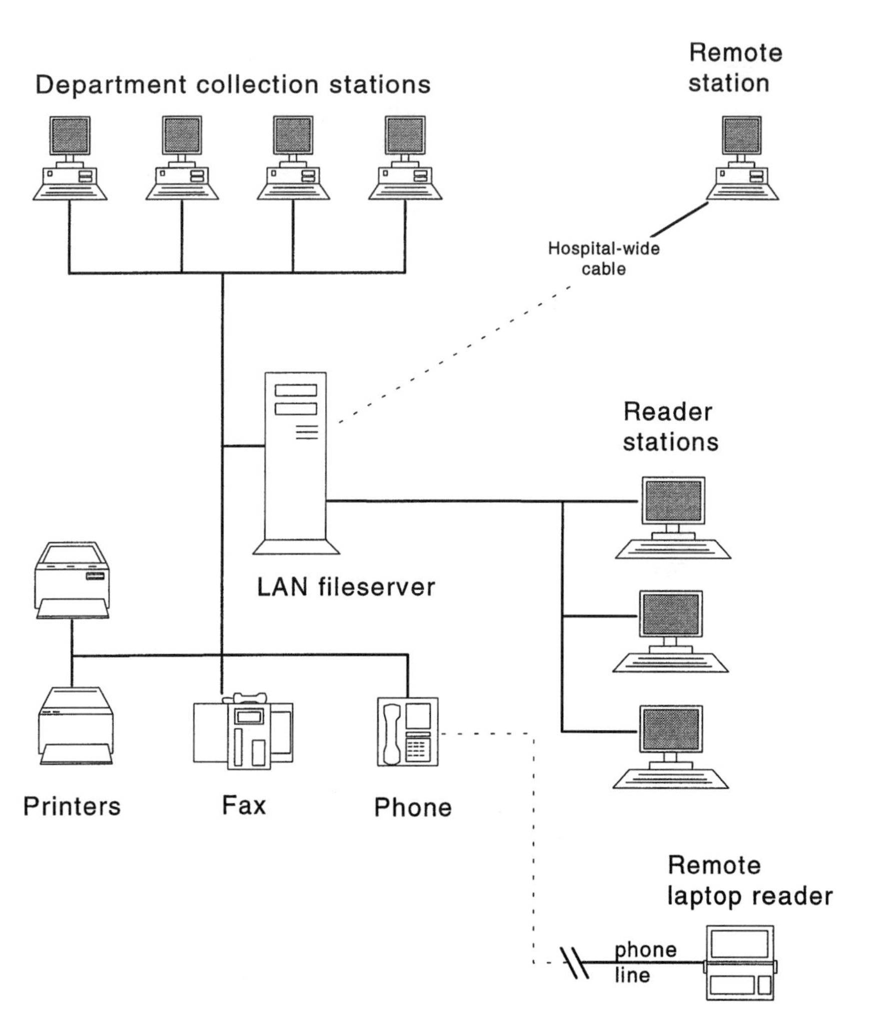

FIG. 3. Departmental network structure.

case it is not reliant upon the network. However, if desired it is just as simple to use the network's hard disk as the collection storage, in which case the EEG being recorded is available simultaneously for review at any other workstation or reader station. This feature is useful if an immediate interpretation is necessary prior to the patient being disconnected, e.g., whether a suspicious episode had ictal EEG changes.

After the recording is completed, the technologist enters any residual annotation (e.g., additional documentation of interesting events during the EEG, demographic information, hospital number, tags to flag interesting EEG segments, etc.) and then initiates file transfer from their local hard drive to the fileserver on the network.

Once the EEG data is copied to the fileserver, it is available for review and interpretation. After this it can be archived onto WORM cartridges and deleted from network storage.

A patient's EEG file can be retrieved from archival storage for any purpose at a fraction of the time needed to retrieve and review paper recordings. Among the many reasons for retrieval are the comparison of findings in several different recordings, research projects, print outs for poster illustration, etc. The patient's data is then retrieved from the CMS Visit database, so that the corresponding WORM cartridge number and filename can be obtained. By reading from the WORM cartridge directly, or by copying the required file back onto the fileserver hard disk, the EEG is again available for review or analysis.

If video data is also kept for some recordings, the VCR tape numbers can be indicated in the EEG file and entered in CMS. An archival tape system can be implemented so that only segments of interest in any given tape are retained by copying onto master tapes. The original tape then would be recycled.

PREFERRED DATA REVIEW FEATURES

The important features for the data review process are listed below.

Clarity of Display. This means large screen (at least 15"), high resolution (at least 1280 ˇ 1024), and stable screen image without flicker (i.e., noninterlaced).

Display Reformatting. This is the ability to use different display settings for the screen image. This includes filter and gain, montage, display speed, grid marks, etc, as well as print-out options.

Speed of Paging. Optimally the screen update of 10-s pages of EEG data can be achieved at 2/s or faster. This should be adjustable.

Windowing. This is the ability to open a second window on the screen for viewing different segments of the EEG reading, e.g., when comparing the discharges at the current moment and a few minutes prior.

Annotation. The interpreter can insert his/her own comment as a reminder for future reference, as feedback to the technologist, or as a question to the technologist (e.g., regarding clinical manifestation or state change during a suspicious EEG segment).

Other desirable features are:

Audio/Video Integration. If a video camera was operational during the EEG recording (e.g., ambulatory intensive monitoring), the interpreter should be able to request viewing of the corresponding video sequence synchronized to the exact time of the EEG being displayed. This is useful during EEG review for electroclinical correlation during a seizure or clinical event.

Portability. It is convenient to have the ability to review the EEG from any station connected to the network. This can be within the laboratory, elsewhere in the hospital, or at a remote site. The only requirement is that the hardware be compatible, and that the network has high speed capability (e.g., fiber-optic cabling is faster than standard wiring). High speed modem or digital telephone wiring (e.g., so-called ISDN [Integrated Services Digital Network] line) may be quite adequate as a reliable and fast linkage from miles or hundreds of miles away. Some modems even work well with cellular telephones, allowing true portability for data review. One can envisage notebook computers being used as portable review stations.

4

Clinical Examples

Each of the examples in this chapter is chosen to illustrate a specific point, whether it is an occurrence peculiar to digital systems, a normal variant, or an abnormality. When necessary, additional information is added for clarity. Where appropriate, the classification code that we used in our laboratory is displayed. The intent always is to present the reader with understandable digital material, hoping that with familiarity even the novice will quickly lose any inhibition or concerns, and begin to think digitally.

Unless otherwise stated, the usual recording parameters are: linked ears reference (A1–A2), 0.3 to 70 Hz filters, 30 mm/s paper speed, 11 bits ADC precision, silver-silver chloride electrodes applied with collodion using the International 10-20 system, electrode impedance less than 3 k Ω. Grid lines are 1 s apart; if absent, the entire page is usually 10 s at a paper speed of 30 mm/s. Paper speed (PS, millimeters/second), sensitivity (SENS, microvolts/millimeter), and amplifier filter settings (low [LF] and high [HF] frequency, hertz), as well as a voltage calibration, are placed next to a vertical line of given length; all are represented by icons at the top left corner.

In the examples below, the figure number (e.g., Fig. 4-1) is listed with explanatory notes. Repeat illustrations (e.g., a, b, c, etc.) reflect the same data but redisplayed under different display settings (montage, sensitivity, paper speed, etc.). The montages used are:

Run 1 referential, parasagittal chain, then temporal chain; right over left;
Run 2 bipolar (double banana), else same as run 1;
Run 3 bipolar coronal, from front of the head; right to left;
Run 4 bipolar posterior halo, parasagittal chain, then posterior halo starting at Fp2;
Neonatal double interelectrode distance, double banana bipolar chain.

ARTIFACTS

Electrode Artifact

FIG. 4-1a,b A left parietal (P3) electrode pop artifact is seen on referential and bipolar montages, runs 1 and 2 (8 bits).
FIG. 4-2a,b An electromyogram contaminating the reference is seen diffusely on the referential montage, but is cleared up quite nicely on the bipolar montage (8 bits).
FIG. 4-3a,b This is similar to the previous example (8 bits).
FIG. 4-4a,b,c An electrocardiogram (EKG) contaminating the reference electrode is seen on the referential montage. Once again the artifact is decreased by using the bipolar montage (shown in 20 and 10 channels; 8 bits).
FIG. 4-5a,b A static electricity artifact is seen on the referential montage (right at the left margin of the page) and not on the bipolar montage.

Reference Contamination

FIG. 4-6a,b A focal spike discharge is seen phase reversing at F7 on Run 2. The same discharges are seen diffusely on Run 1 due to reference contamination. The rhythmicity of the discharges suggests an ongoing seizure.
FIG. 4-7a,b A high amplitude discharge is clearly seen at the right temporal area on Run 2. Run 1 shows it contaminating the reference also.
FIG. 4-8a,b,c A right temporal/frontal discharge contaminating the reference looks diffuse on Run 1, phase reversals on Run 2 suggest maximum involvement at F8 and T4. This discharge is further clarified by using a vertex reference.
FIG. 4-9a,b Complex discharges arising from the bitemporal regions look generalized on Run 1, but Run 2 enhances focality at the temporal lobes and shows left central involvement also.

Electrode Artifact

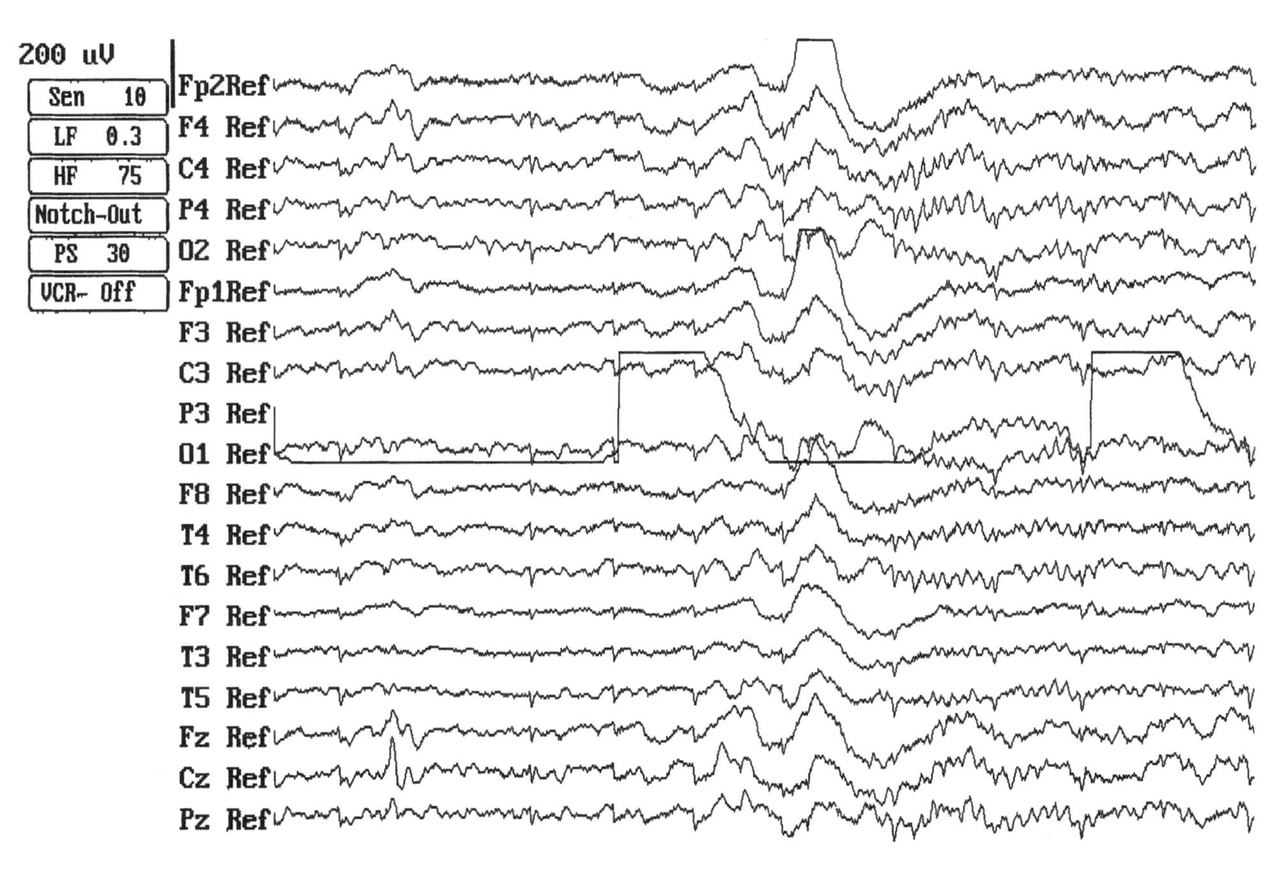

FIG. 4-1a,b A left parietal (P3) electrode pop artifact is seen on referential and bipolar montages, runs 1 and 2 (8 bits).

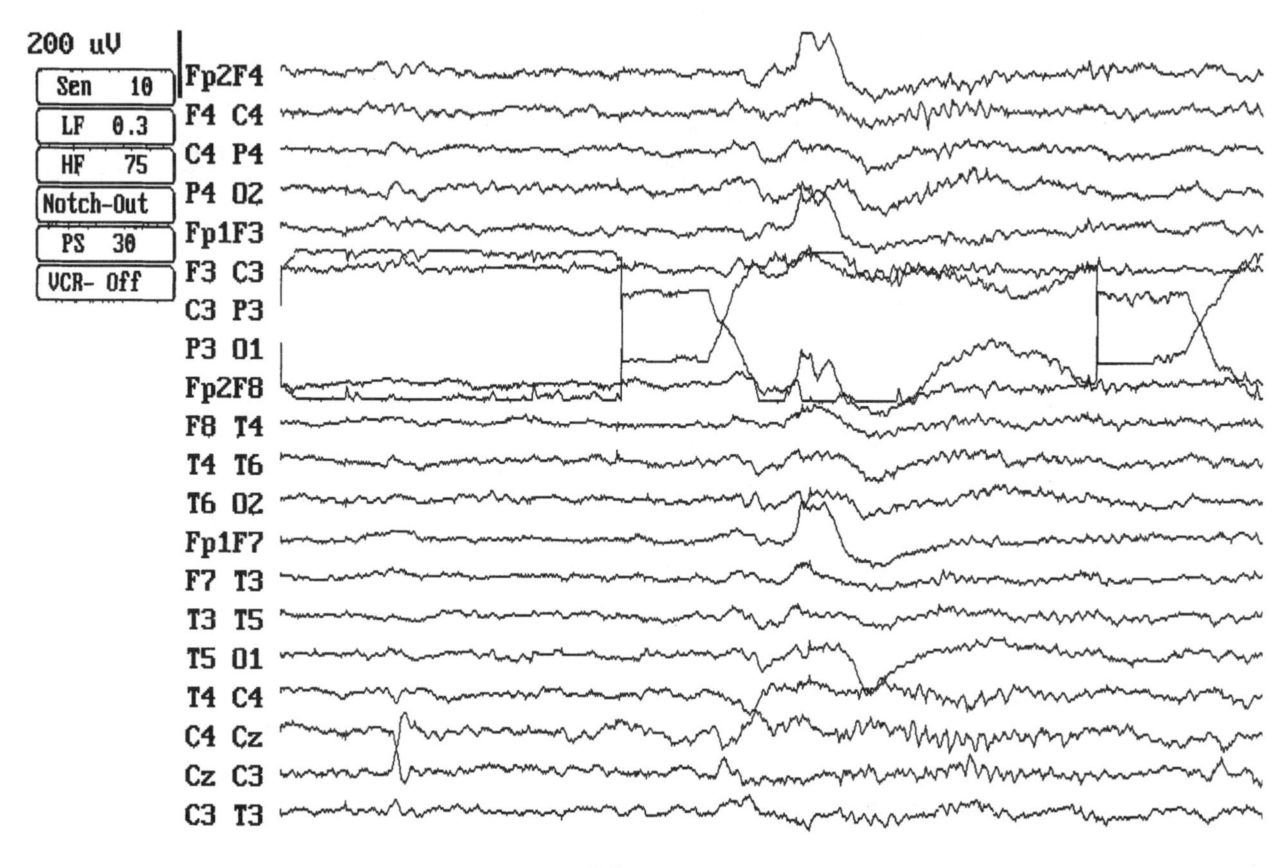
200 uV
Sen 10
LF 0.3
HF 75
Notch-Out
PS 30
VCR- Off
Fp2F4
F4 C4
C4 P4
P4 O2
Fp1F3
F3 C3
C3 P3
P3 O1
Fp2F8
F8 T4
T4 T6
T6 O2
Fp1F7
F7 T3
T3 T5
T5 O1
T4 C4
C4 Cz
Cz C3
C3 T3

FIG. 4-1 b

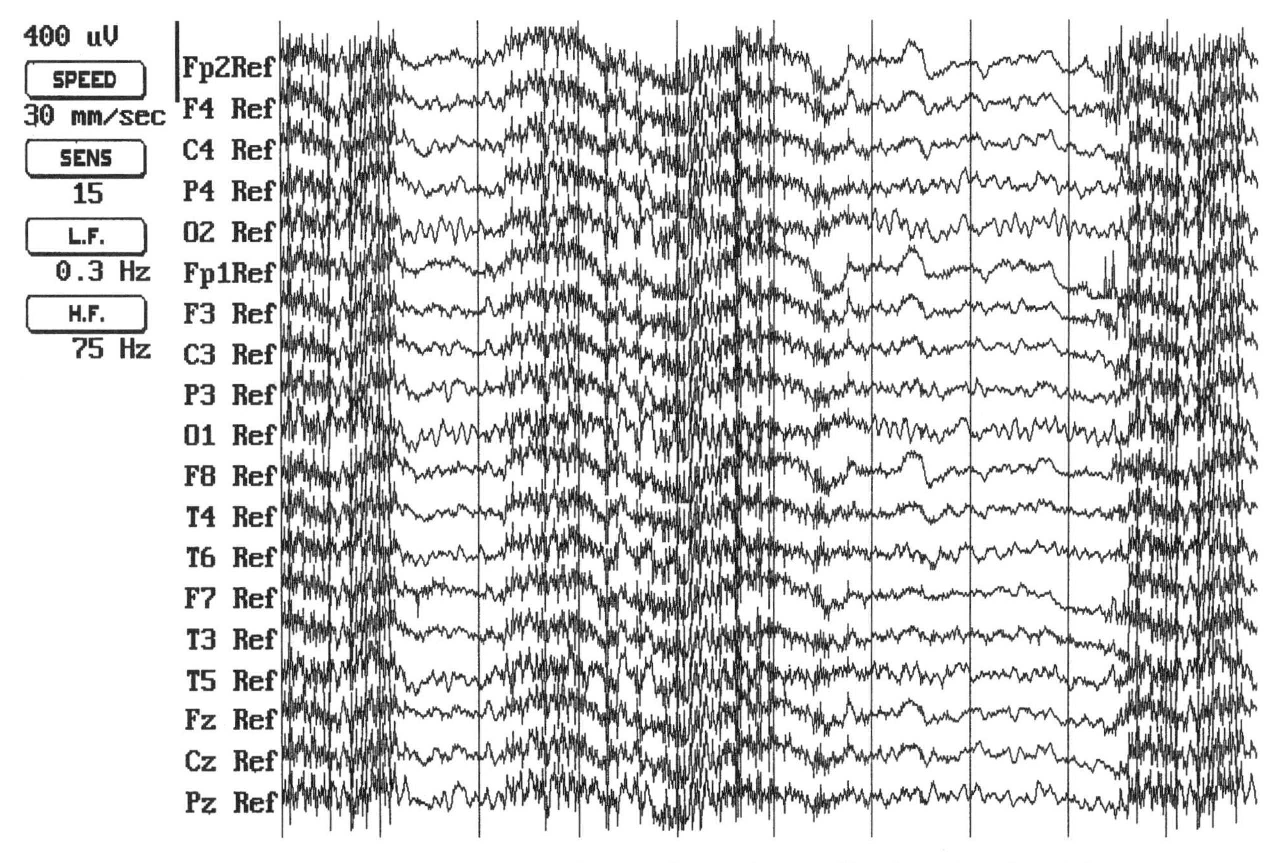

FIG. 4-2a,b An electromyogram contaminating the reference is seen diffusely on the referential montage, but is cleared up quite nicely on the bipolar montage (8 bits).

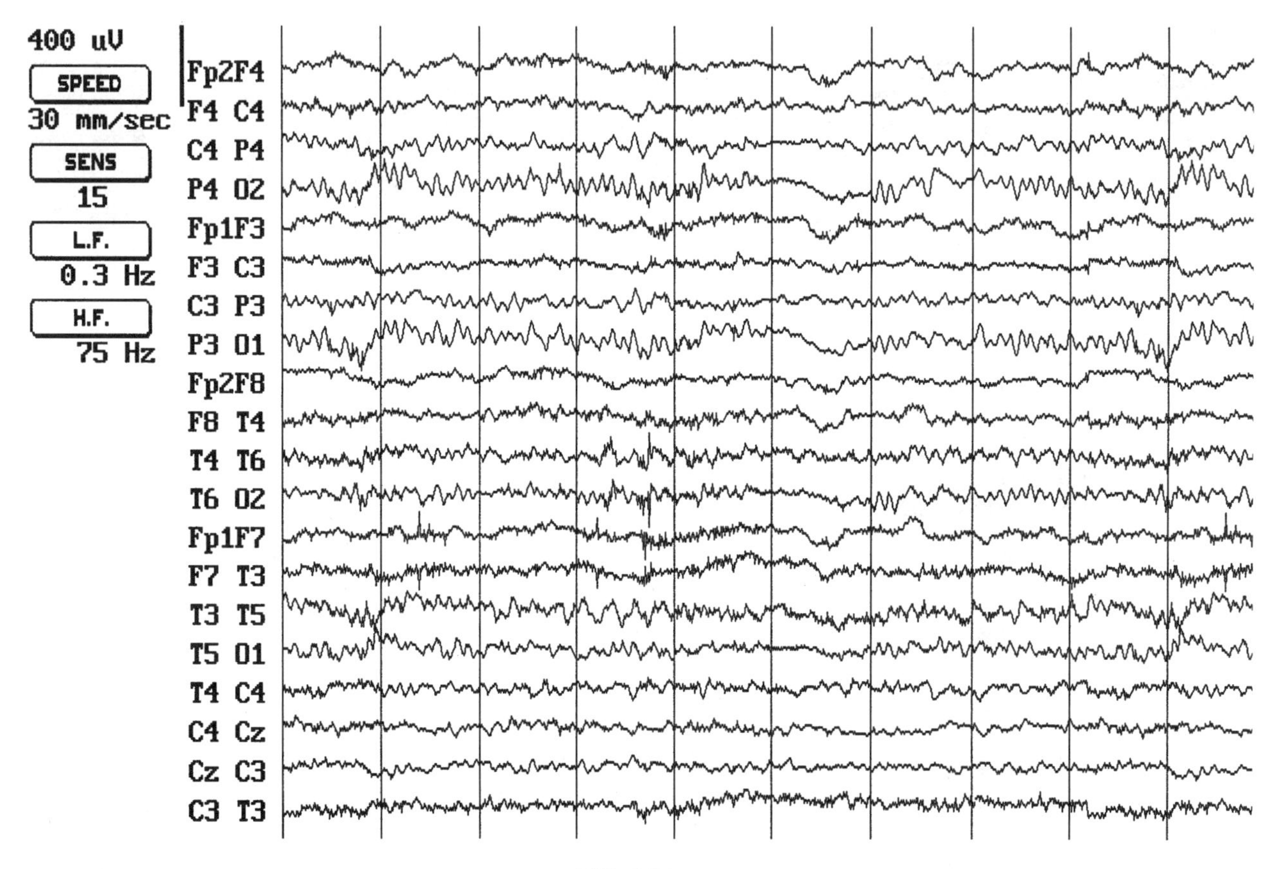
400 uV
SPEED
30 mm/sec
SENS
15
L.F.
0.3 Hz
H.F.
75 Hz
Fp2F4
F4 C4
C4 P4
P4 O2
Fp1F3
F3 C3
C3 P3
P3 O1
Fp2F8
F8 T4
T4 T6
T6 O2
Fp1F7
F7 T3
T3 T5
T5 O1
T4 C4
C4 Cz
Cz C3
C3 T3

FIG. 4-2 b

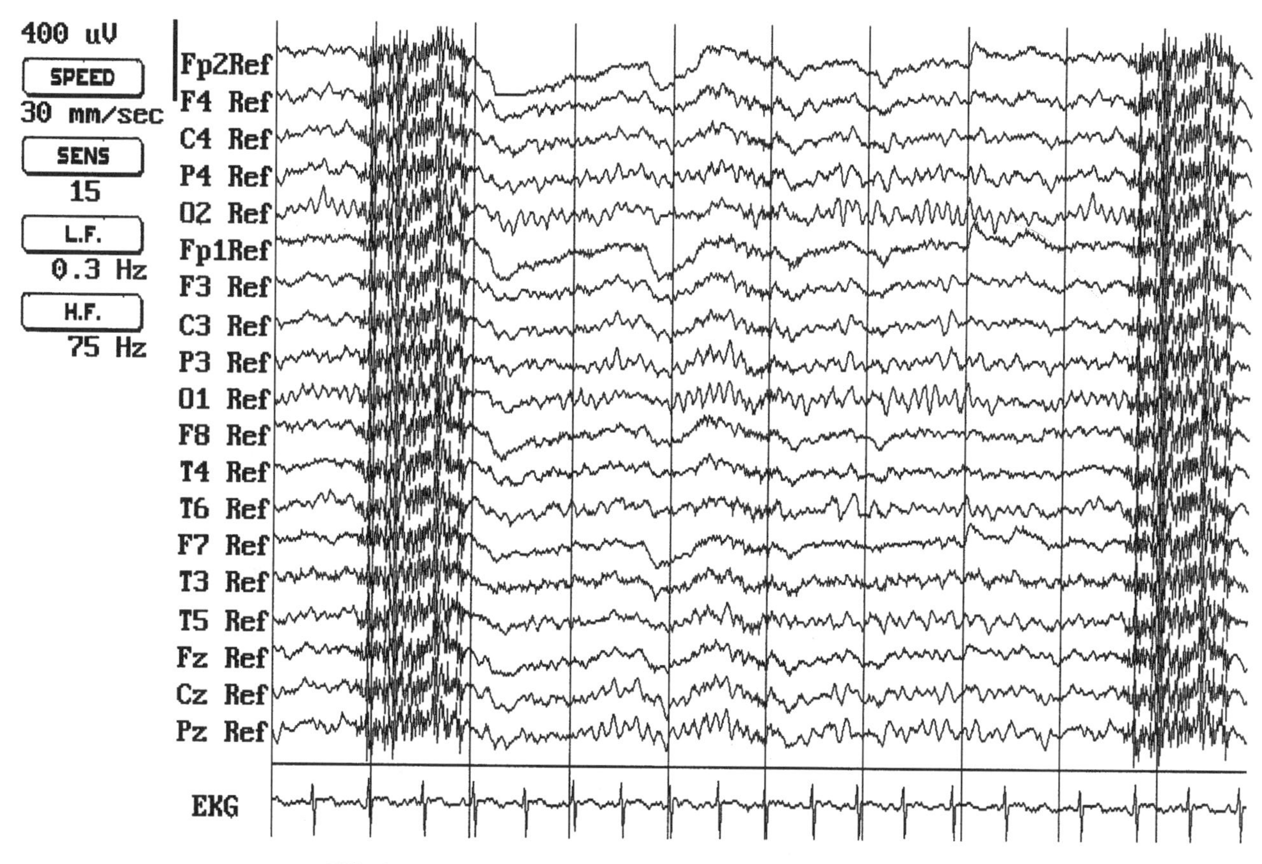

FIG. 4-3a,b This is similar to the previous example (8 bits).

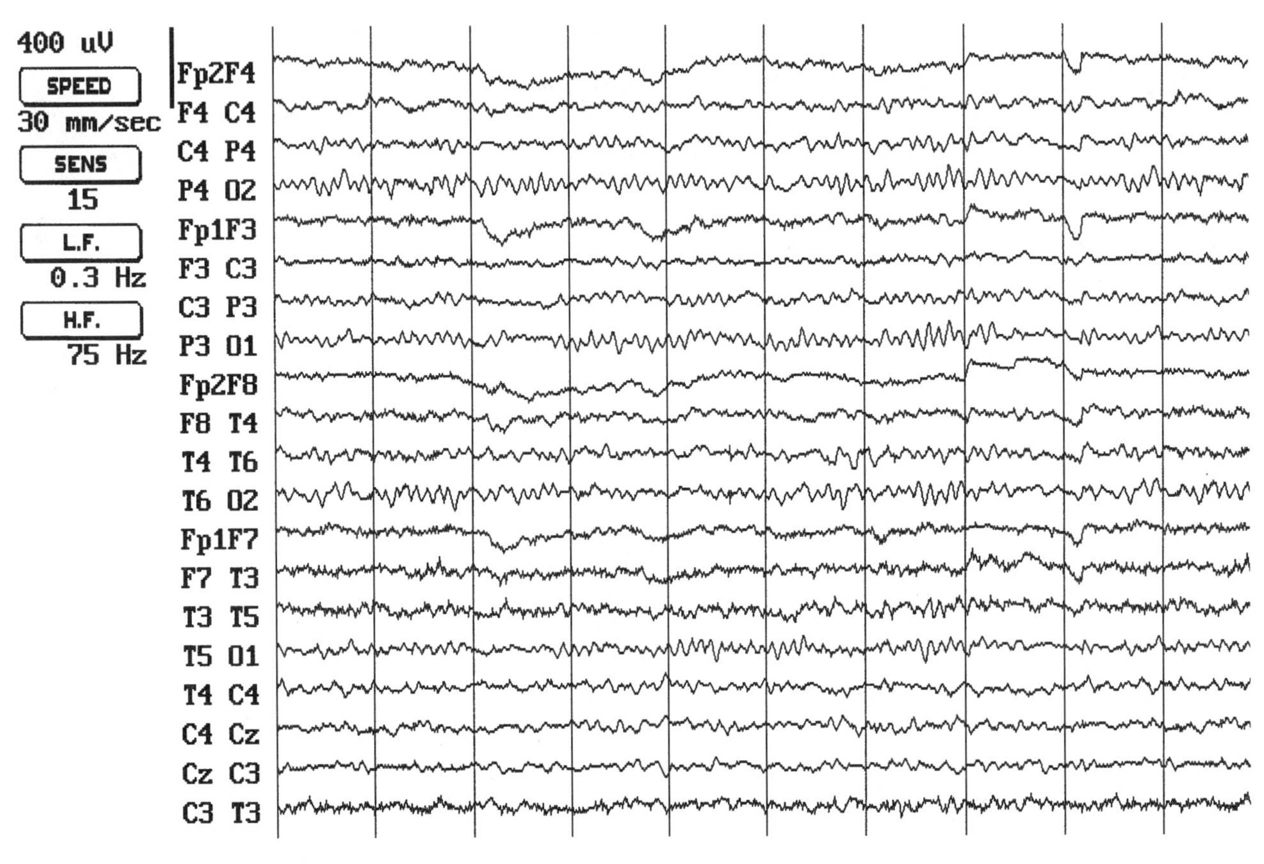
400 uV
SPEED
30 mm/sec
SENS
15
L.F.
0.3 Hz
H.F.
75 Hz
Fp2F4
F4 C4
C4 P4
P4 O2
Fp1F3
F3 C3
C3 P3
P3 O1
Fp2F8
F8 T4
T4 T6
T6 O2
Fp1F7
F7 T3
T3 T5
T5 O1
T4 C4
C4 Cz
Cz C3
C3 T3

FIG. 4-3 b

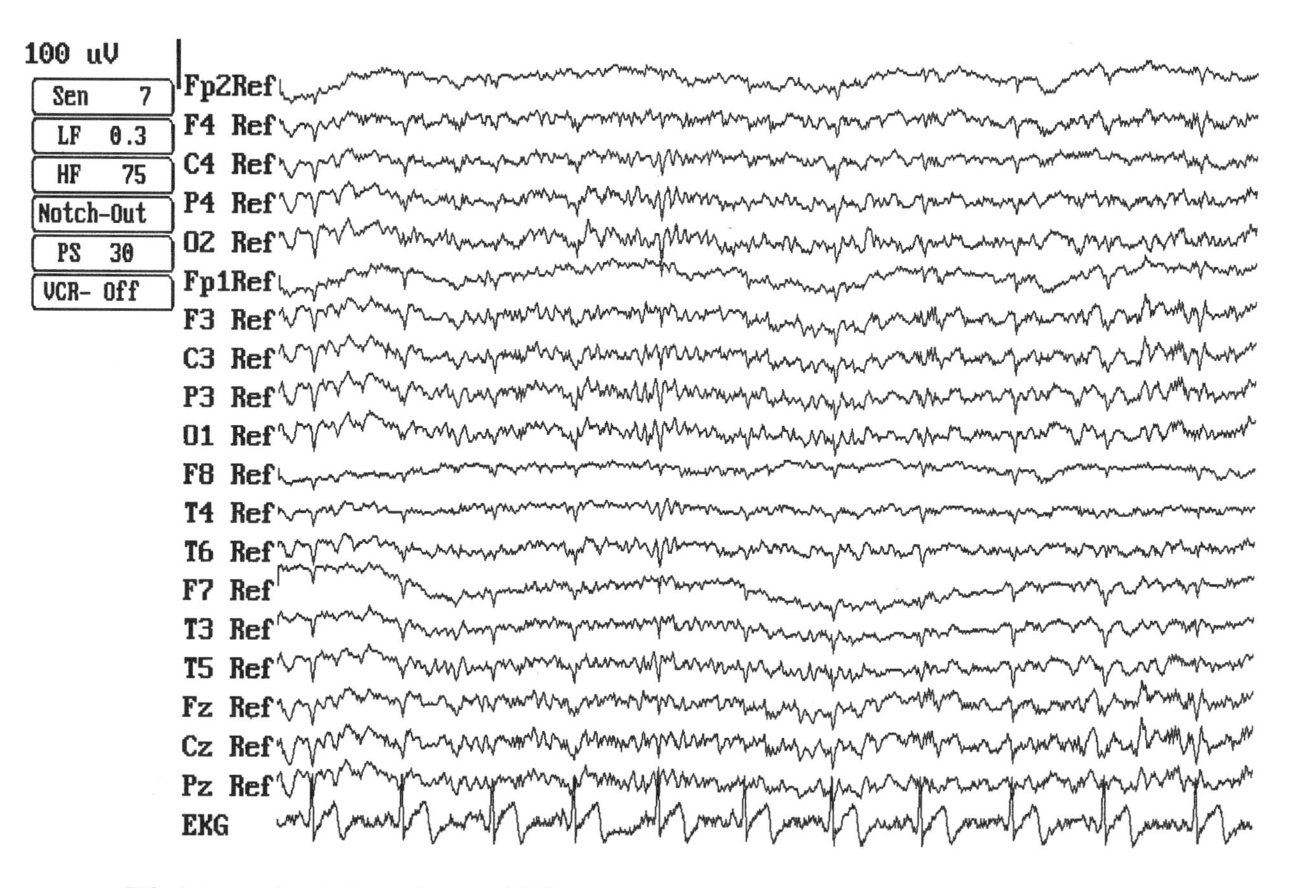

FIG. 4-4a,b,c An electrocardiogram (EKG) contaminating the reference electrode is seen on the referential montage. Once again the artifact is decreased by using the bipolar montage (shown in 20 and 10 channels; 8 bits).

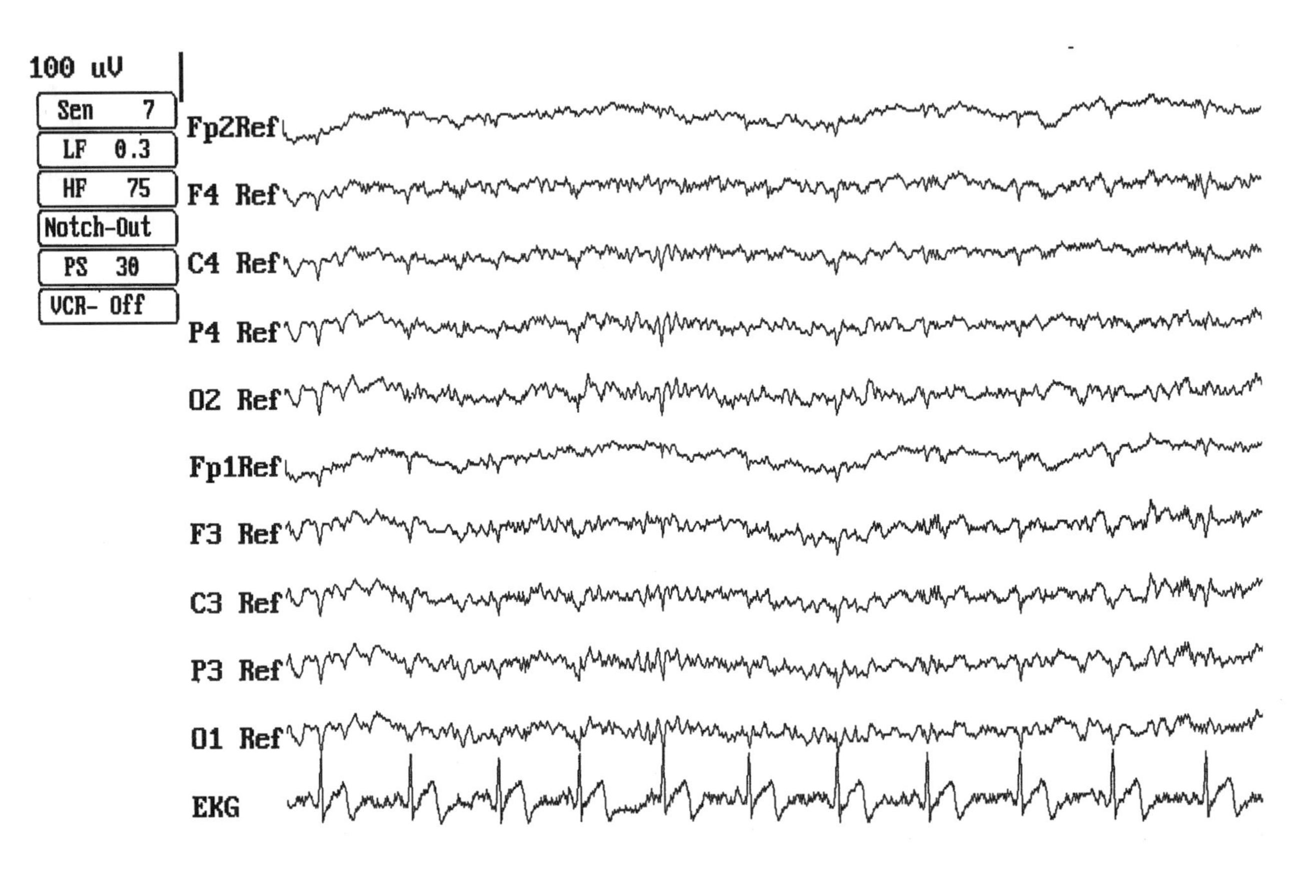
100 uV
Sen 7
LF 0.3
HF 75
Notch-Out
PS 30
VCR- Off
Fp2Ref
F4 Ref
C4 Ref
P4 Ref
O2 Ref
Fp1Ref
F3 Ref
C3 Ref
P3 Ref
O1 Ref
EKG

FIG. 4-4 b

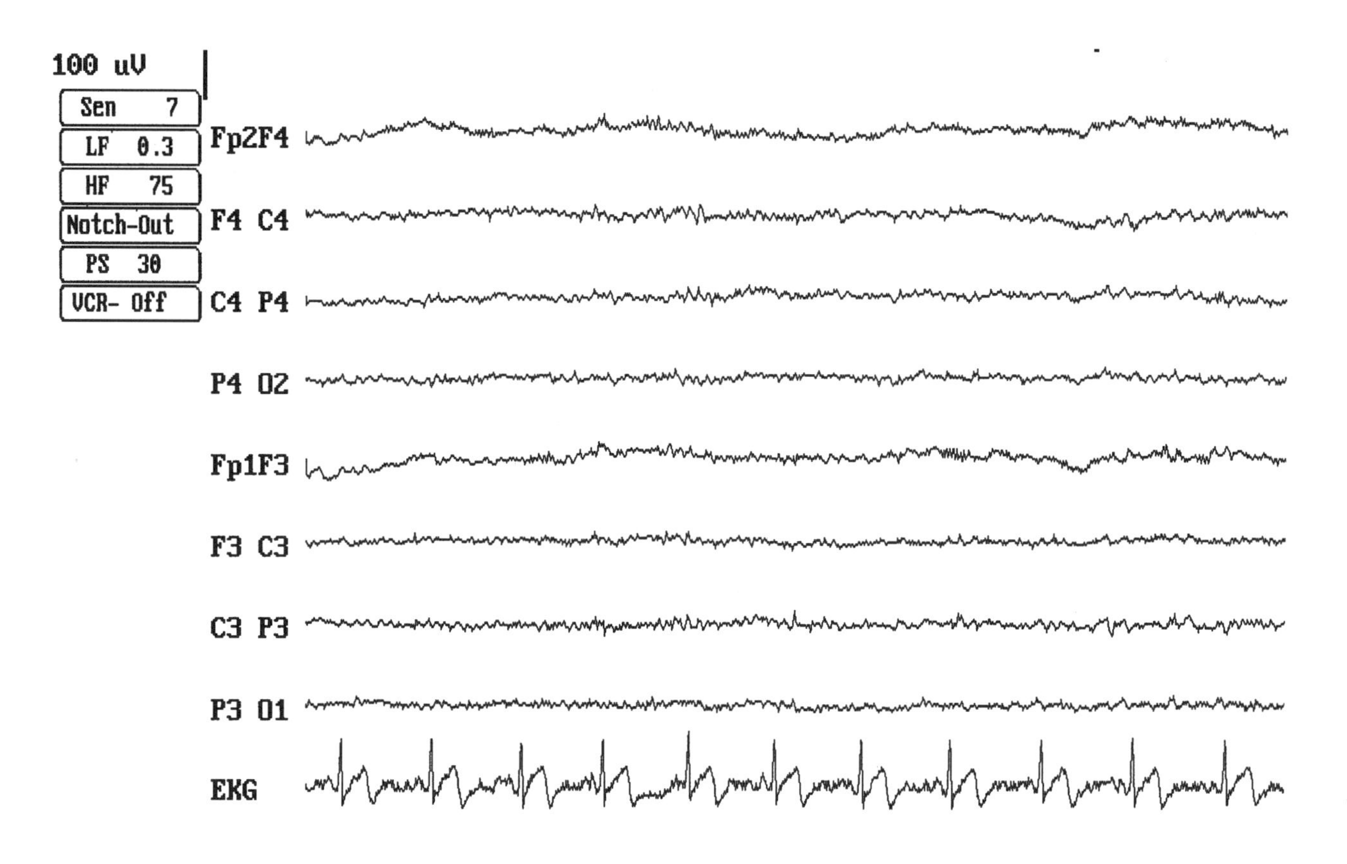
100 uV
Sen 7
LF 0.3
HF 75
Notch-Out
PS 30
VCR- Off
Fp2F4
F4 C4
C4 P4
P4 O2
Fp1F3
F3 C3
C3 P3
P3 O1
EKG

FIG. 4-4c

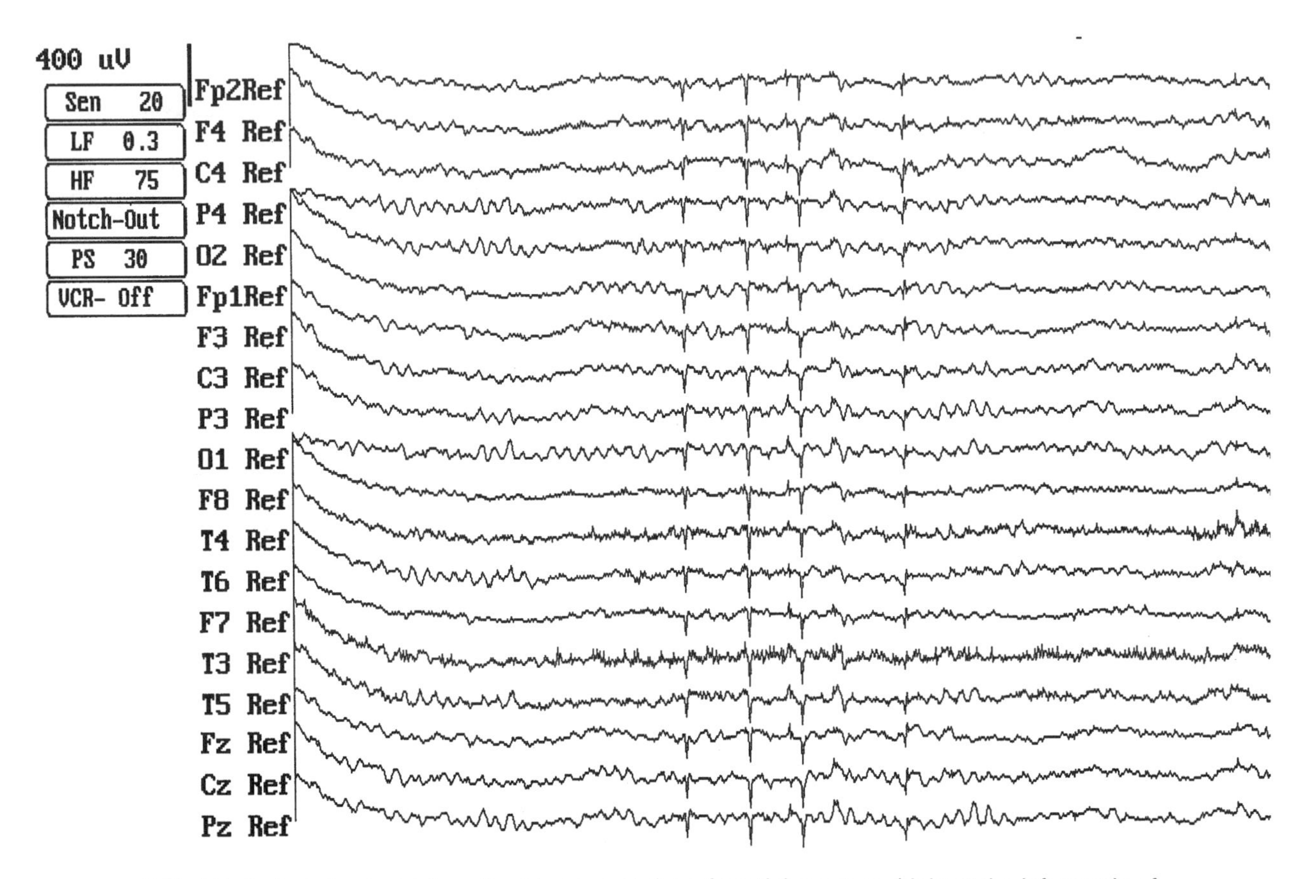

FIG. 4-5a,b A static electricity artifact is seen on the referential montage (right at the left margin of the page) and not on the bipolar montage.

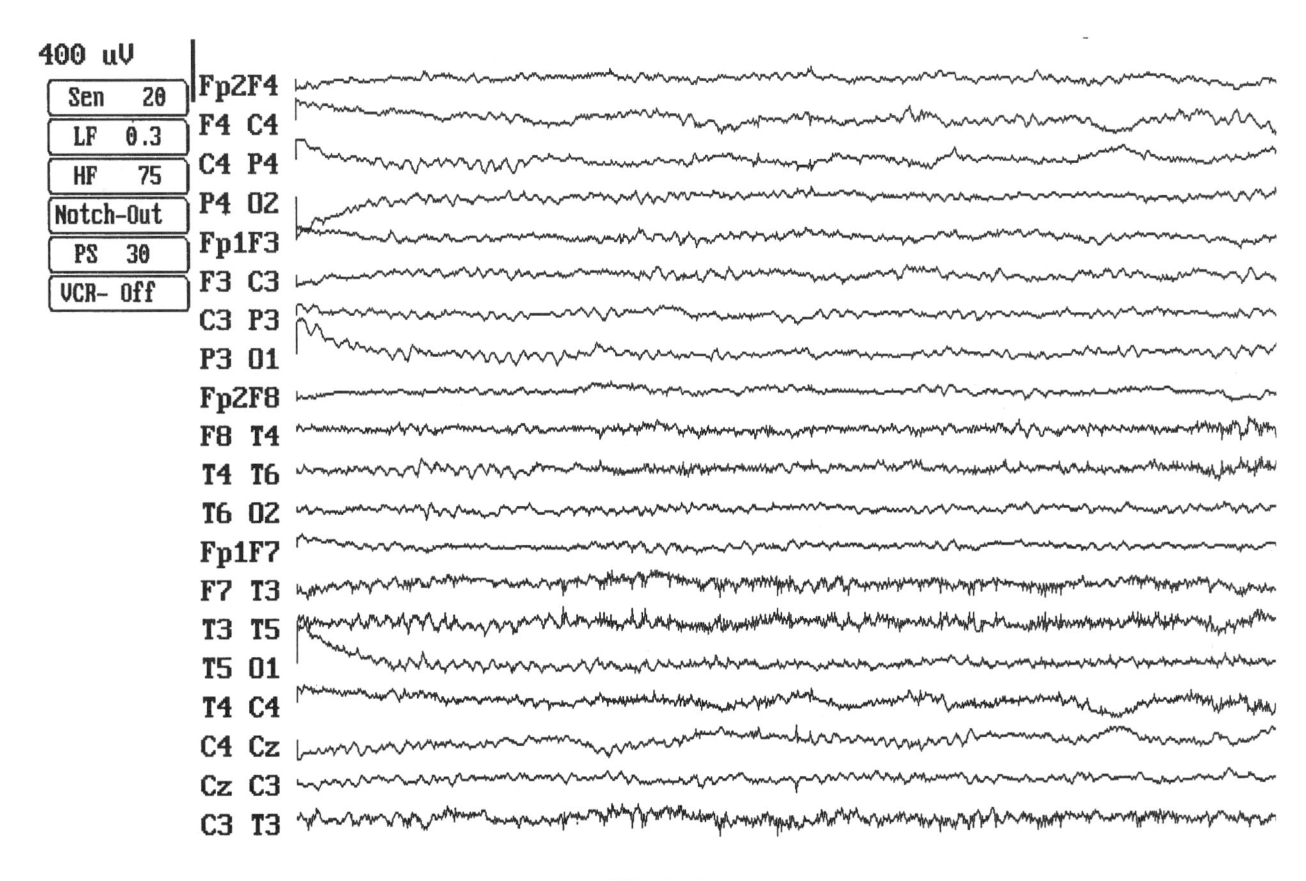
400 uV
Sen 20
LF 0.3
HF 75
Notch-Out
PS 30
VCR- Off
Fp2F4
F4 C4
C4 P4
P4 O2
Fp1F3
F3 C3
C3 P3
P3 O1
Fp2F8
F8 T4
T4 T6
T6 O2
Fp1F7
F7 T3
T3 T5
T5 O1
T4 C4
C4 Cz
Cz C3
C3 T3

FIG. 4-5b

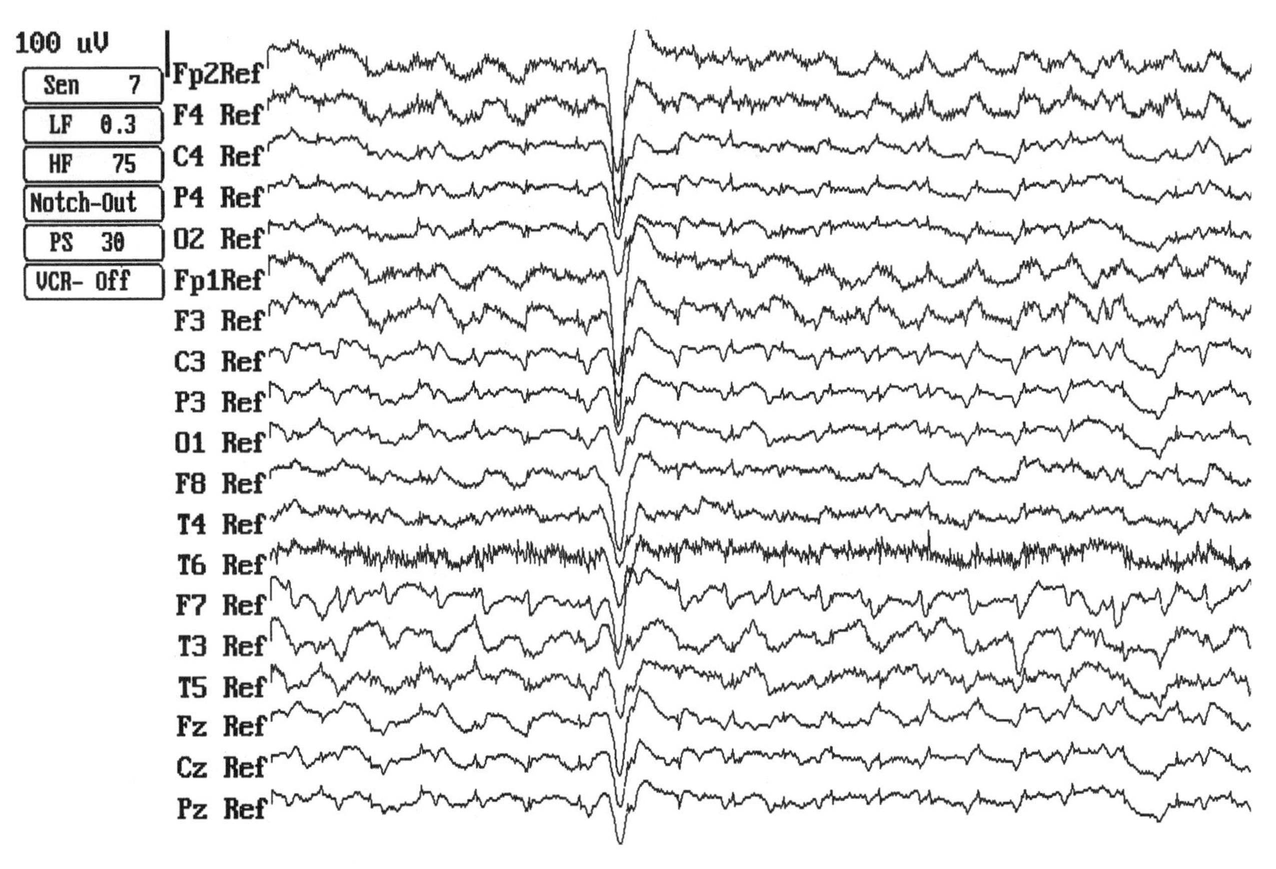

FIG. 4-6a,b A focal spike discharge is seen phase reversing at F7 on Run 2. The same discharges are seen diffusely on Run 1 due to reference contamination. The rhythmicity of the discharges suggests an ongoing seizure.

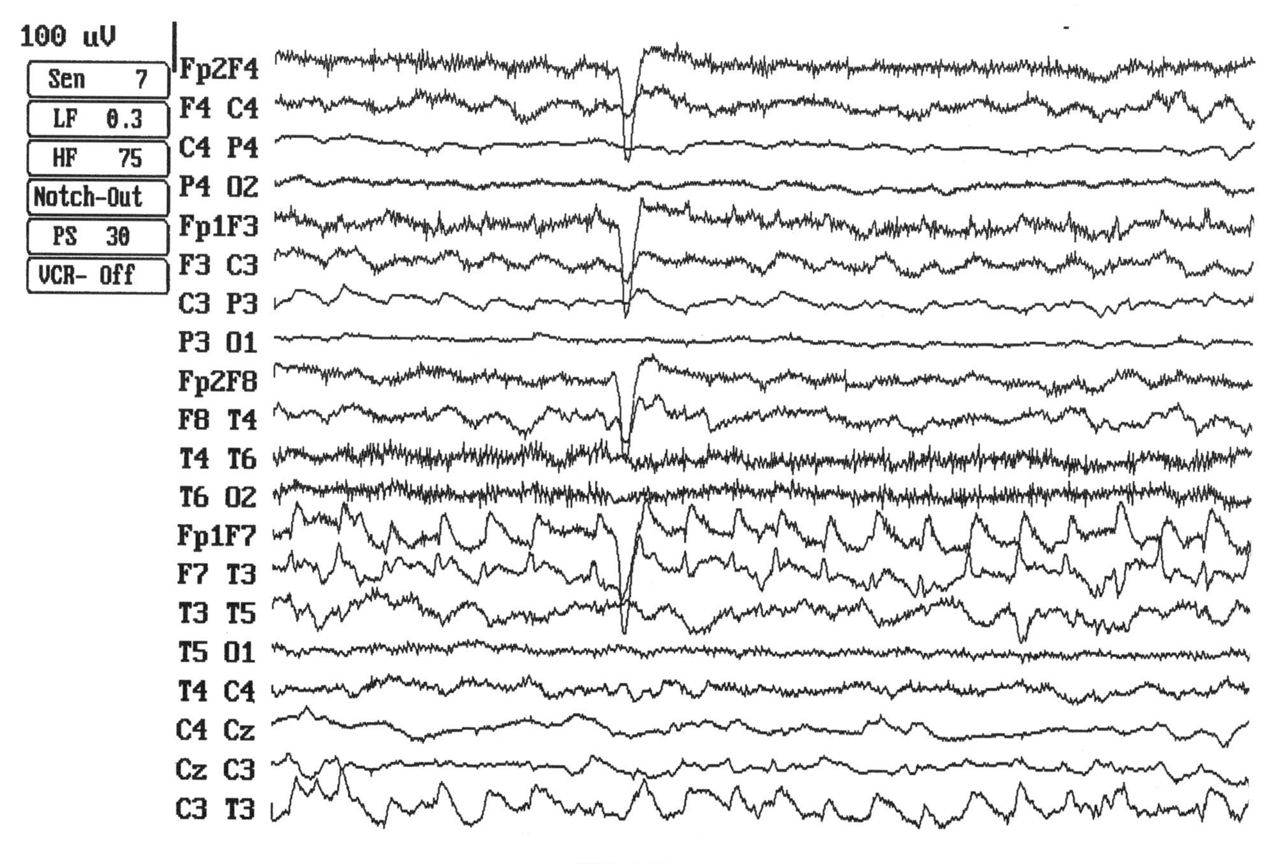
100 uV
Sen 7
LF 0.3
HF 75
Notch-Out
PS 30
VCR- Off
Fp2F4
F4 C4
C4 P4
P4 O2
Fp1F3
F3 C3
C3 P3
P3 O1
Fp2F8
F8 T4
T4 T6
T6 O2
Fp1F7
F7 T3
T3 T5
T5 O1
T4 C4
C4 Cz
Cz C3
C3 T3

FIG. 4-6 b

Reference Contamination

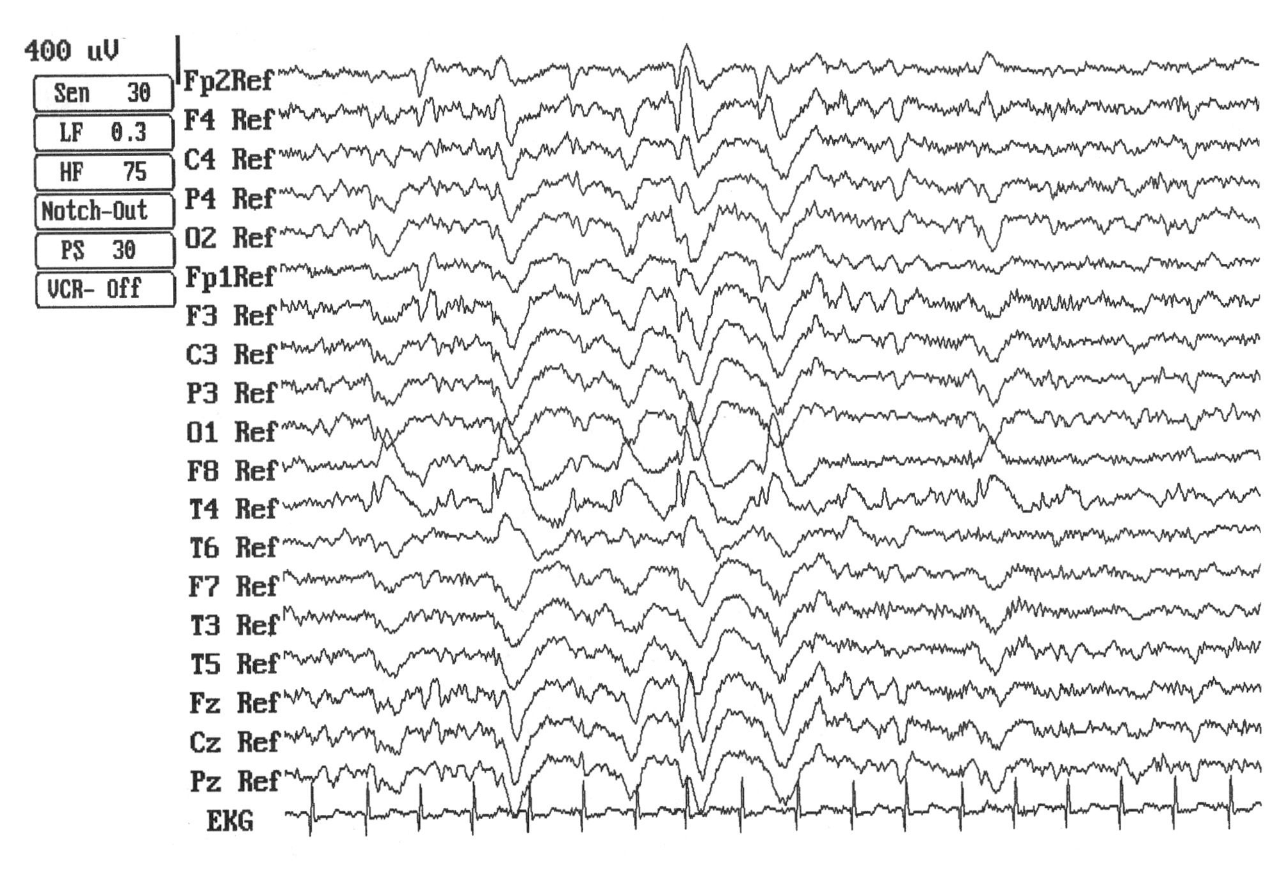

FIG. 4-7a,b A high amplitude discharge is clearly seen at the right temporal area on Run 2. Run 1 shows contaminating the reference also.

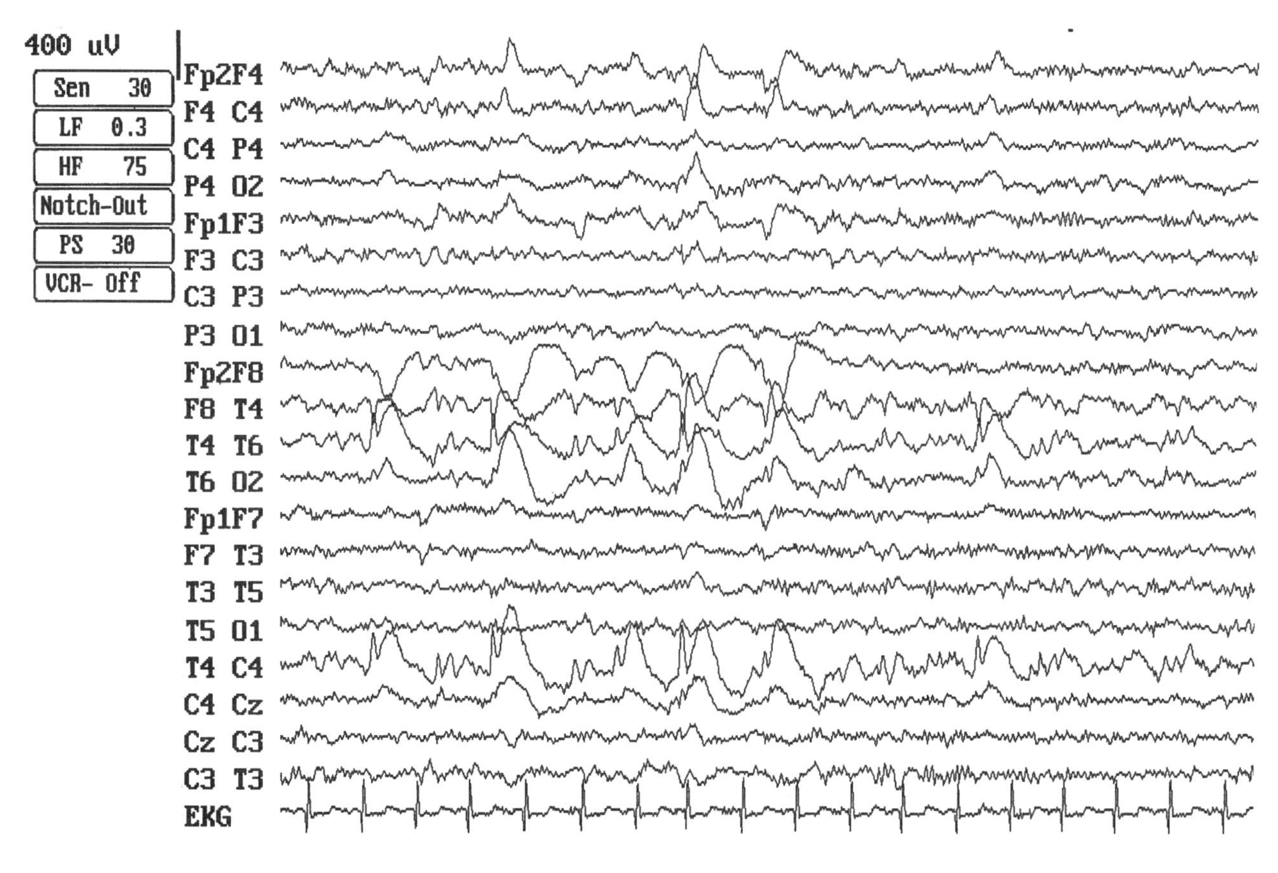
400 uV
Sen 30
LF 0.3
HF 75
Notch-Out
PS 30
VCR- Off
Fp2F4
F4 C4
C4 P4
P4 O2
Fp1F3
F3 C3
C3 P3
P3 O1
Fp2F8
F8 T4
T4 T6
T6 O2
Fp1F7
F7 T3
T3 T5
T5 O1
T4 C4
C4 Cz
Cz C3
C3 T3
EKG

FIG. 4-7 b

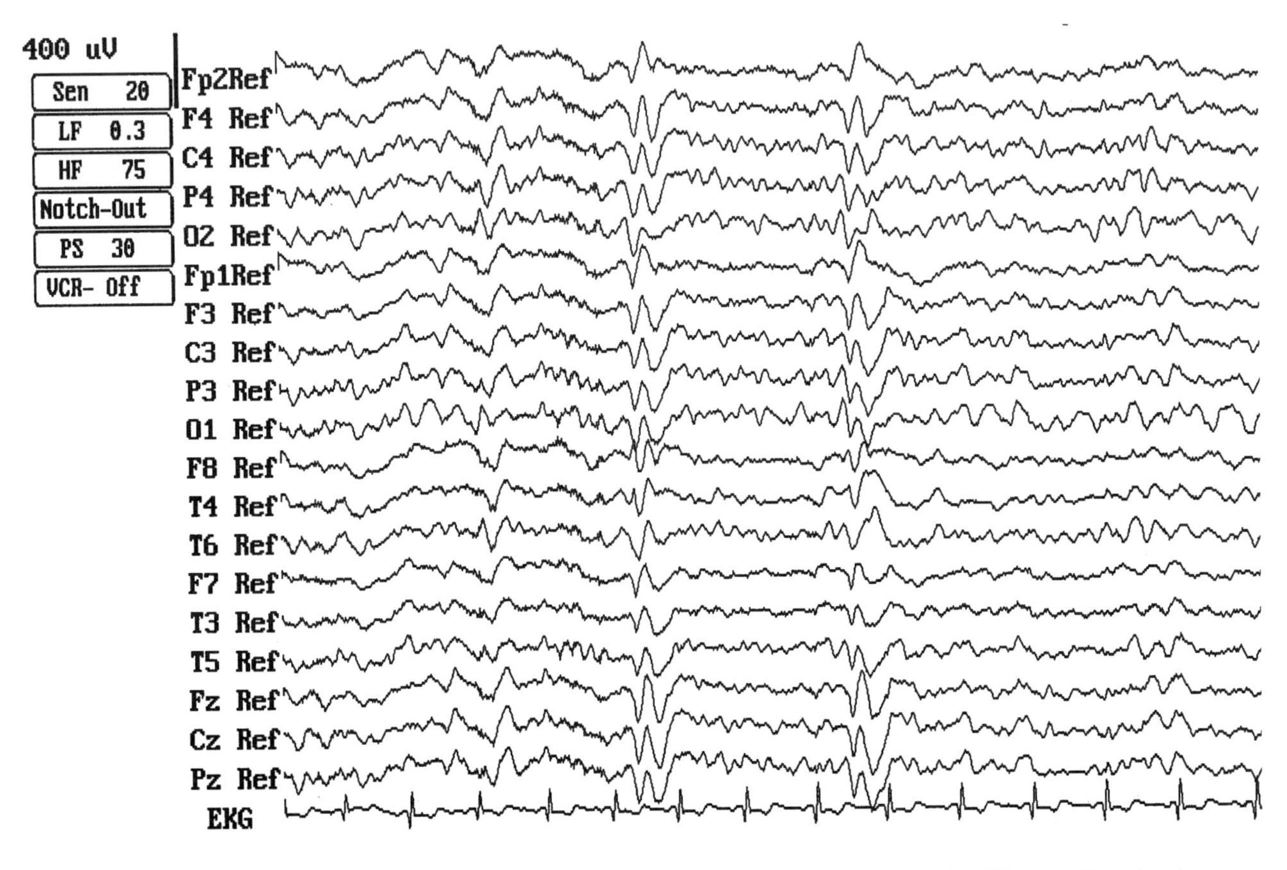

FIG. 4-8a,b,c A right temporal/frontal discharge contaminating the reference looks diffuse on Run 1, phase reversals on Run 2 suggest maximum involvement at F8 and T4. This discharge is further clarified by using a vertex reference.

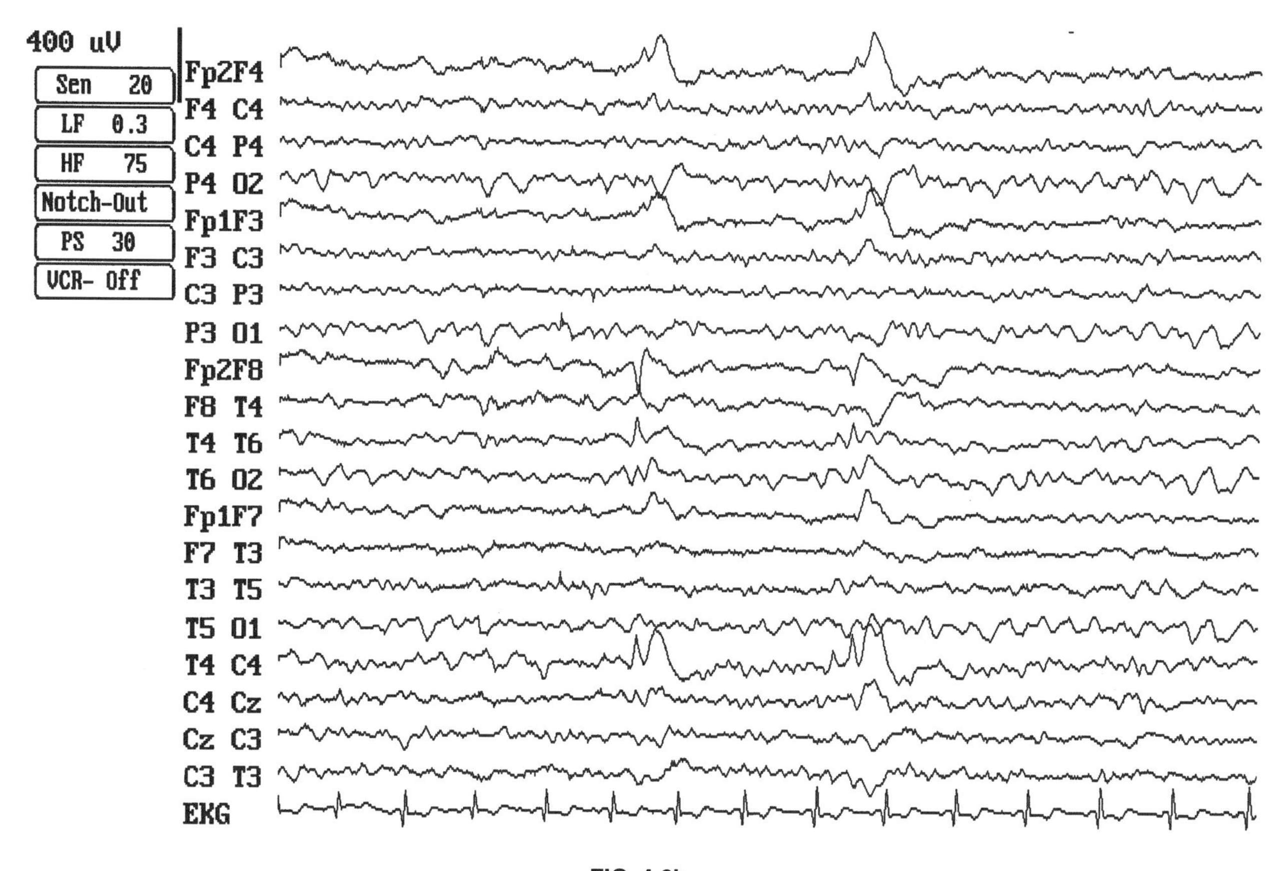
400 uV
Sen 20
LF 0.3
HF 75
Notch-Out
PS 30
VCR- Off
Fp2F4
F4 C4
C4 P4
P4 O2
Fp1F3
F3 C3
C3 P3
P3 O1
Fp2F8
F8 T4
T4 T6
T6 O2
Fp1F7
F7 T3
T3 T5
T5 O1
T4 C4
C4 Cz
Cz C3
C3 T3
EKG

FIG. 4-8b

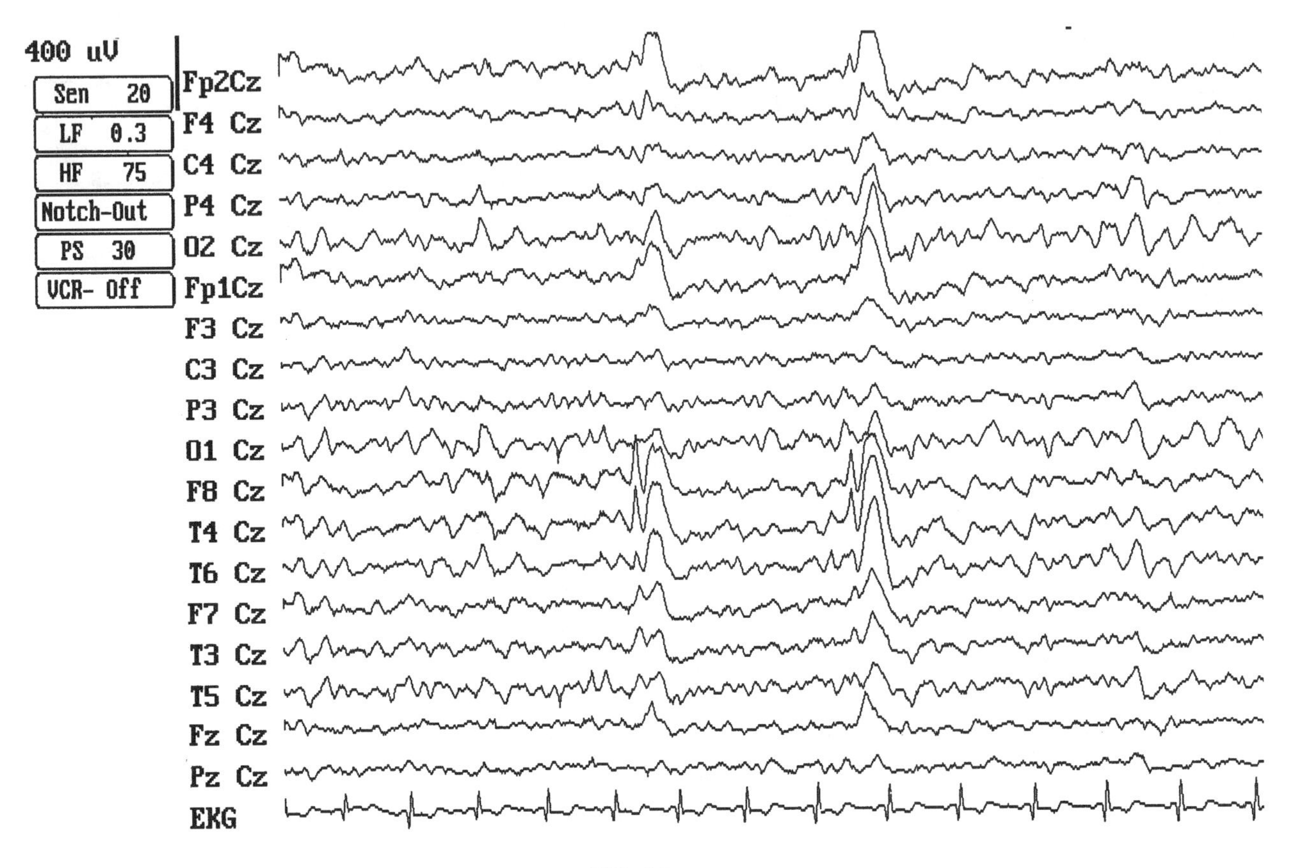
400 uV
Sen 20
LF 0.3
HF 75
Notch-Out
PS 30
VCR- Off
Fp2Cz
F4 Cz
C4 Cz
P4 Cz
O2 Cz
Fp1Cz
F3 Cz
C3 Cz
P3 Cz
O1 Cz
F8 Cz
T4 Cz
T6 Cz
F7 Cz
T3 Cz
T5 Cz
Fz Cz
Pz Cz
EKG

FIG. 4-8 c

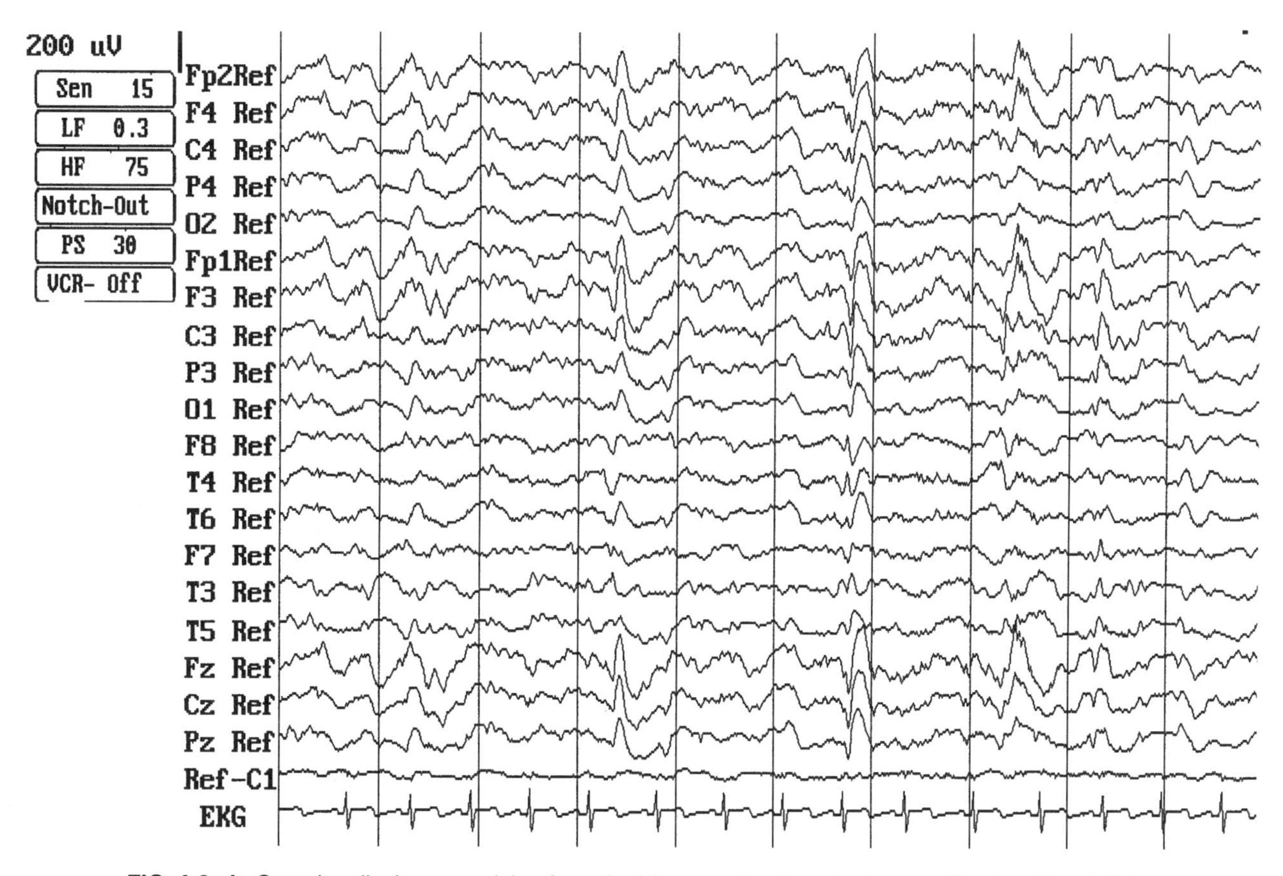

FIG. 4-9a,b Complex discharges arising from the bitemporal regions look generalized on Run 1, but Run 2 enhances focality at the temporal lobes and shows left central involvement also.

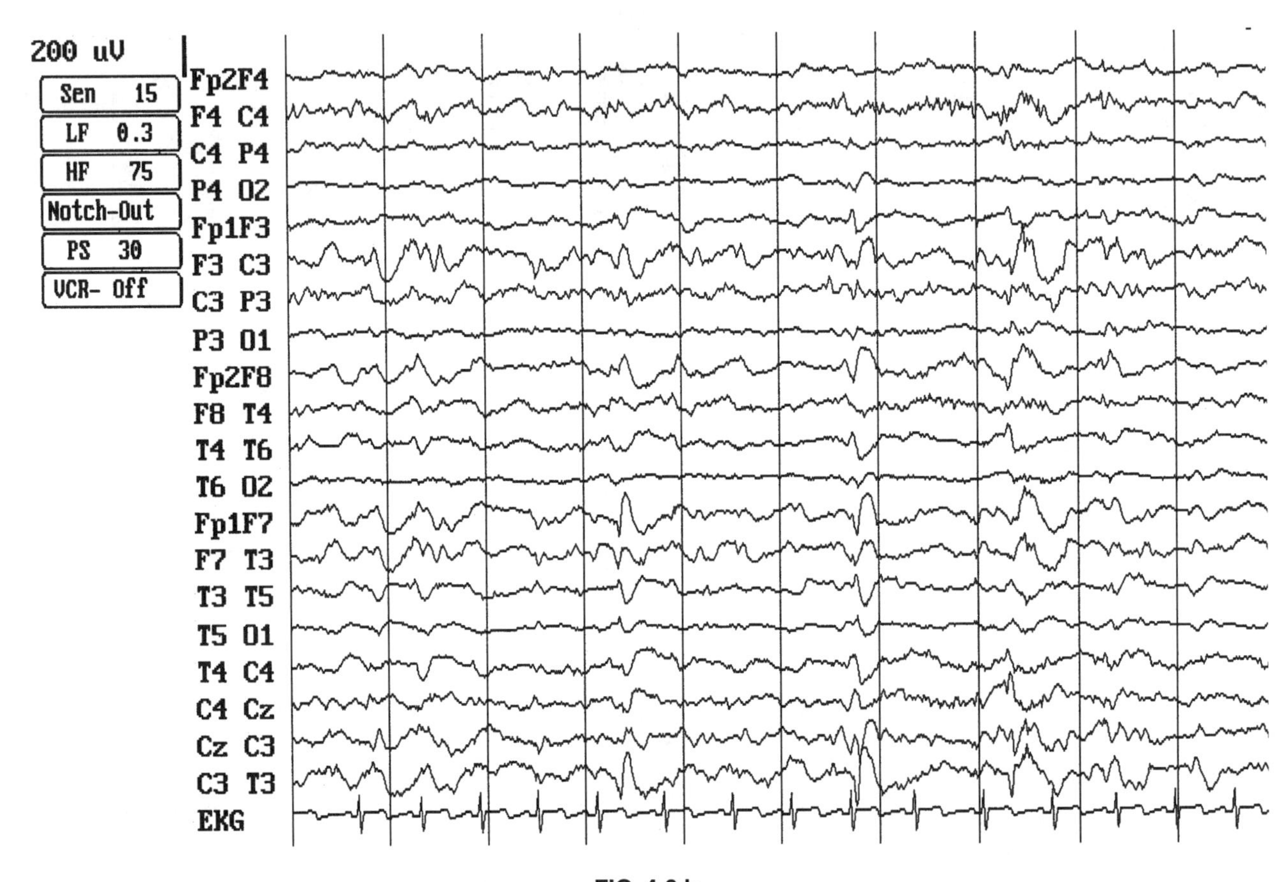
200 uV
Sen 15
LF 0.3
HF 75
Notch-Out
PS 30
VCR- Off
Fp2F4
F4 C4
C4 P4
P4 O2
Fp1F3
F3 C3
C3 P3
P3 O1
Fp2F8
F8 T4
T4 T6
T6 O2
Fp1F7
F7 T3
T3 T5
T5 O1
T4 C4
C4 Cz
Cz C3
C3 T3
EKG

FIG. 4-9 b

NORMAL EXAMPLES

Sleep

FIG. 4-10a,b A diffuse drowsy pattern consisting of theta is seen on two different runs.
FIG. 4-11a,b,c A high amplitude hypnagogic hypersynchrony burst (normal variant) seen at sensitivity 15 μV/mm looks ominous. The same sample with a lower sensitivity shows the burst better. A paper speed of 7.5 mm/sec shows the frequency of the bursts.
FIG. 4-12a,b Normal symmetrical vertex waves seen on two different runs.
FIG. 4-13a,b,c Asymmetric vertex waves show higher amplitude on the right as seen on three different runs.
FIG. 4-14a,b Asymmetric sleep spindles as seen on two different runs.

Normal Variants

FIG. 4-15a,b,c A normal symmetrical background with a 9 to 10 Hz posterior dominant rhythm seen on three different montages.
FIG. 4-16a,b,c An asymmetric posterior dominant rhythm shows a lower amplitude at O1 and more so at T5, as seen on run 1. On run 2 it appears to be symmetrical and on run 3 it appears to be only at T6.
FIG. 4-17a,b,c A burst of alpha frequency activity seen at both occipital areas on eye closure—commonly known as alpha squeak—is seen on run 1 and 2. A paper speed of 60 mm/s illustrates morphology the best.
FIG. 4-18a,b,c An independent bitemporal psychomotor variant is seen phase reversing on runs 2 and 3. On run 1 it appears to be diffuse theta activity.
FIG. 4-19a,b This is another example of a psychomotor variant similar to Fig. 4-18.
FIG. 4-20a,b,c,d This example shows an unusual 5 Hz theta seen at the central leads on three different runs. The slower paper speed (15 mm/s) shows a longer trend.
FIG. 4-21a,b,c The 14 and 6 positive spikes (ctenoids) seen over the right parasagittal area on run 1 are eliminated by cancellation on run 2. The paper speed of 60 mm/s further magnifies this normal variant.
FIG. 4-22a,b Another sample of 14 and 6 positive spikes that are asynchronous are clearly seen on the referential run but poorly on the bipolar run.
FIG. 4-23a,b,c,d Normal bioccipital delta in light sleep is seen on three different runs. The delta is best seen on run 4 due to the phase reversals. The paper speed of 15 mm/s further enhances the delta. Also of note is the arrhythmic EKG contaminating the reference on run 1 that is eliminated by runs 2 and 3.
FIG. 4-24a,b,c A well regulated drowsy burst is seen better on run 1 than 2. The paper speed, 15 mm/s, further enhances the rhythmicity of the burst.
FIG. 4-25a,b Central mu rhythm, which is slightly higher on the left, is seen on runs 1 and 2.
FIG. 4-26a,b A low amplitude right sided small sharp spike is seen clearly on run 1 but disappears on run 2.
FIG. 4-27a,b High amplitude symmetrical lambda is seen equally well on runs 1 and 2.
FIG. 4-28a,b Sharp transients are seen with eye closure at the bioccipital area in the first and last second of this sample. This transient is seen well on both runs. Also an asymmetric mu rhythm is seen at the right central.

Neonatal Examples

FIG. 4-29a,b This shows a sleep EEG in a neonate 39 weeks conceptional age (CA). The paper speed, 15 mm/s, demonstrates the periodicity of bursts.
FIG. 4-30a,b An example of a sleep EEG in a neonate 40 weeks CA is shown.
FIG. 4-31a,b This example shows a sleep EEG in a neonate 42 weeks CA.
FIG. 4-32a,b A sleep EEG in a neonate 46 weeks CA is shown.
FIG. 4-33a,b,c This sleep EEG in a 3 month old shows Vertex waves and sleep spindles.

Apparent Delta Focus

FIG. 4-34a,b,c Run 3 shows a focal delta at T6; on run 2 it appears to be bilateral. Run 1 shows the slow wave to be lower voltage at T5; therefore the apparent focality at T6 is due to the lower amplitude delta at T5. This delta activity has the characteristics of benign posterior slow waves of youth.
FIG. 4-35a,b,c This example is similar to the previous one but the slowing is of higher frequency (4 to 5 Hz).
FIG. 4-36a,b,c This is similar to FIG. 4-34.
FIG. 4-37a,b,c This example is similar to FIG. 4-34 except that the slowing is at theta frequency.
FIG. 4-38a,b,c Run 3 shows an irregular posterior head delta that is maximum at T6. There also appears to be a sharp wave at T6. Run 2 shows the bilateral nature of the slowing. Run 1 further clarifies that indeed there is a posterior head delta, but that it is not focal to T6. It is lower amplitude at T5. Also the appearance of the "sharp wave" at T6 was merely a random occurrence from subtracting two relatively large slow waves.
FIG. 4-39a,b,c This is similar to the previous sample.
FIG. 4-40a,b,c This is similar to the previous sample.

Sleep

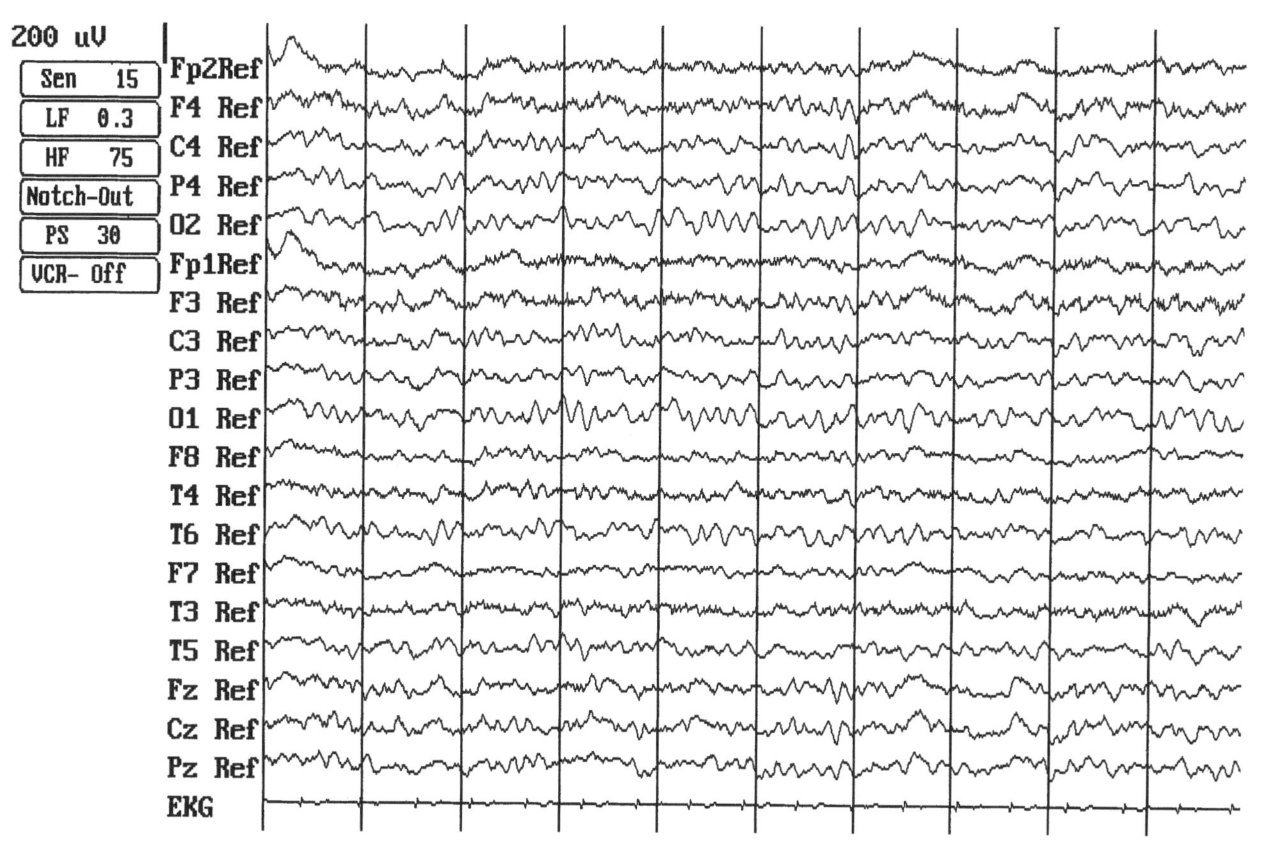

FIG. 4-10a,b A diffuse drowsy pattern consisting of theta is seen on two different runs.

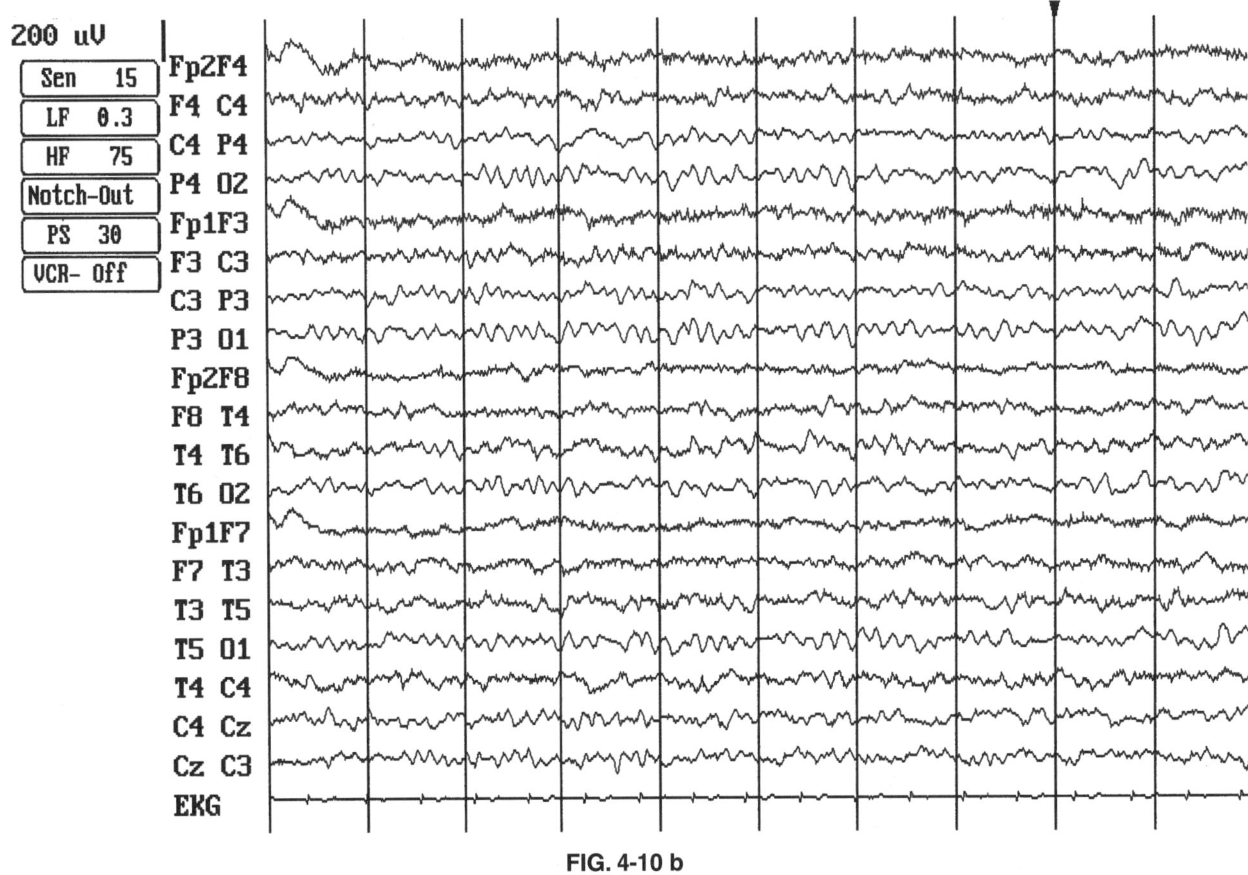
200 uV
Sen 15
LF 0.3
HF 75
Notch-Out
PS 30
VCR- Off
Fp2F4
F4 C4
C4 P4
P4 O2
Fp1F3
F3 C3
C3 P3
P3 O1
Fp2F8
F8 T4
T4 T6
T6 O2
Fp1F7
F7 T3
T3 T5
T5 O1
T4 C4
C4 Cz
Cz C3
EKG

FIG. 4-10 b

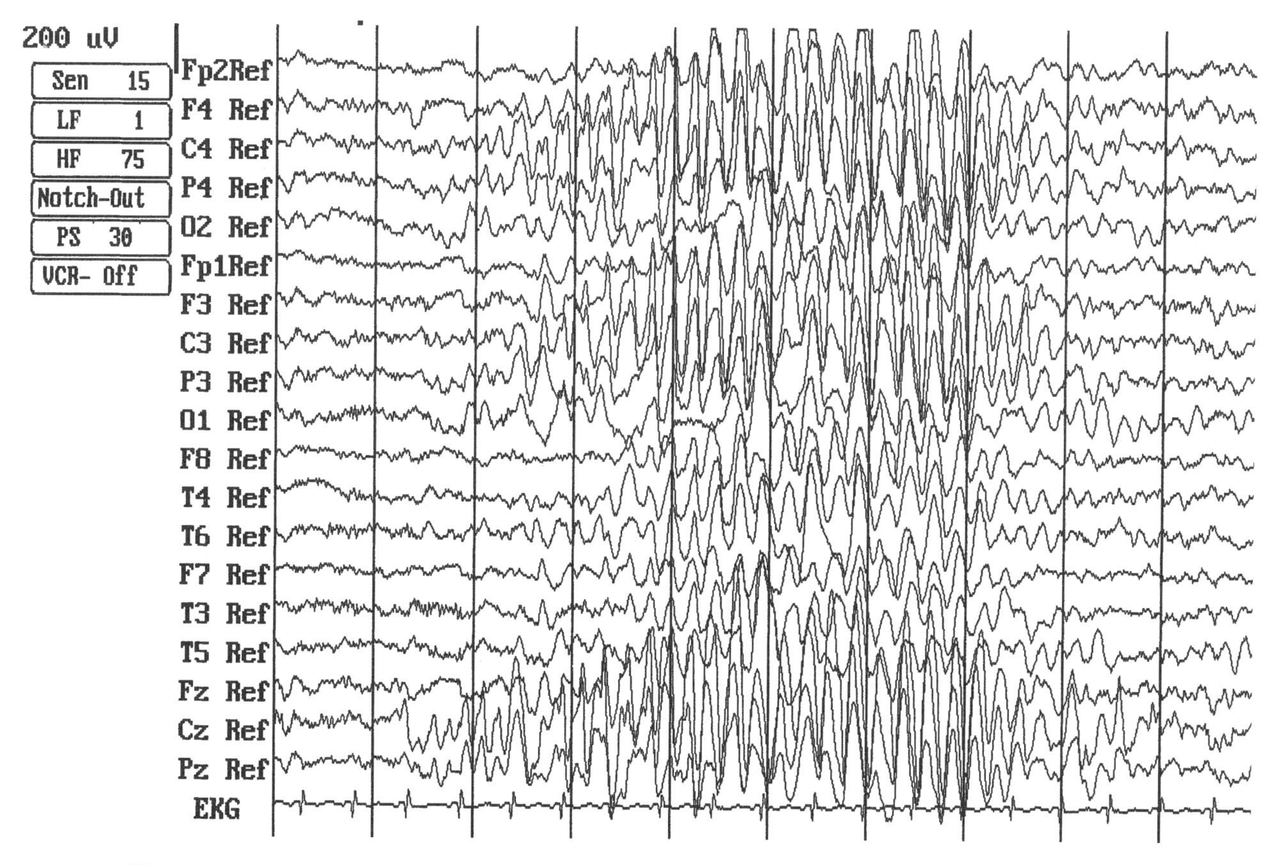

FIG. 4-11a,b,c A high amplitude hypnagogic hypersynchrony burst (normal variant) seen at sensitivity 15 μV/mm looks ominous. The same sample with a lower sensitivity shows the burst better. A paper speed of 7.5 mm/sec shows the frequency of the bursts.

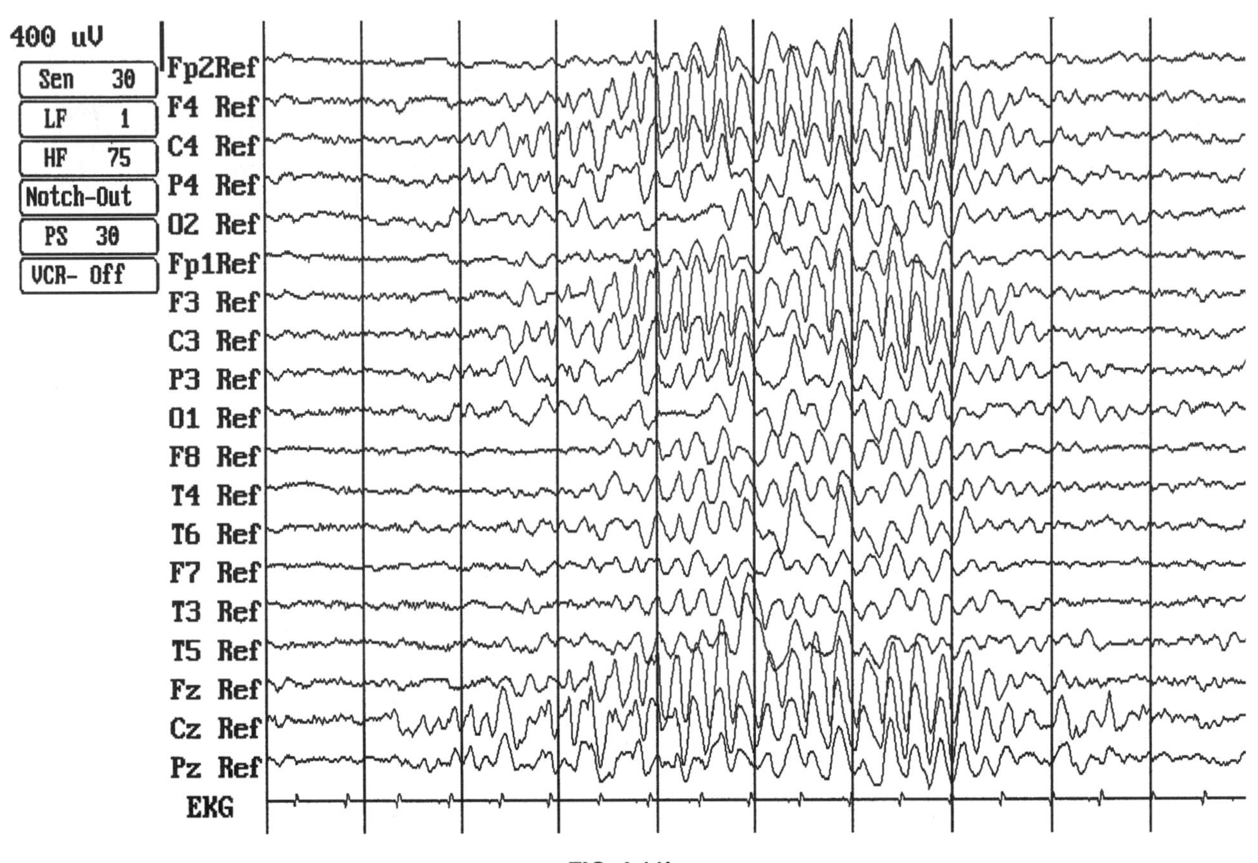
400 uV
Sen 30
LF 1
HF 75
Notch-Out
PS 30
VCR- Off
Fp2Ref
F4 Ref
C4 Ref
P4 Ref
O2 Ref
Fp1Ref
F3 Ref
C3 Ref
P3 Ref
O1 Ref
F8 Ref
T4 Ref
T6 Ref
F7 Ref
T3 Ref
T5 Ref
Fz Ref
Cz Ref
Pz Ref
EKG

FIG. 4-11b

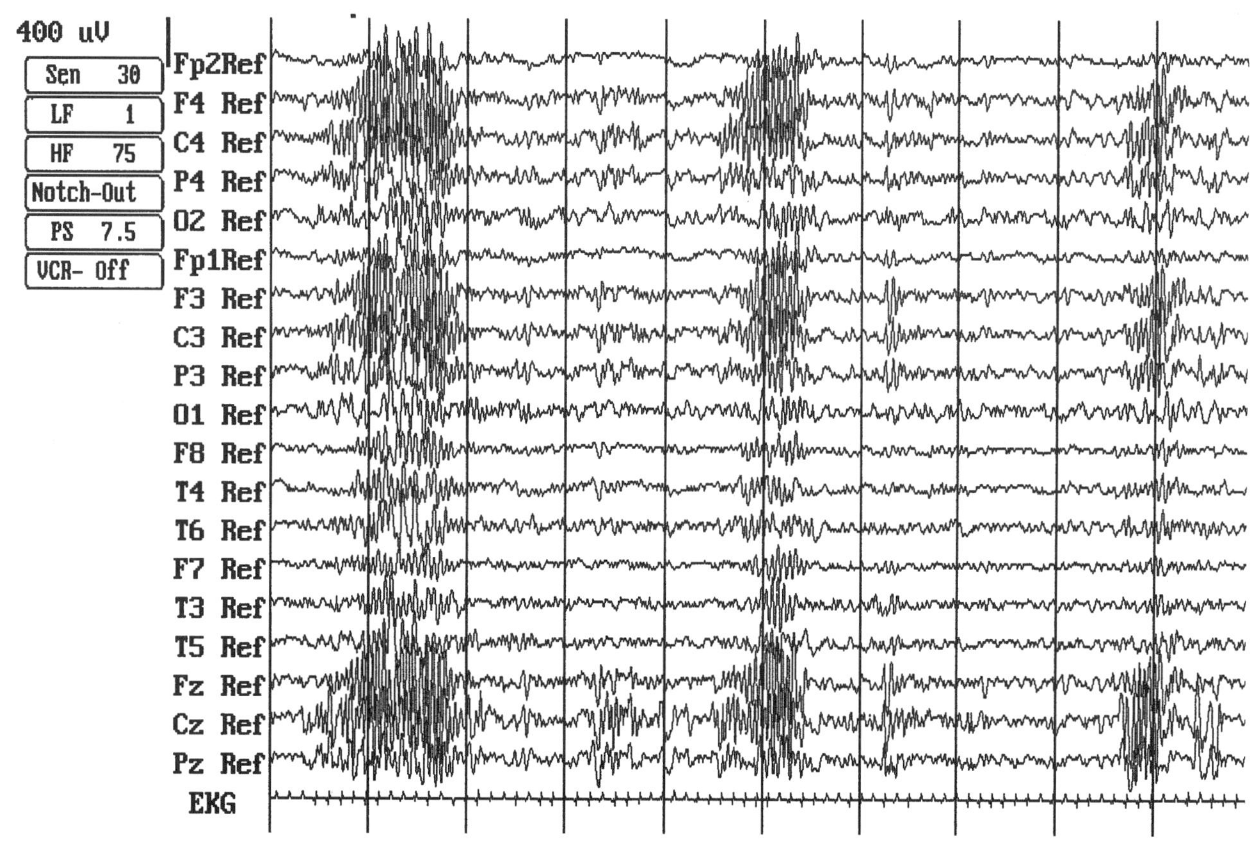
400 uV
Sen 30
LF 1
HF 75
Notch-Out
PS 7.5
VCR- Off
Fp2Ref
F4 Ref
C4 Ref
P4 Ref
O2 Ref
Fp1Ref
F3 Ref
C3 Ref
P3 Ref
O1 Ref
F8 Ref
T4 Ref
T6 Ref
F7 Ref
T3 Ref
T5 Ref
Fz Ref
Cz Ref
Pz Ref
EKG

FIG. 4-11c

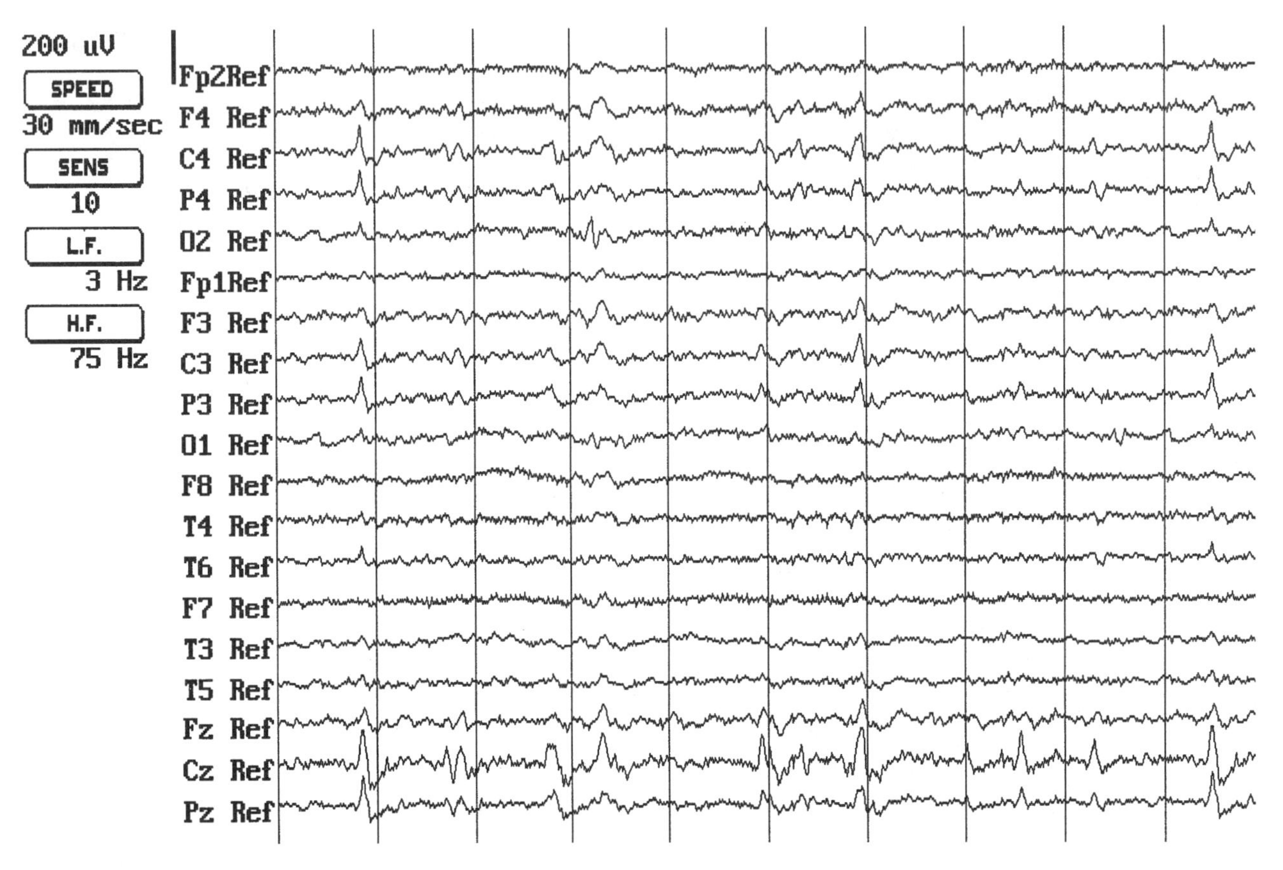

FIG. 4-12a,b Normal symmetrical vertex waves seen on two different runs.

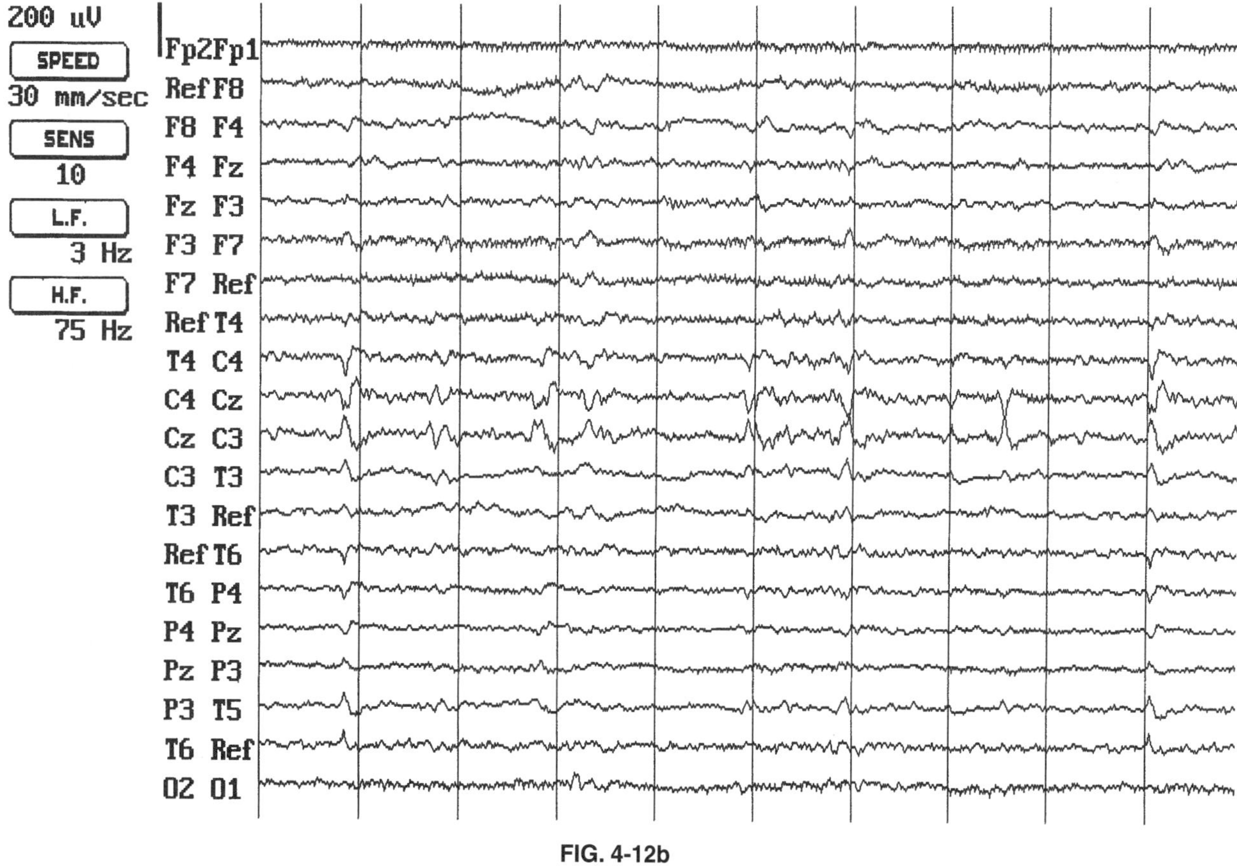
200 uV
SPEED
30 mm/sec
SENS
10
L.F.
3 Hz
H.F.
75 Hz
Fp2Fp1
Ref F8
F8 F4
F4 Fz
Fz F3
F3 F7
F7 Ref
Ref T4
T4 C4
C4 Cz
Cz C3
C3 T3
T3 Ref
Ref T6
T6 P4
P4 Pz
Pz P3
P3 T5
T6 Ref
O2 O1

FIG. 4-12b

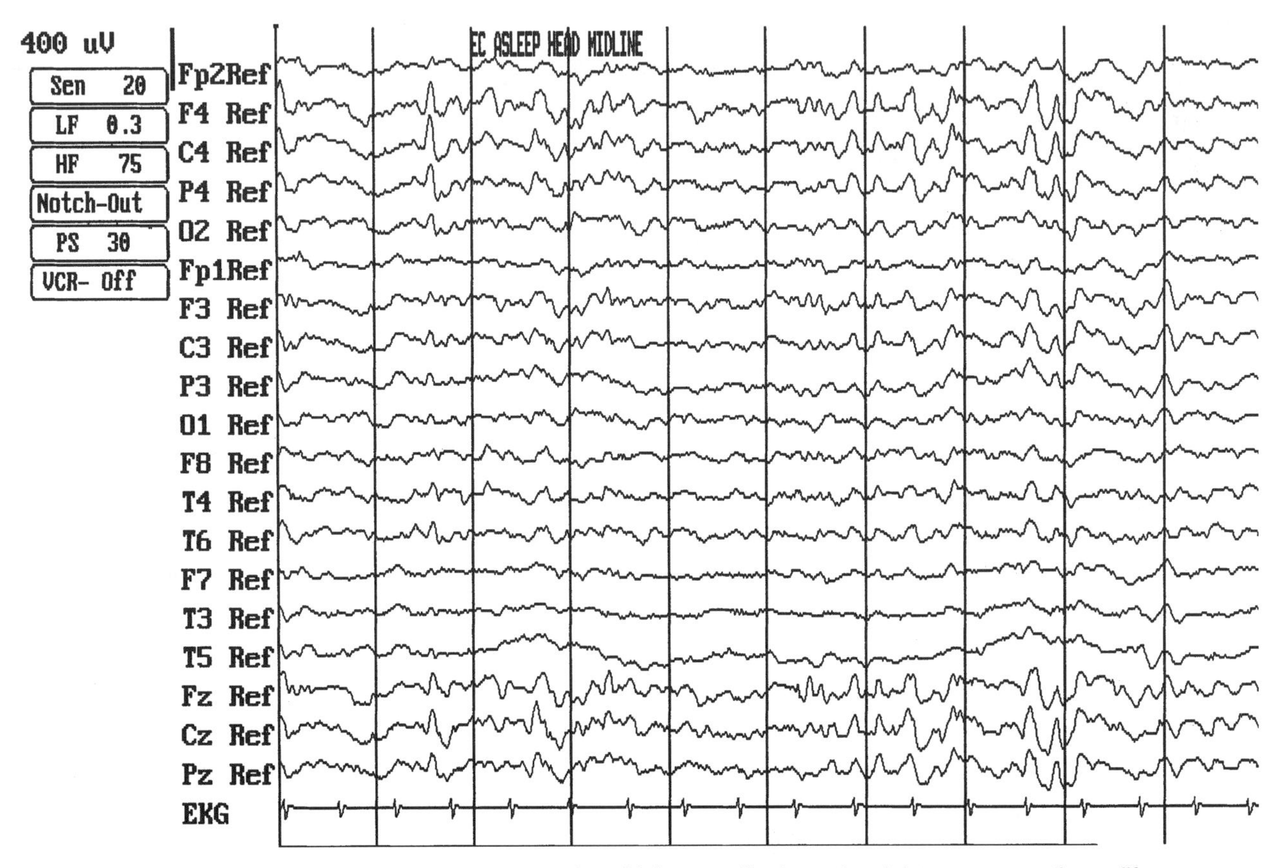

FIG. 4-13a,b,c Asymmetric vertex waves show higher amplitude on the right as seen on three different runs.

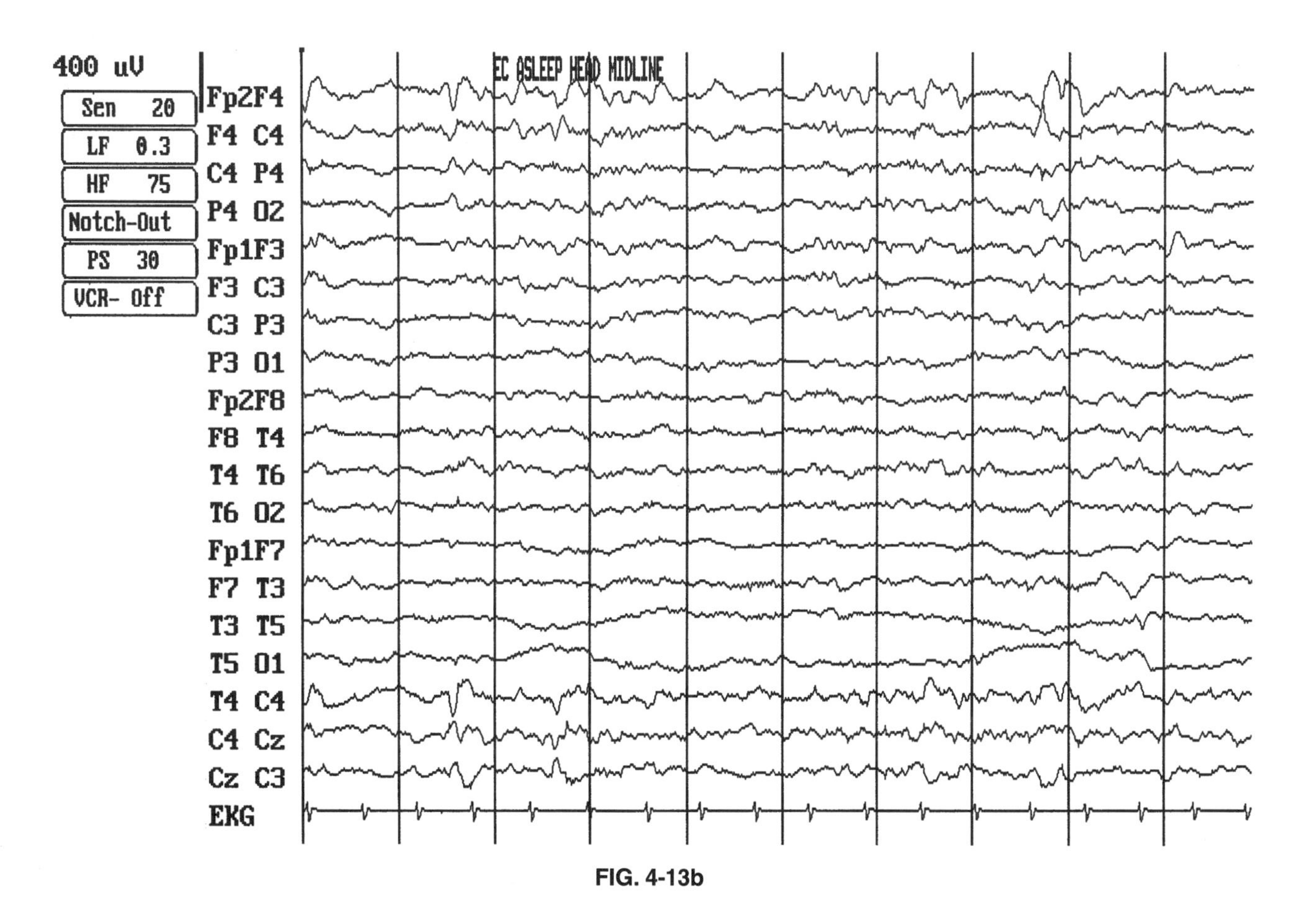
400 uV
Sen 20
LF 0.3
HF 75
Notch-Out
PS 30
VCR- Off
EC ASLEEP HEAD MIDLINE
Fp2F4
F4 C4
C4 P4
P4 O2
Fp1F3
F3 C3
C3 P3
P3 O1
Fp2F8
F8 T4
T4 T6
T6 O2
Fp1F7
F7 T3
T3 T5
T5 O1
T4 C4
C4 Cz
Cz C3
EKG

FIG. 4-13b

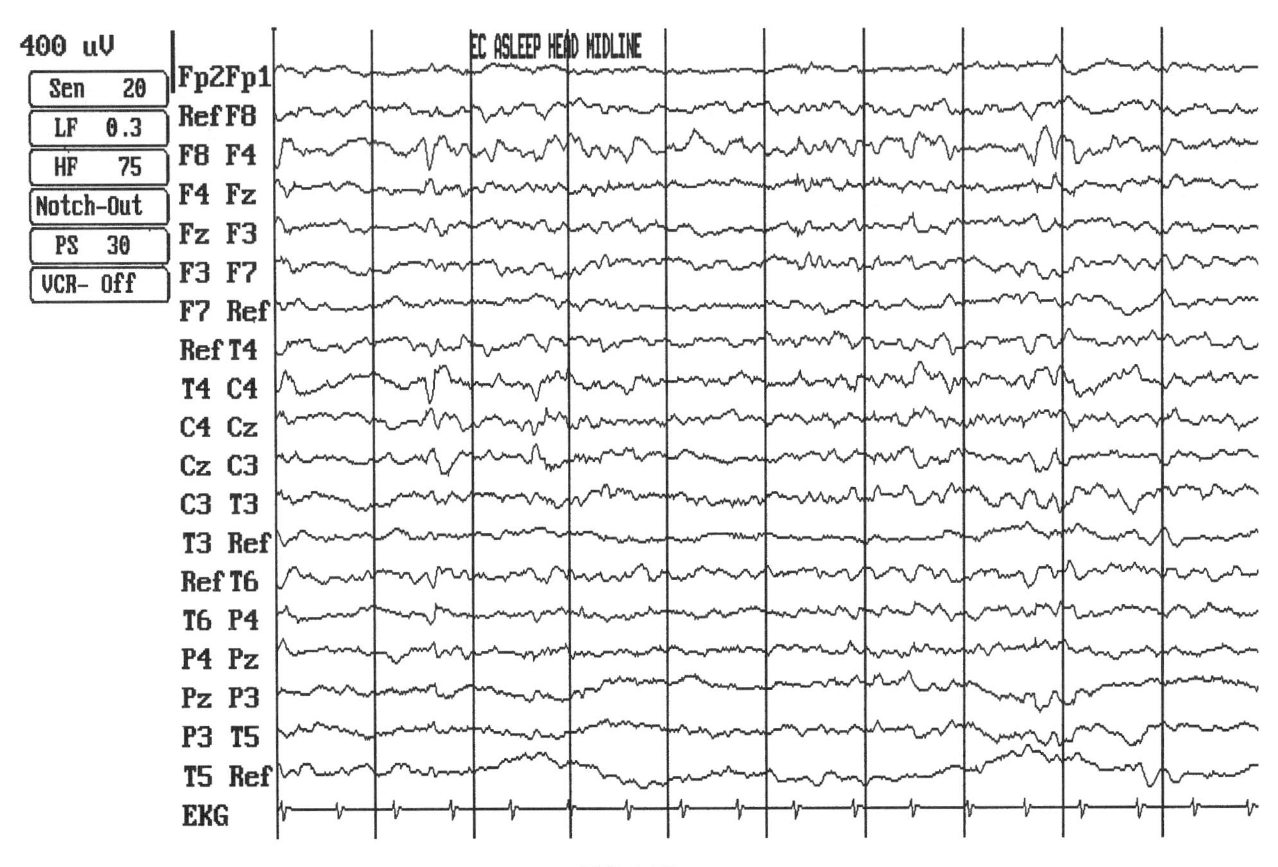
400 uV
Sen 20
LF 0.3
HF 75
Notch-Out
PS 30
VCR- Off
EC ASLEEP HEAD MIDLINE
Fp2Fp1
Ref F8
F8 F4
F4 Fz
Fz F3
F3 F7
F7 Ref
Ref T4
T4 C4
C4 Cz
Cz C3
C3 T3
T3 Ref
Ref T6
T6 P4
P4 Pz
Pz P3
P3 T5
T5 Ref
EKG

FIG. 4-13c

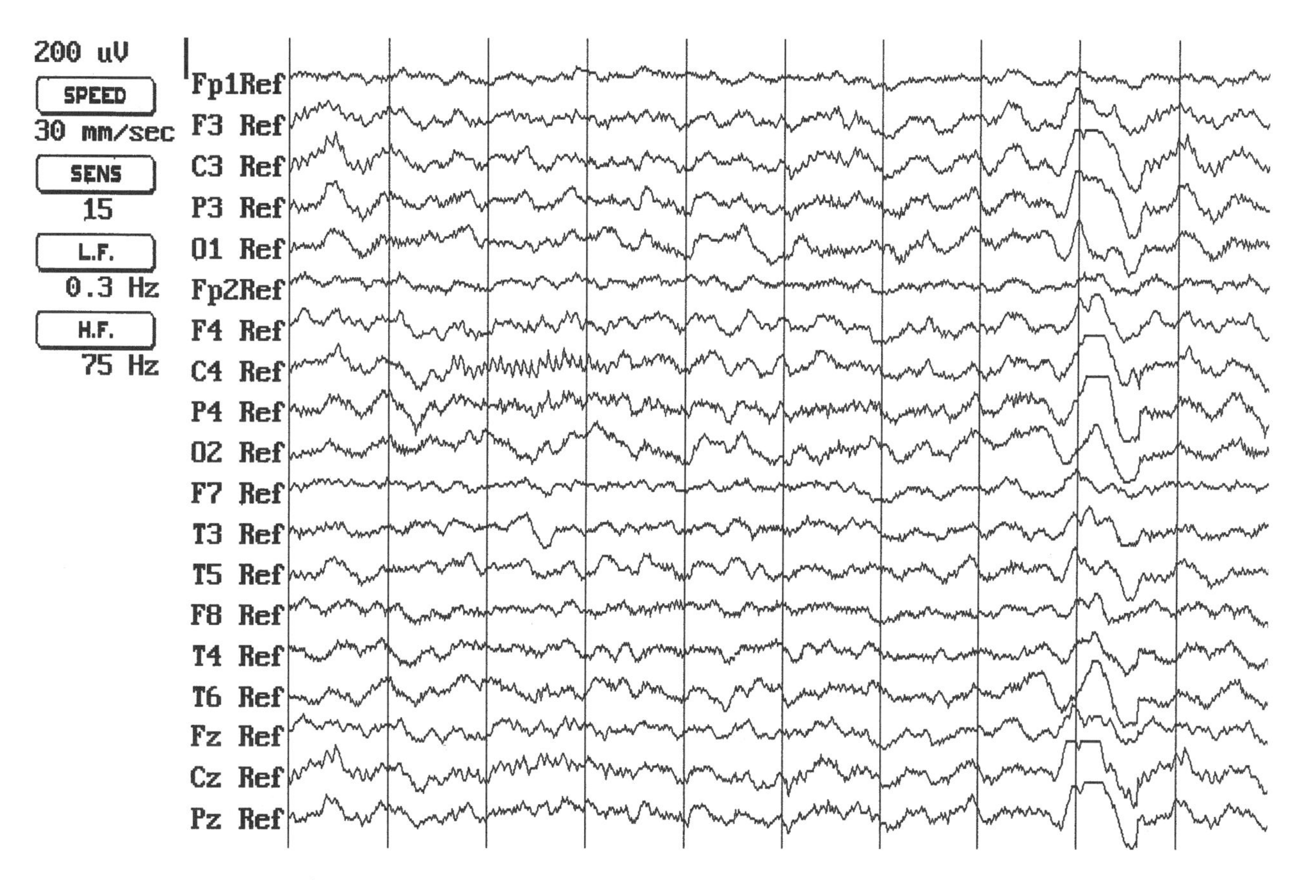

FIG. 4-14a,b Asymmetric sleep spindles as seen on two different runs.

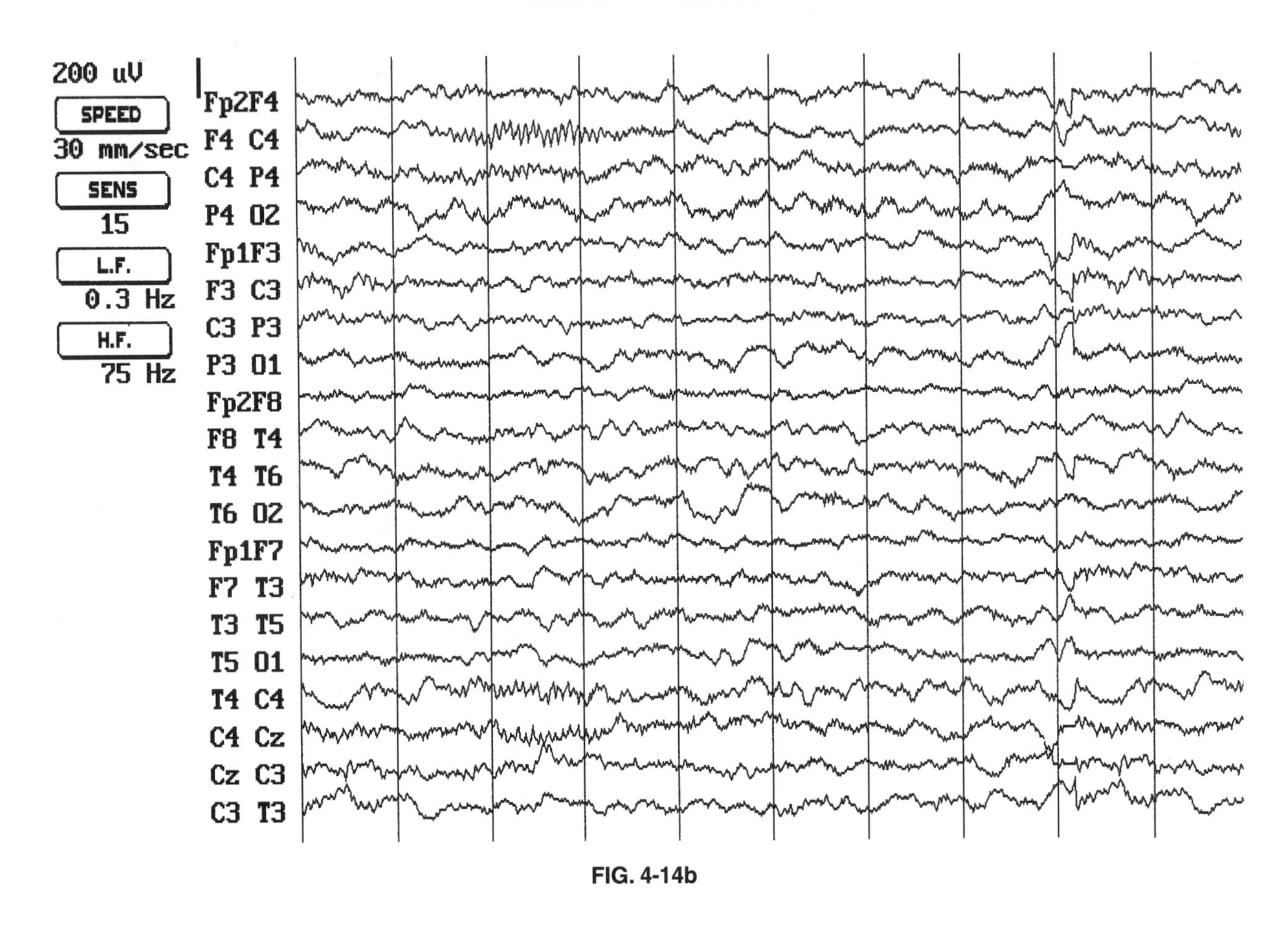
200 uV
SPEED
30 mm/sec
SENS
15
L.F.
0.3 Hz
H.F.
75 Hz
Fp2F4
F4 C4
C4 P4
P4 O2
Fp1F3
F3 C3
C3 P3
P3 O1
Fp2F8
F8 T4
T4 T6
T6 O2
Fp1F7
F7 T3
T3 T5
T5 O1
T4 C4
C4 Cz
Cz C3
C3 T3

FIG. 4-14b

Normal Variants

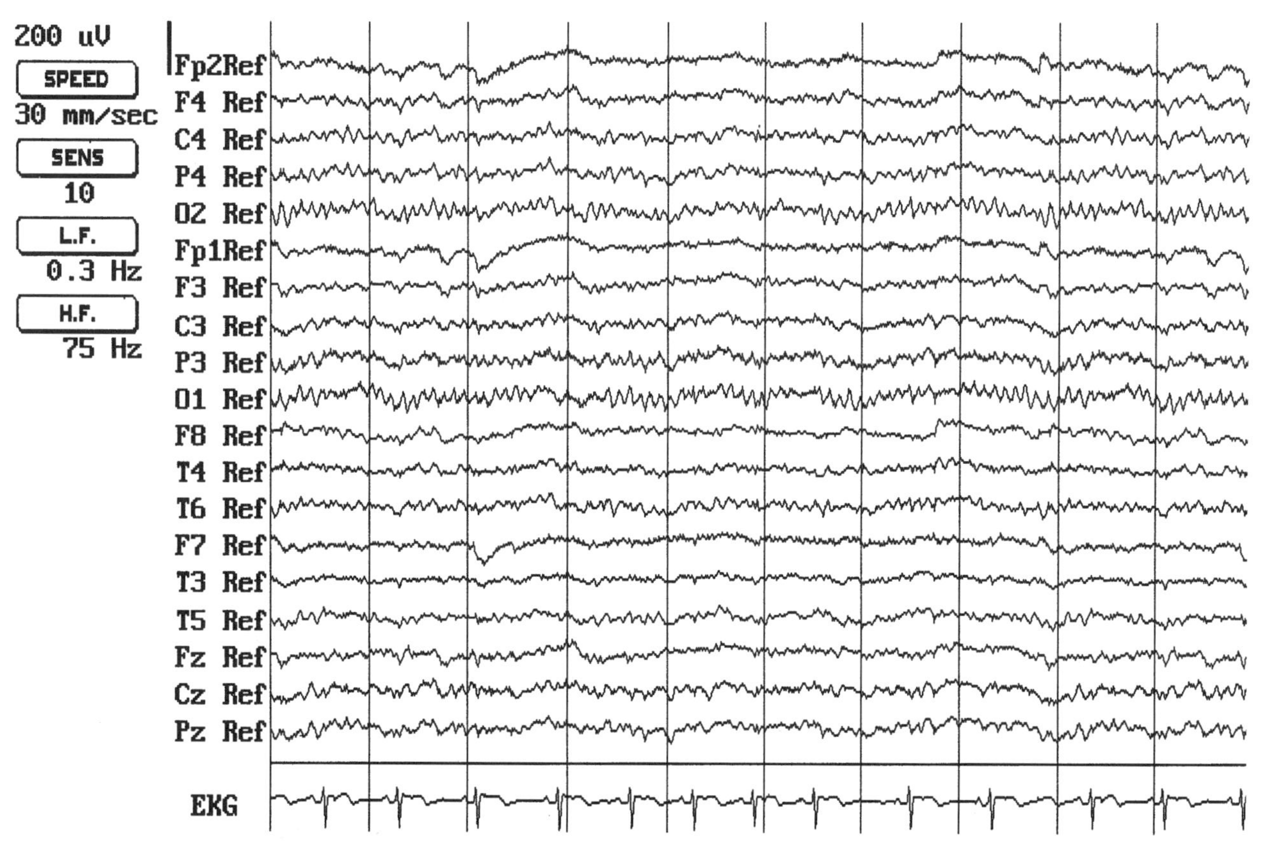

FIG. 4-15a,b,c A normal symmetrical background with a 9 to 10 Hz posterior dominant rhythm seen on three different montages.

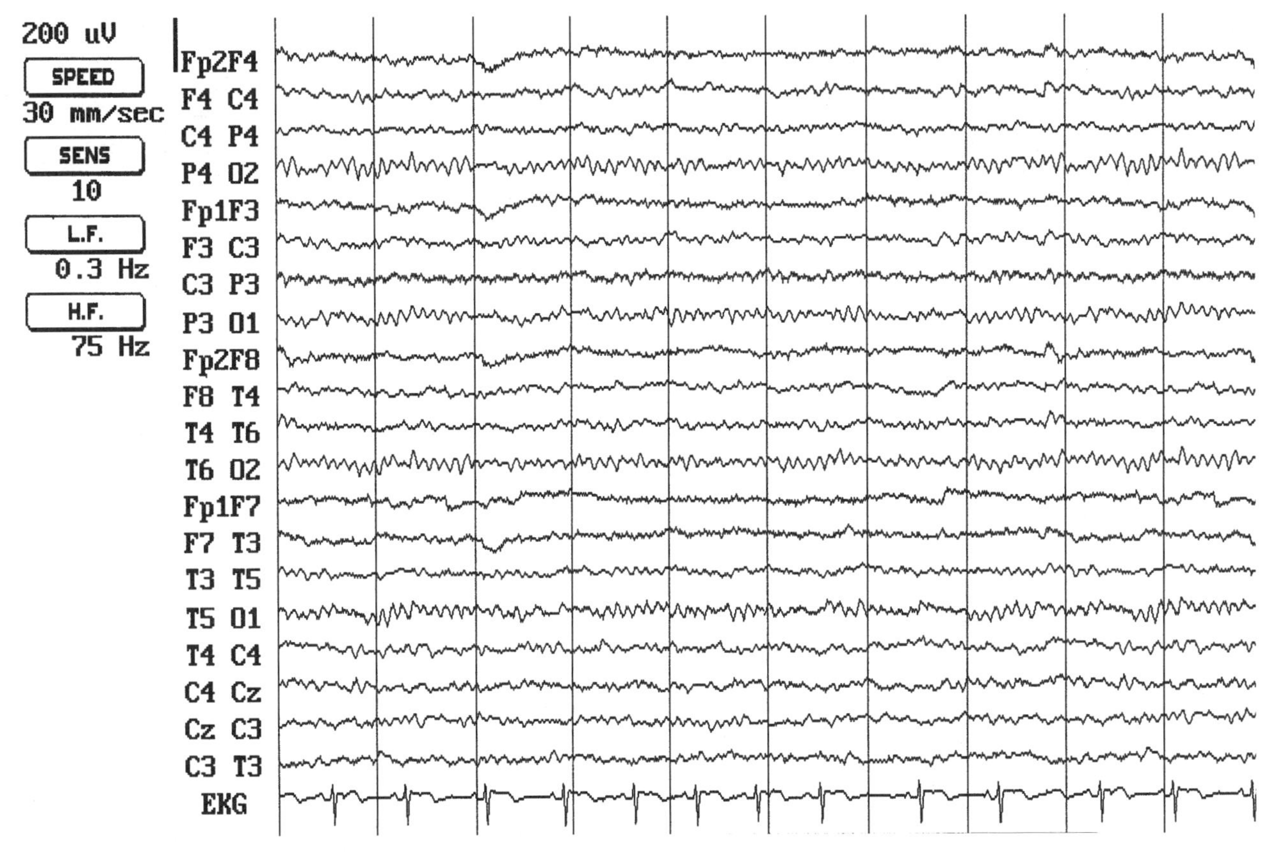
200 uV
SPEED
30 mm/sec
SENS
10
L.F.
0.3 Hz
H.F.
75 Hz
Fp2F4
F4 C4
C4 P4
P4 O2
Fp1F3
F3 C3
C3 P3
P3 O1
Fp2F8
F8 T4
T4 T6
T6 O2
Fp1F7
F7 T3
T3 T5
T5 O1
T4 C4
C4 Cz
Cz C3
C3 T3
EKG

FIG. 4-15b

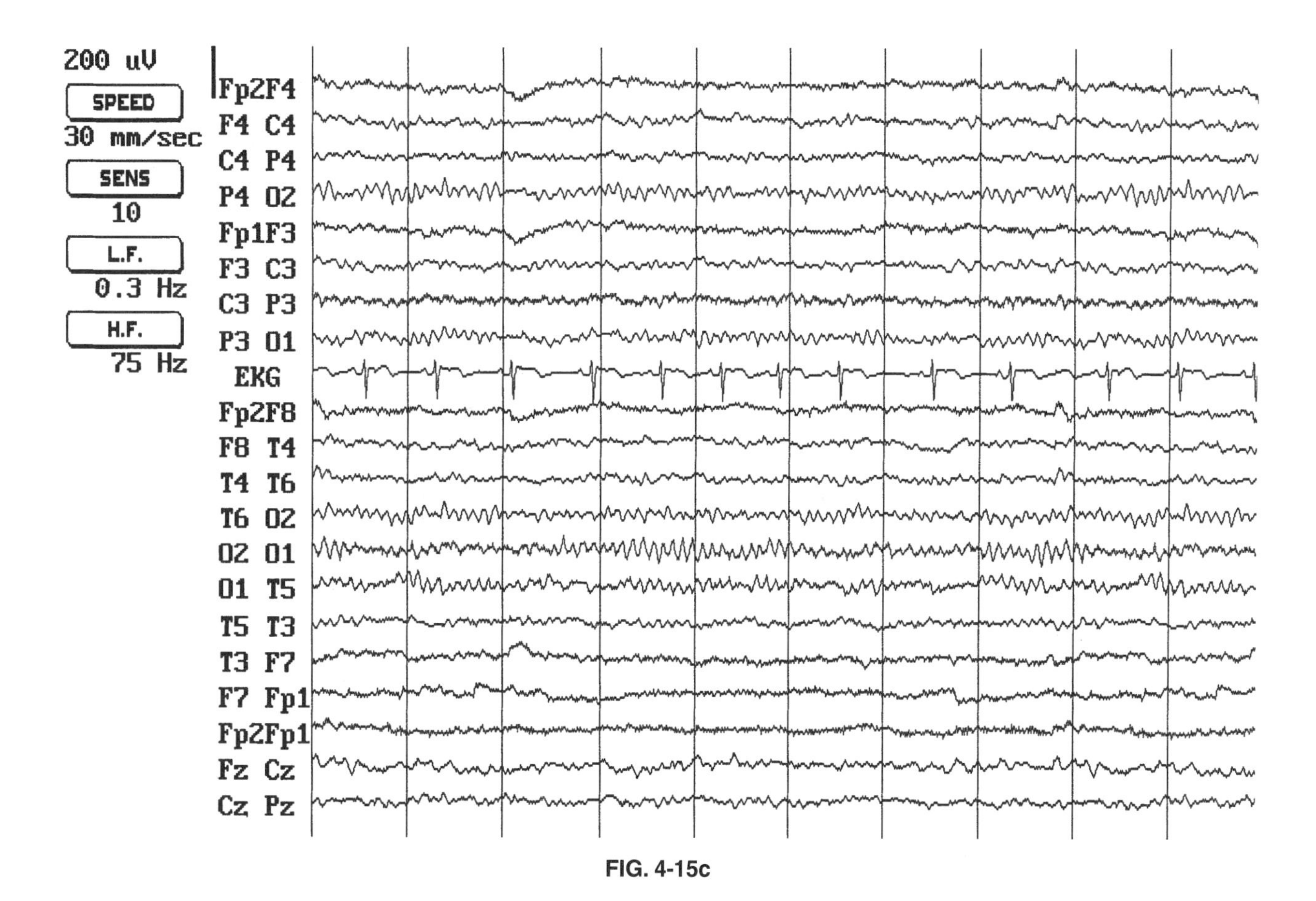
200 uV
SPEED
30 mm/sec
SENS
10
L.F.
0.3 Hz
H.F.
75 Hz
Fp2F4
F4 C4
C4 P4
P4 O2
Fp1F3
F3 C3
C3 P3
P3 O1
EKG
Fp2F8
F8 T4
T4 T6
T6 O2
O2 O1
O1 T5
T5 T3
T3 F7
F7 Fp1
Fp2Fp1
Fz Cz
Cz Pz

FIG. 4-15c

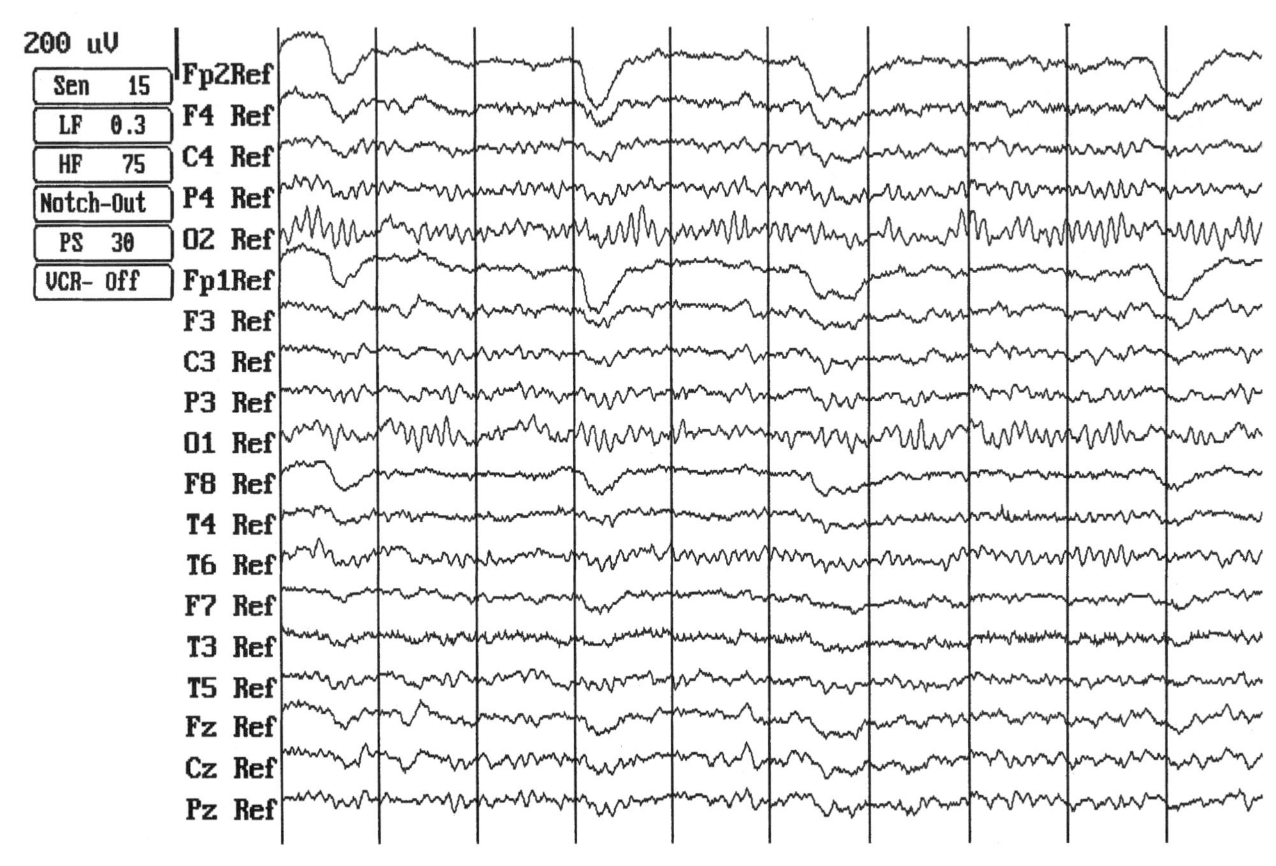

FIG. 4-16a,b,c An asymmetric posterior dominant rhythm shows a lower amplitude at O1 and more so at T5, as seen on run 1. On run 2 it appears to be symmetrical and on run 3 it appears to be only at T6.

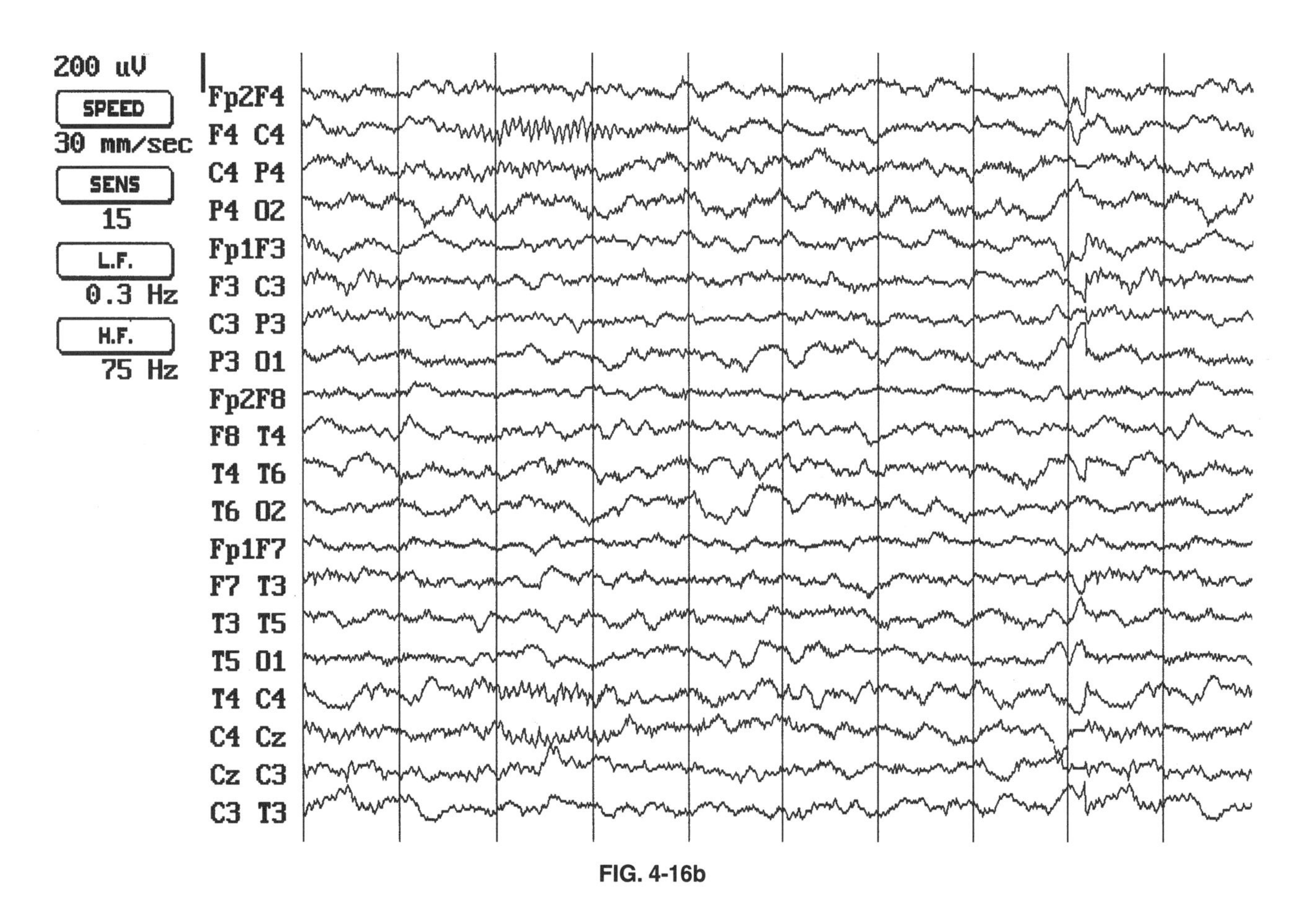
200 uV
SPEED
30 mm/sec
SENS
15
L.F.
0.3 Hz
H.F.
75 Hz
Fp2F4
F4 C4
C4 P4
P4 O2
Fp1F3
F3 C3
C3 P3
P3 O1
Fp2F8
F8 T4
T4 T6
T6 O2
Fp1F7
F7 T3
T3 T5
T5 O1
T4 C4
C4 Cz
Cz C3
C3 T3

FIG. 4-16b

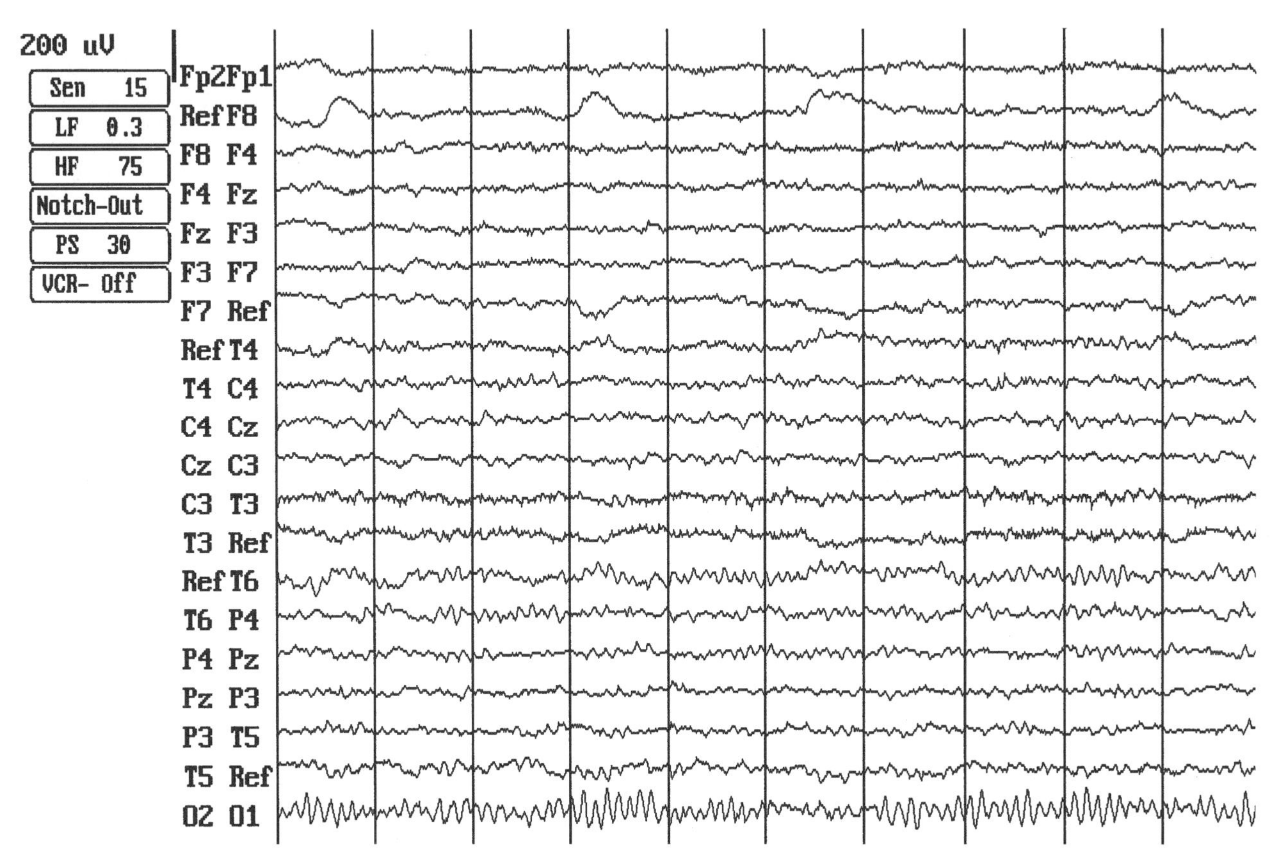
200 uV
Sen 15
LF 0.3
HF 75
Notch-Out
PS 30
VCR- Off
Fp2Fp1
Ref F8
F8 F4
F4 Fz
Fz F3
F3 F7
F7 Ref
Ref T4
T4 C4
C4 Cz
Cz C3
C3 T3
T3 Ref
Ref T6
T6 P4
P4 Pz
Pz P3
P3 T5
T5 Ref
O2 O1

FIG. 4-16c

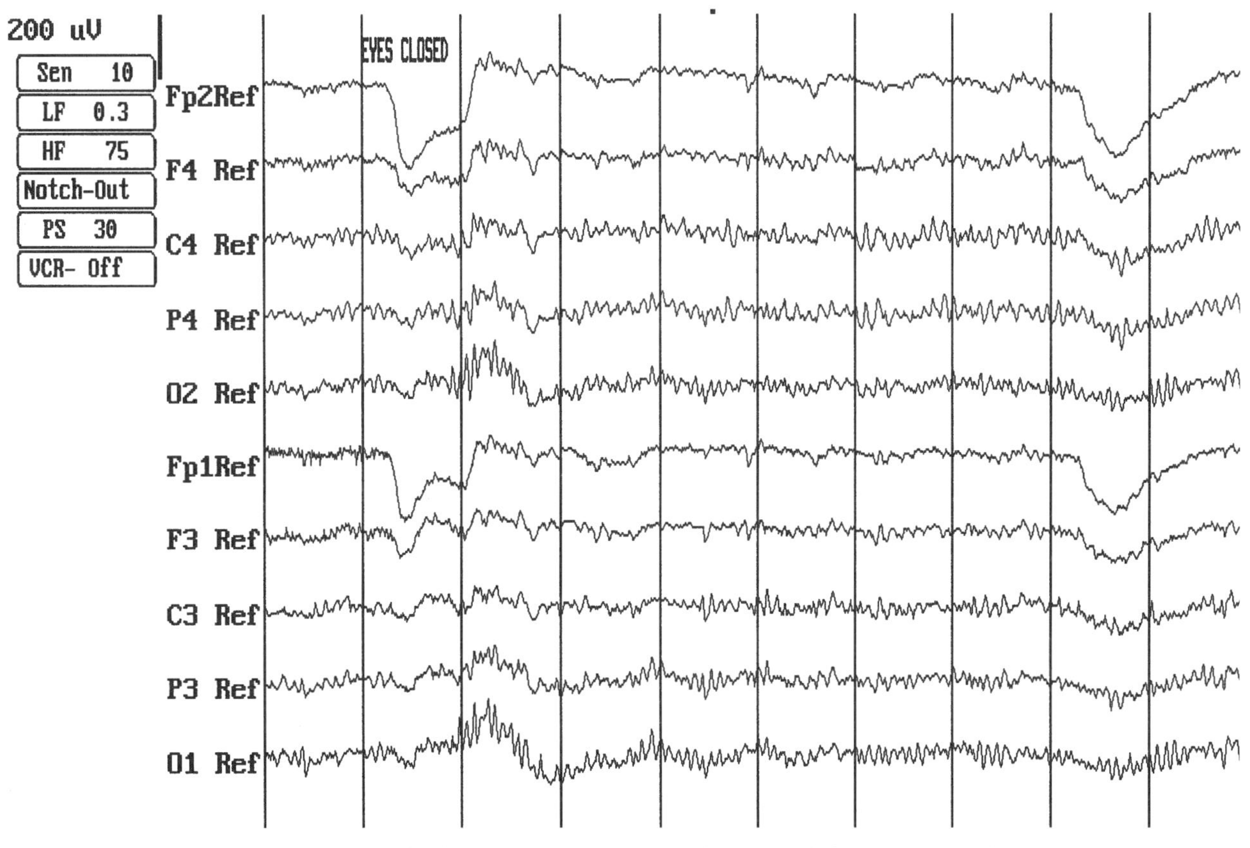

FIG. 4-17a,b,c A burst of alpha frequency activity seen at both occipital areas on eye closure—commonly known as alpha squeak—is seen on run 1 and 2. A paper speed of 60 mm/s illustrates morphology the best.

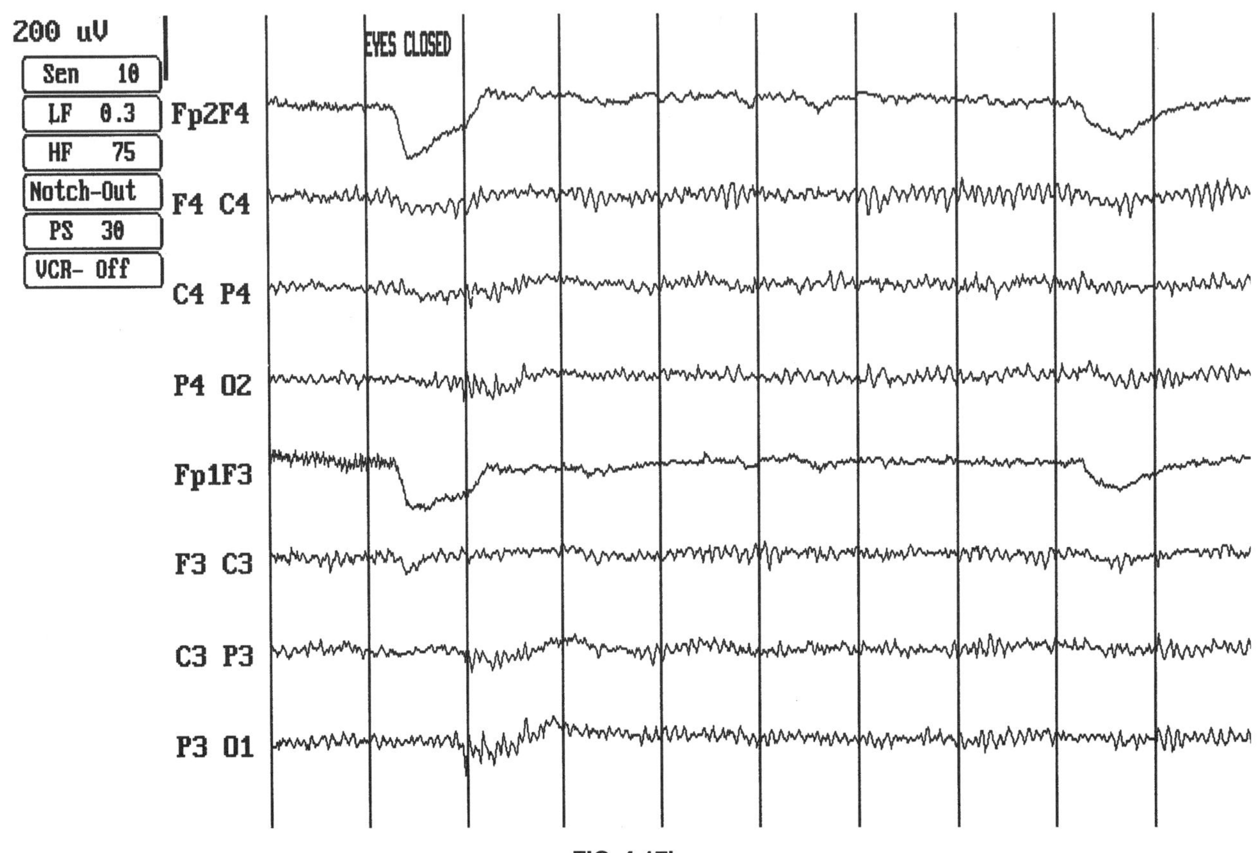
200 uV
Sen 10
LF 0.3
HF 75
Notch-Out
PS 30
VCR- Off
EYES CLOSED
Fp2F4
F4 C4
C4 P4
P4 O2
Fp1F3
F3 C3
C3 P3
P3 O1

FIG. 4-17b

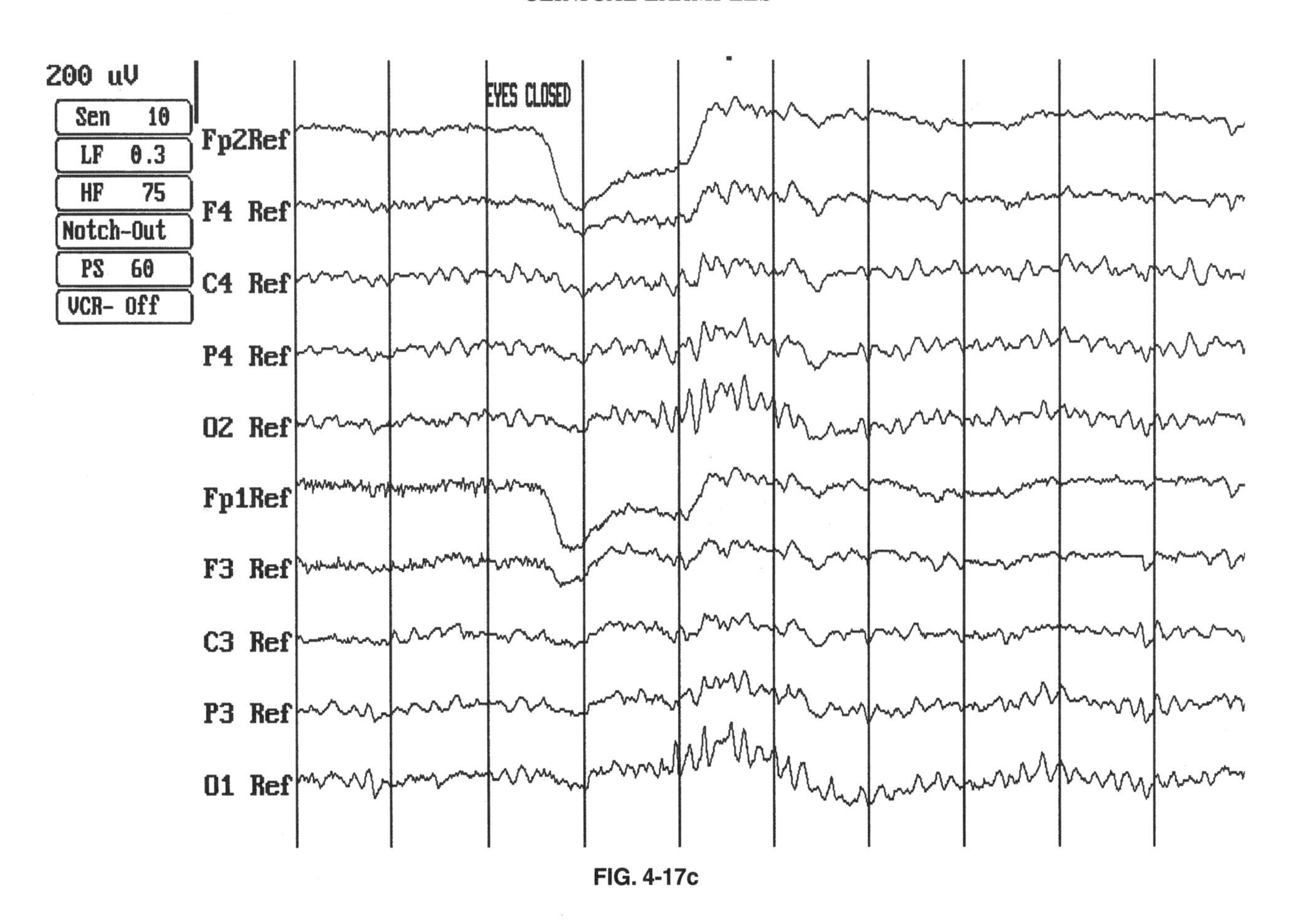
200 uV
Sen 10
LF 0.3
HF 75
Notch-Out
PS 60
VCR- Off
EYES CLOSED
Fp2Ref
F4 Ref
C4 Ref
P4 Ref
O2 Ref
Fp1Ref
F3 Ref
C3 Ref
P3 Ref
O1 Ref

FIG. 4-17c

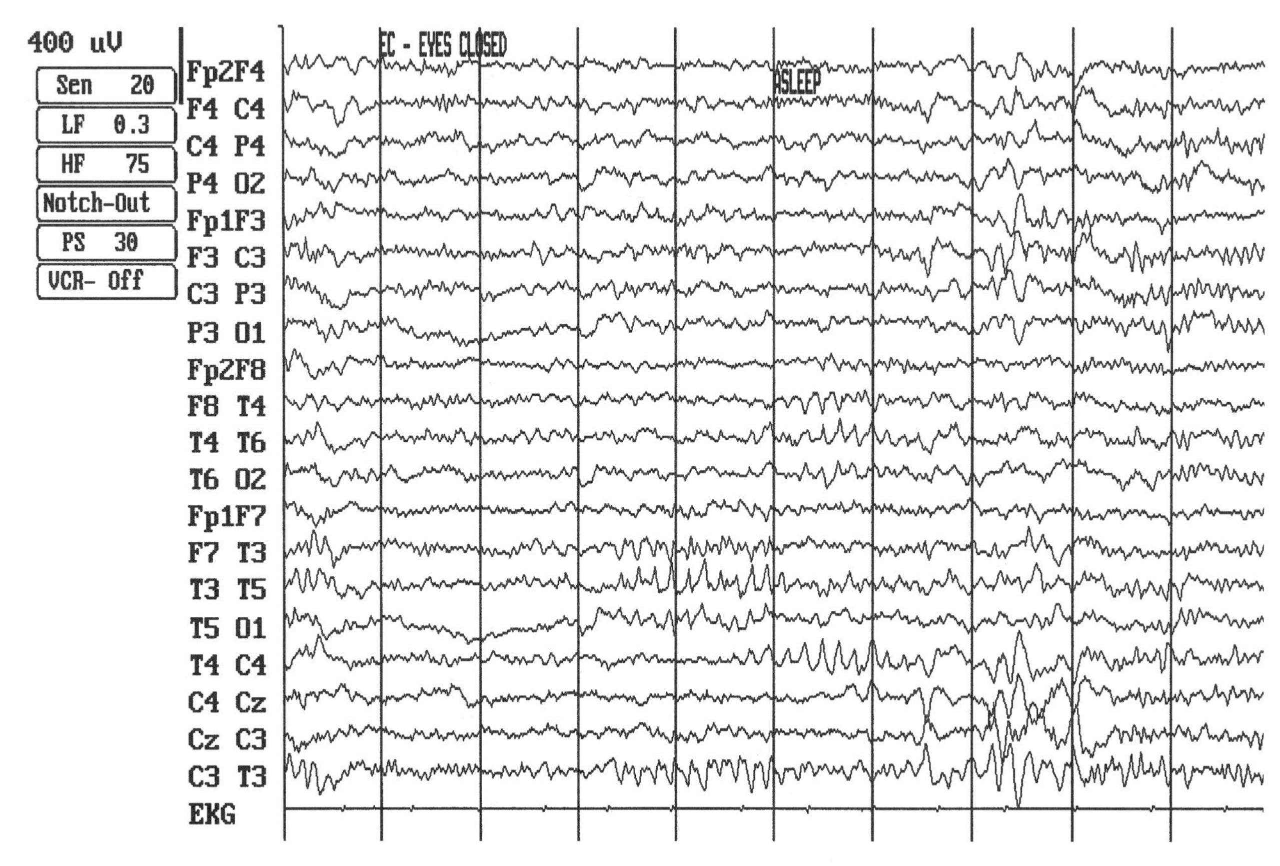

FIG. 4-18a,b,c An independent bitemporal psychomotor variant is seen phase reversing on runs 2 and 3. On run 1 it appears to be diffuse theta activity.

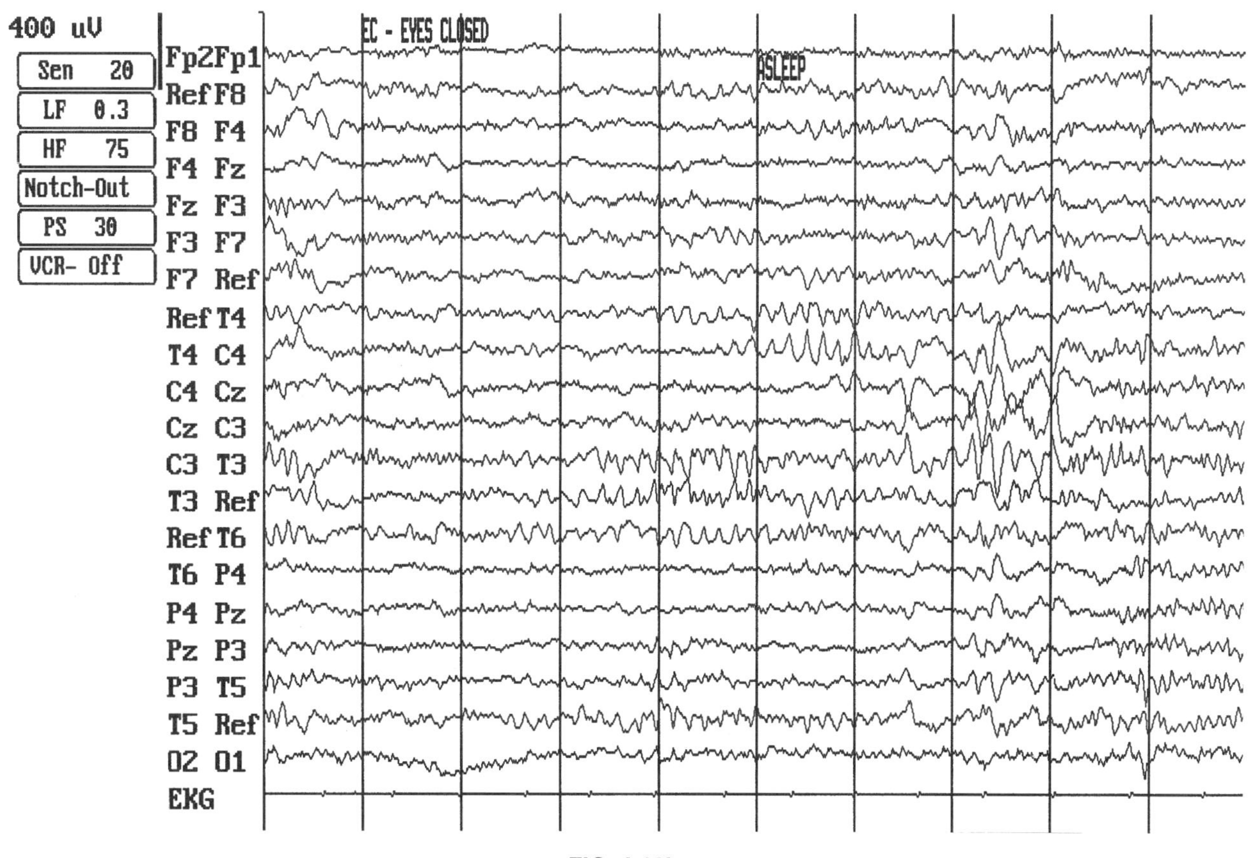
400 uV
Sen 20
LF 0.3
HF 75
Notch-Out
PS 30
VCR- Off
Fp2Fp1
Ref F8
F8 F4
F4 Fz
Fz F3
F3 F7
F7 Ref
Ref T4
T4 C4
C4 Cz
Cz C3
C3 T3
T3 Ref
Ref T6
T6 P4
P4 Pz
Pz P3
P3 T5
T5 Ref
O2 O1
EKG
EC - EYES CLOSED
ASLEEP

FIG. 4-18b

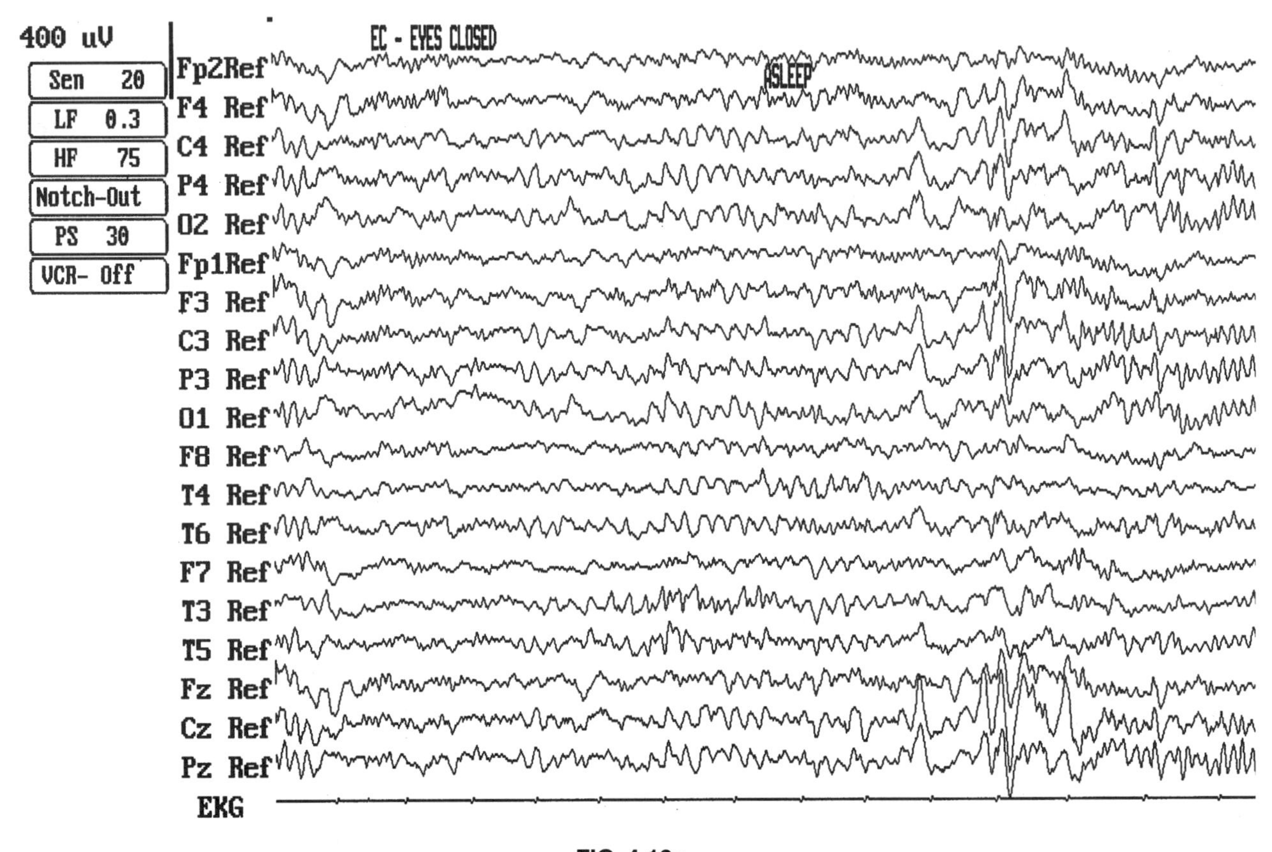
400 uV
Sen 20
LF 0.3
HF 75
Notch-Out
PS 30
VCR- Off
EC - EYES CLOSED
ASLEEP
Fp2Ref
F4 Ref
C4 Ref
P4 Ref
O2 Ref
Fp1Ref
F3 Ref
C3 Ref
P3 Ref
O1 Ref
F8 Ref
T4 Ref
T6 Ref
F7 Ref
T3 Ref
T5 Ref
Fz Ref
Cz Ref
Pz Ref
EKG

FIG. 4-18c

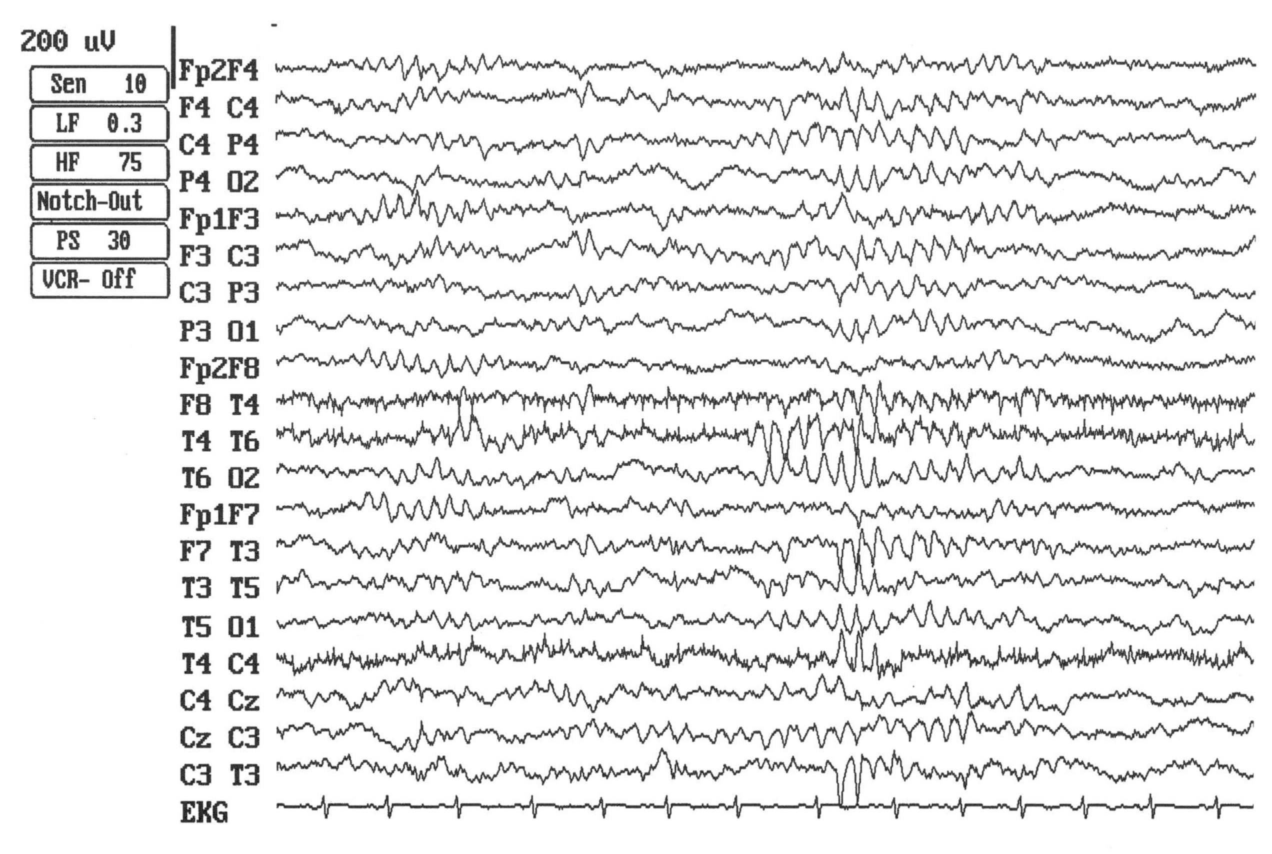

FIG. 4-19a,b This is another example of a psychomotor variant similar to Fig. 4-18.

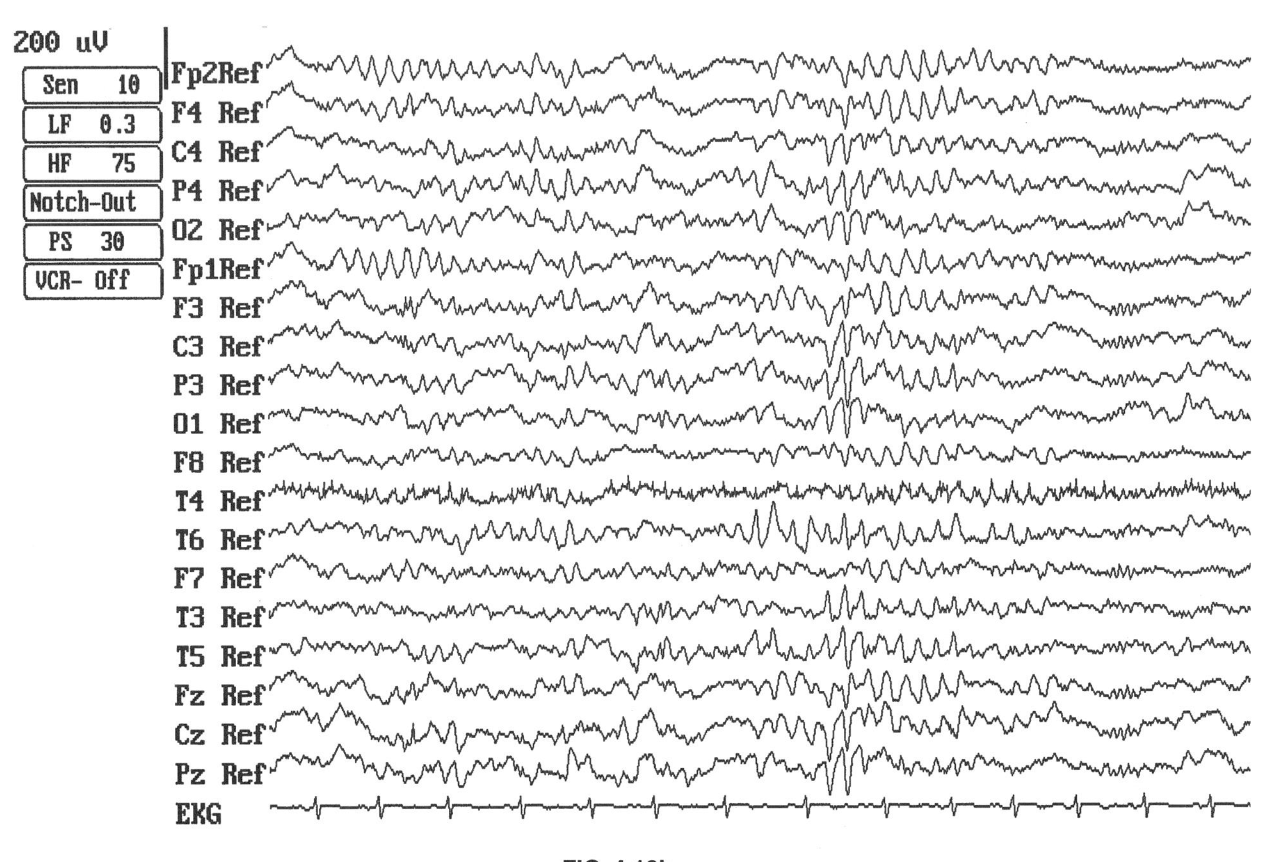
200 uV
Sen 10
LF 0.3
HF 75
Notch-Out
PS 30
VCR- Off
Fp2Ref
F4 Ref
C4 Ref
P4 Ref
O2 Ref
Fp1Ref
F3 Ref
C3 Ref
P3 Ref
O1 Ref
F8 Ref
T4 Ref
T6 Ref
F7 Ref
T3 Ref
T5 Ref
Fz Ref
Cz Ref
Pz Ref
EKG

FIG. 4-19b

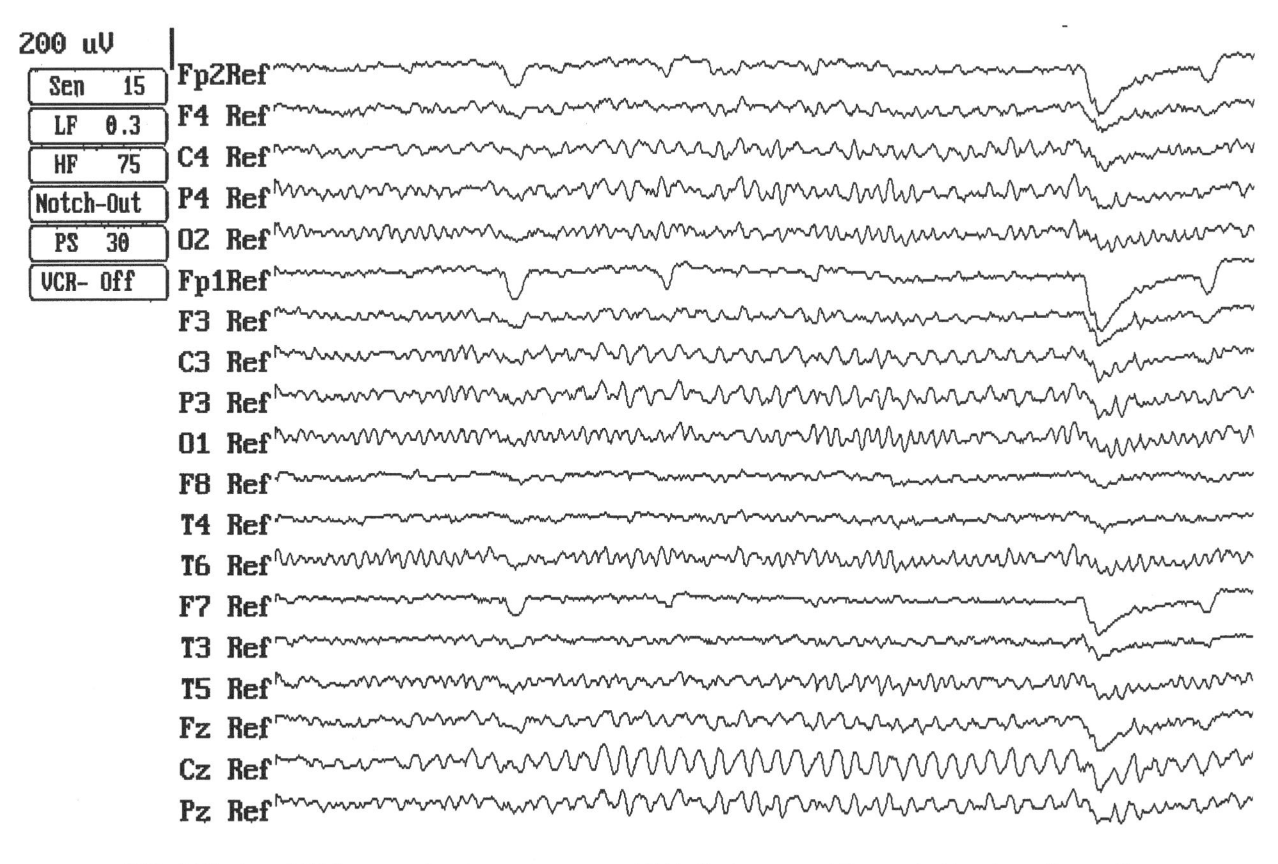

FIG. 4-20a,b,c,d This example shows an unusual 5 Hz theta seen at the central leads on three different runs. The slower paper speed (15 mm/s) shows a longer trend.

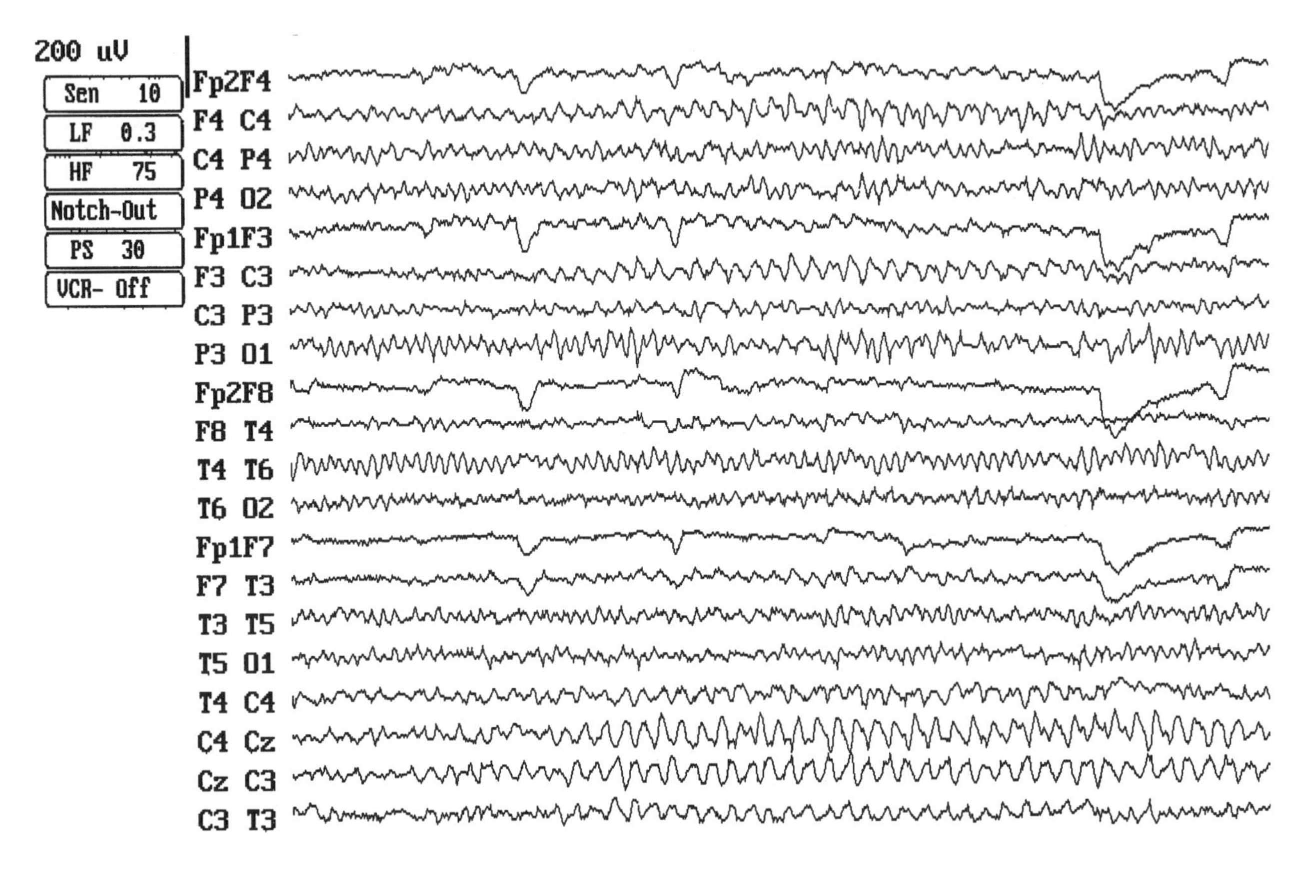
200 uV
Sen 10
LF 0.3
HF 75
Notch-Out
PS 30
VCR- Off
Fp2F4
F4 C4
C4 P4
P4 O2
Fp1F3
F3 C3
C3 P3
P3 O1
Fp2F8
F8 T4
T4 T6
T6 O2
Fp1F7
F7 T3
T3 T5
T5 O1
T4 C4
C4 Cz
Cz C3
C3 T3

FIG. 4-20b

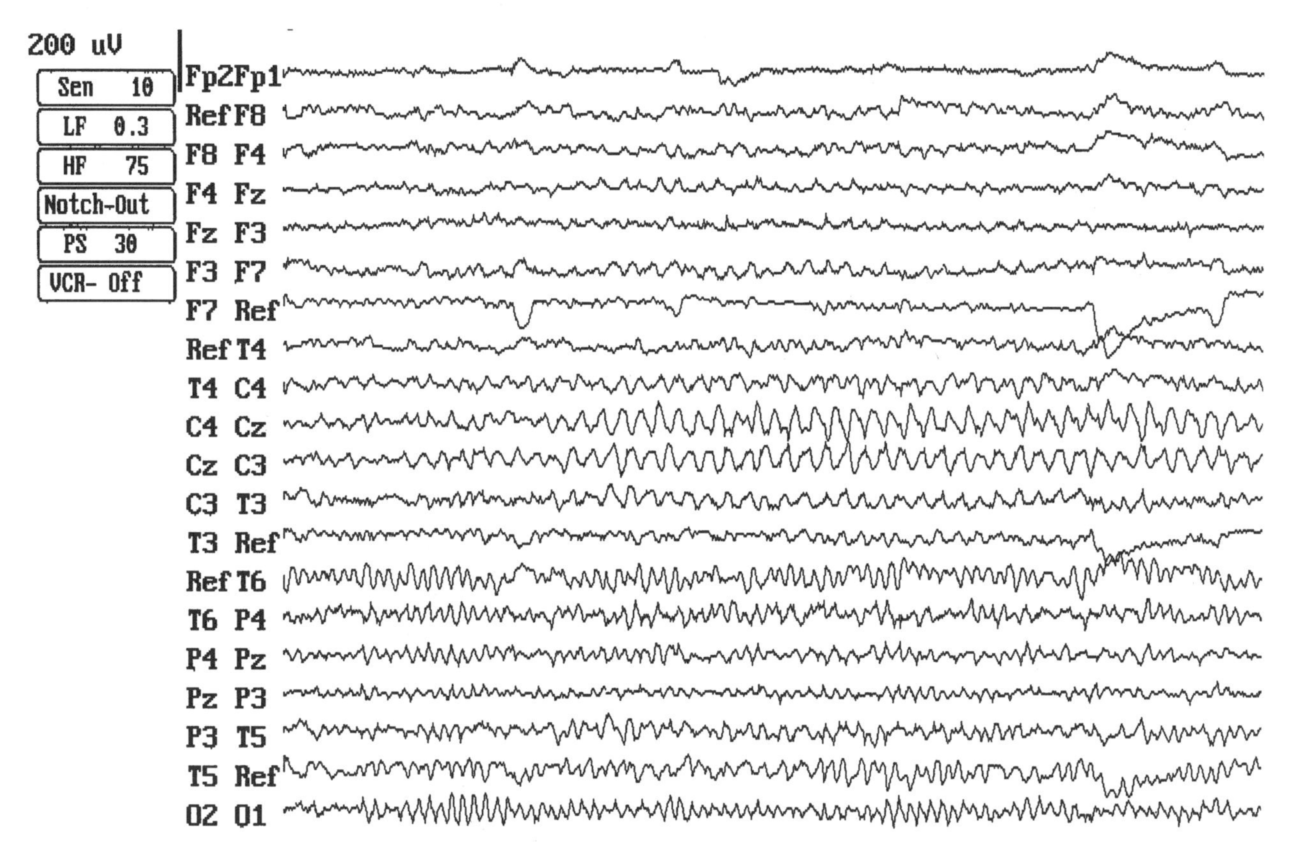
200 uV
Sen 10
LF 0.3
HF 75
Notch-Out
PS 30
VCR- Off
Fp2Fp1
Ref F8
F8 F4
F4 Fz
Fz F3
F3 F7
F7 Ref
Ref T4
T4 C4
C4 Cz
Cz C3
C3 T3
T3 Ref
Ref T6
T6 P4
P4 Pz
Pz P3
P3 T5
T5 Ref
O2 O1

FIG. 4-20c

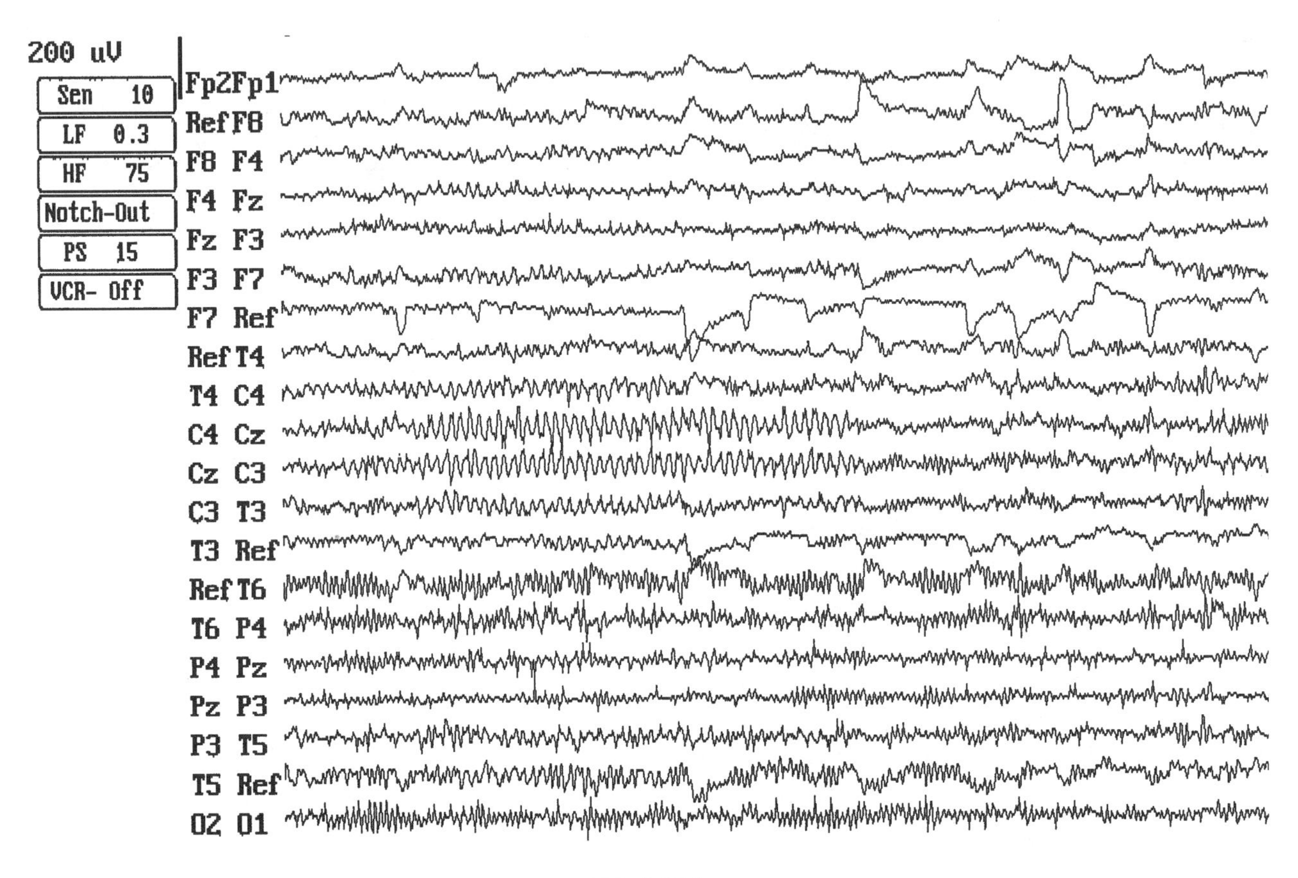
200 uV
Sen 10
LF 0.3
HF 75
Notch-Out
PS 15
VCR- Off
Fp2Fp1
Ref F8
F8 F4
F4 Fz
Fz F3
F3 F7
F7 Ref
Ref T4
T4 C4
C4 Cz
Cz C3
C3 T3
T3 Ref
Ref T6
T6 P4
P4 Pz
Pz P3
P3 T5
T5 Ref
O2 O1

FIG. 4-20d

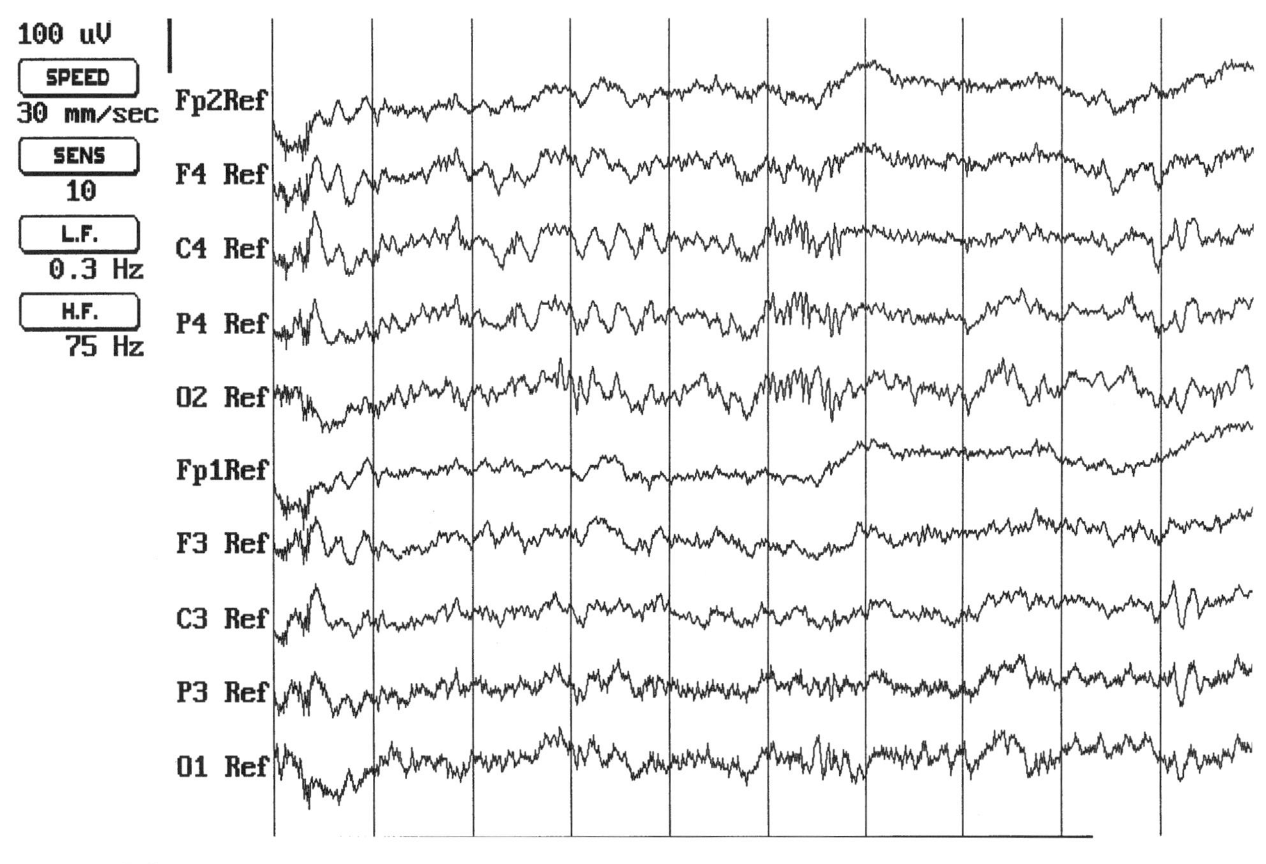

FIG. 4-21a,b,c The 14 and 6 positive spikes (ctenoids) seen over the right parasagittal area on run 1 are eliminated by cancellation on run 2. The paper speed of 60 mm/s further magnifies this normal variant.

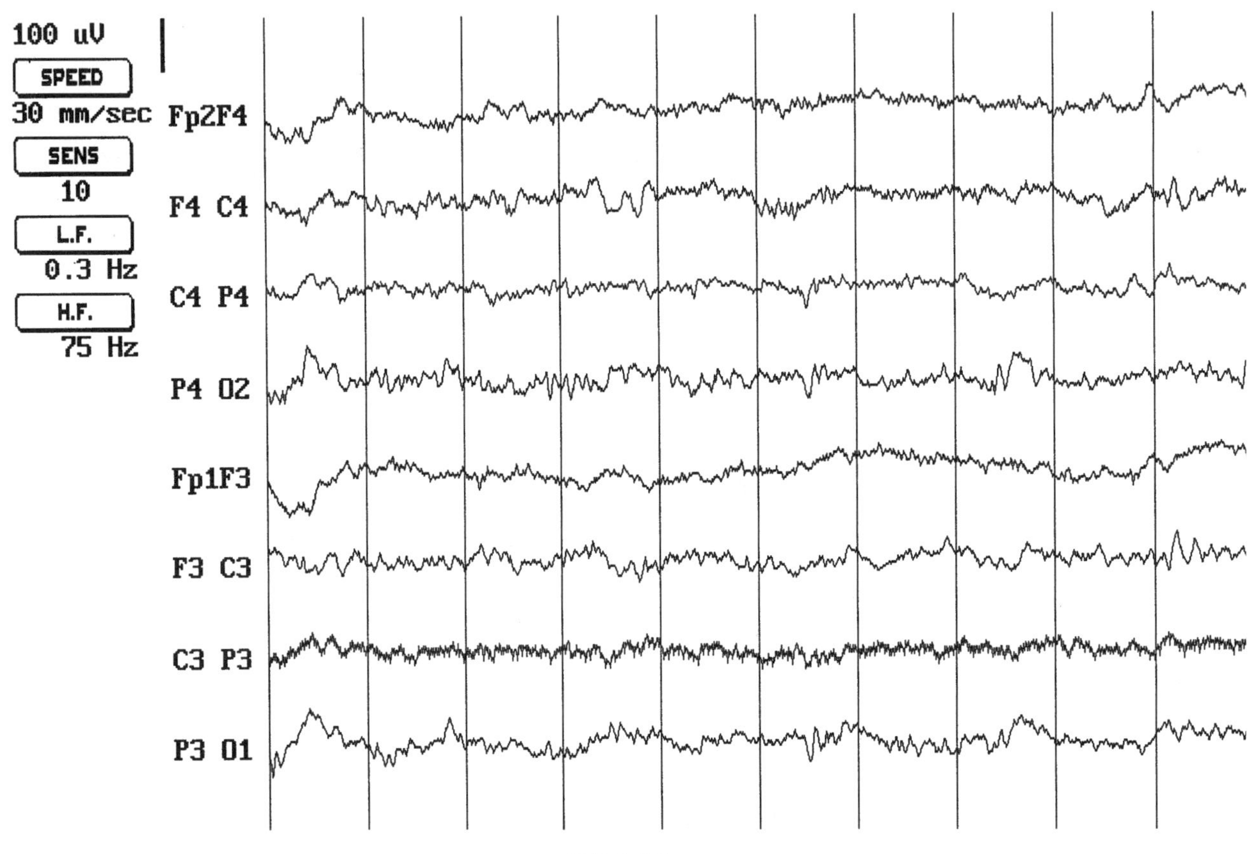
100 uV
SPEED
30 mm/sec
SENS
10
L.F.
0.3 Hz
H.F.
75 Hz
Fp2F4
F4 C4
C4 P4
P4 O2
Fp1F3
F3 C3
C3 P3
P3 O1

FIG. 4-21b

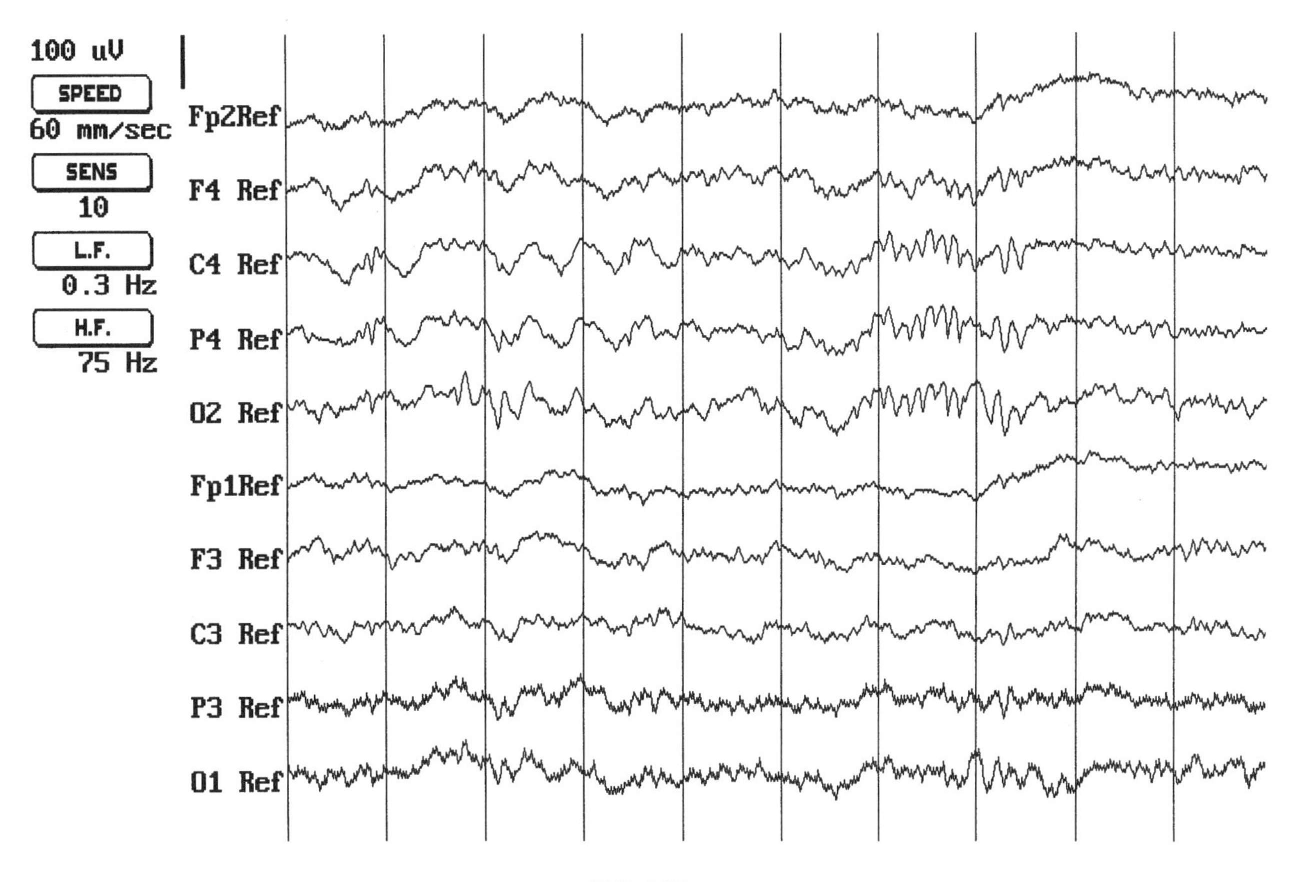
100 uV
SPEED
60 mm/sec
SENS
10
L.F.
0.3 Hz
H.F.
75 Hz
Fp2Ref
F4 Ref
C4 Ref
P4 Ref
O2 Ref
Fp1Ref
F3 Ref
C3 Ref
P3 Ref
O1 Ref

FIG. 4-21c

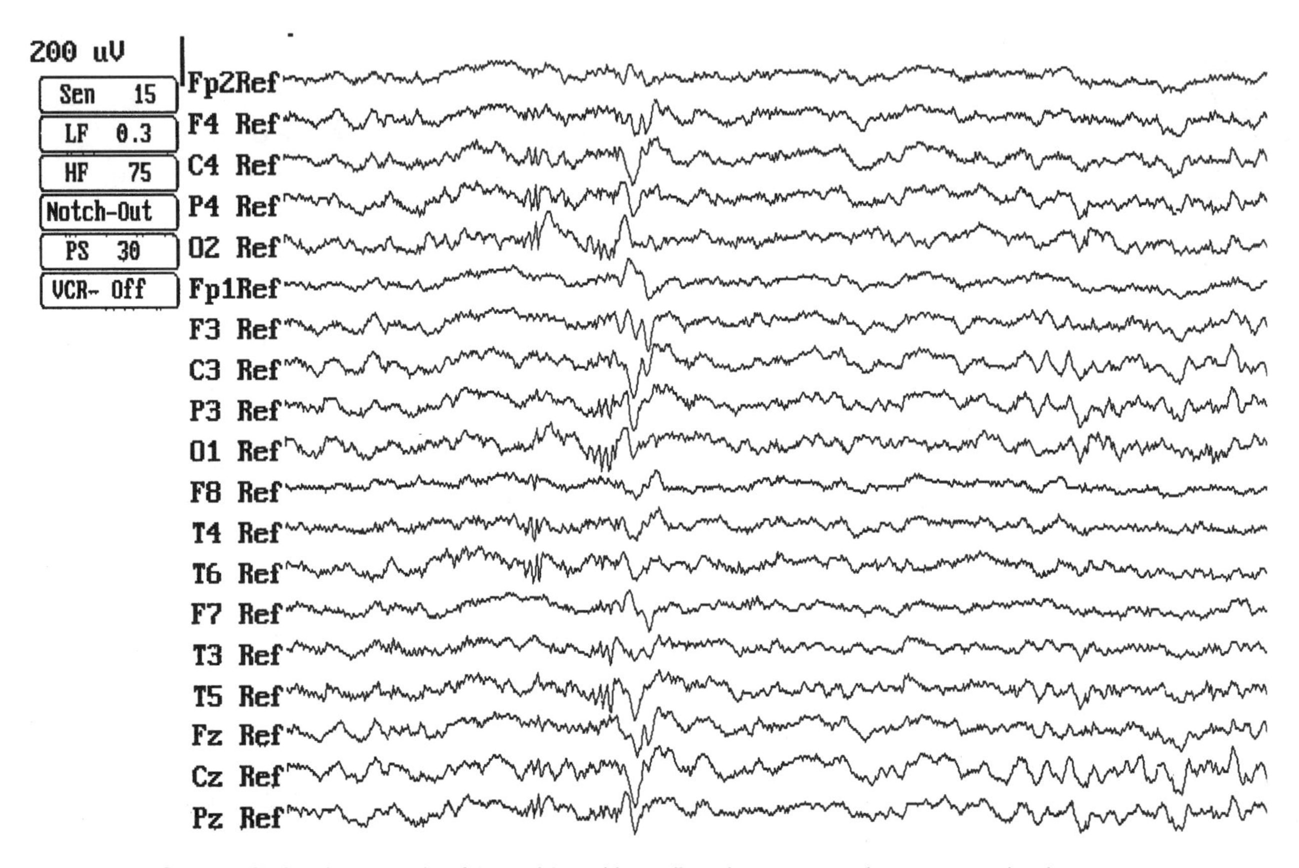

FIG. 4-22a,b Another sample of 14 and 6 positive spikes that are asynchronous are clearly seen on the referential run but poorly on the bipolar run.

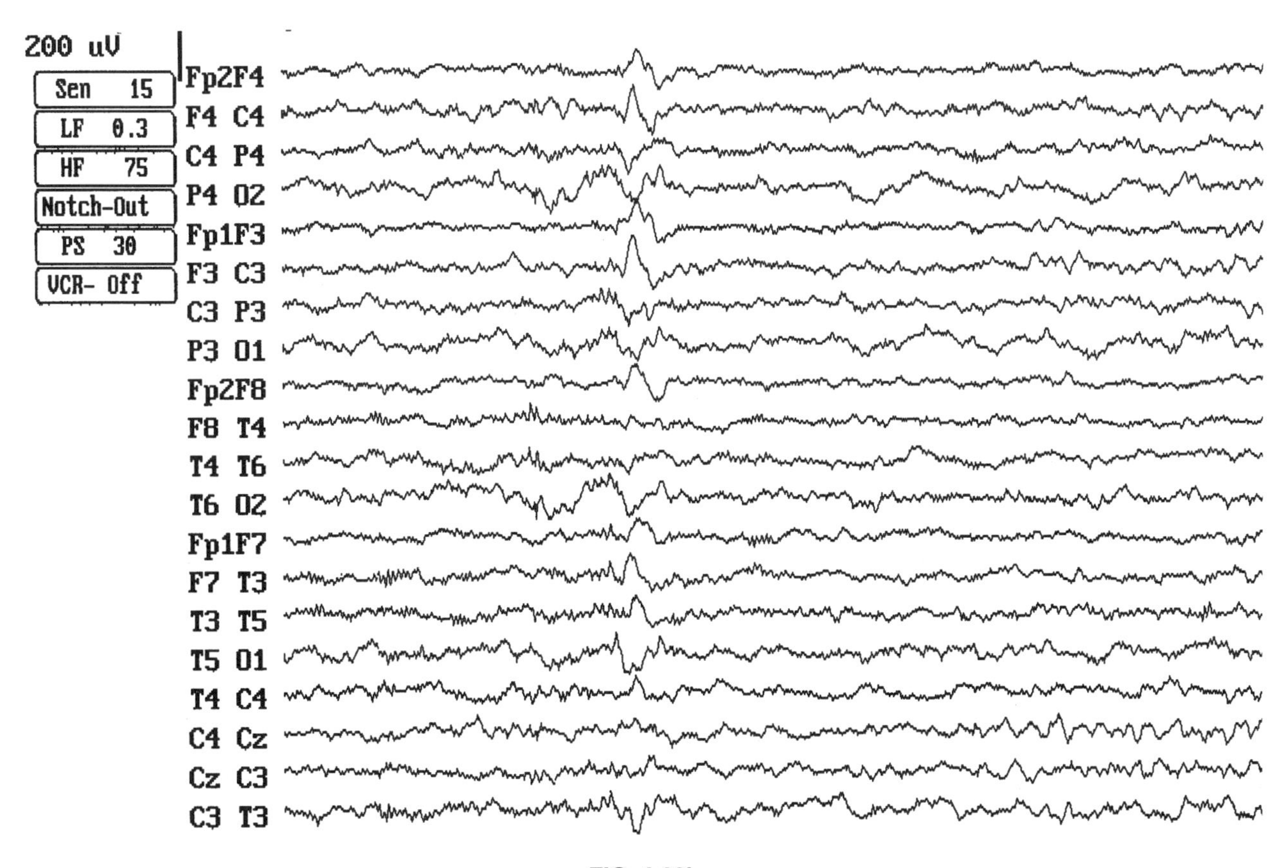
200 uV
Sen 15
LF 0.3
HF 75
Notch-Out
PS 30
VCR- Off
Fp2F4
F4 C4
C4 P4
P4 O2
Fp1F3
F3 C3
C3 P3
P3 O1
Fp2F8
F8 T4
T4 T6
T6 O2
Fp1F7
F7 T3
T3 T5
T5 O1
T4 C4
C4 Cz
Cz C3
C3 T3

FIG. 4-22b

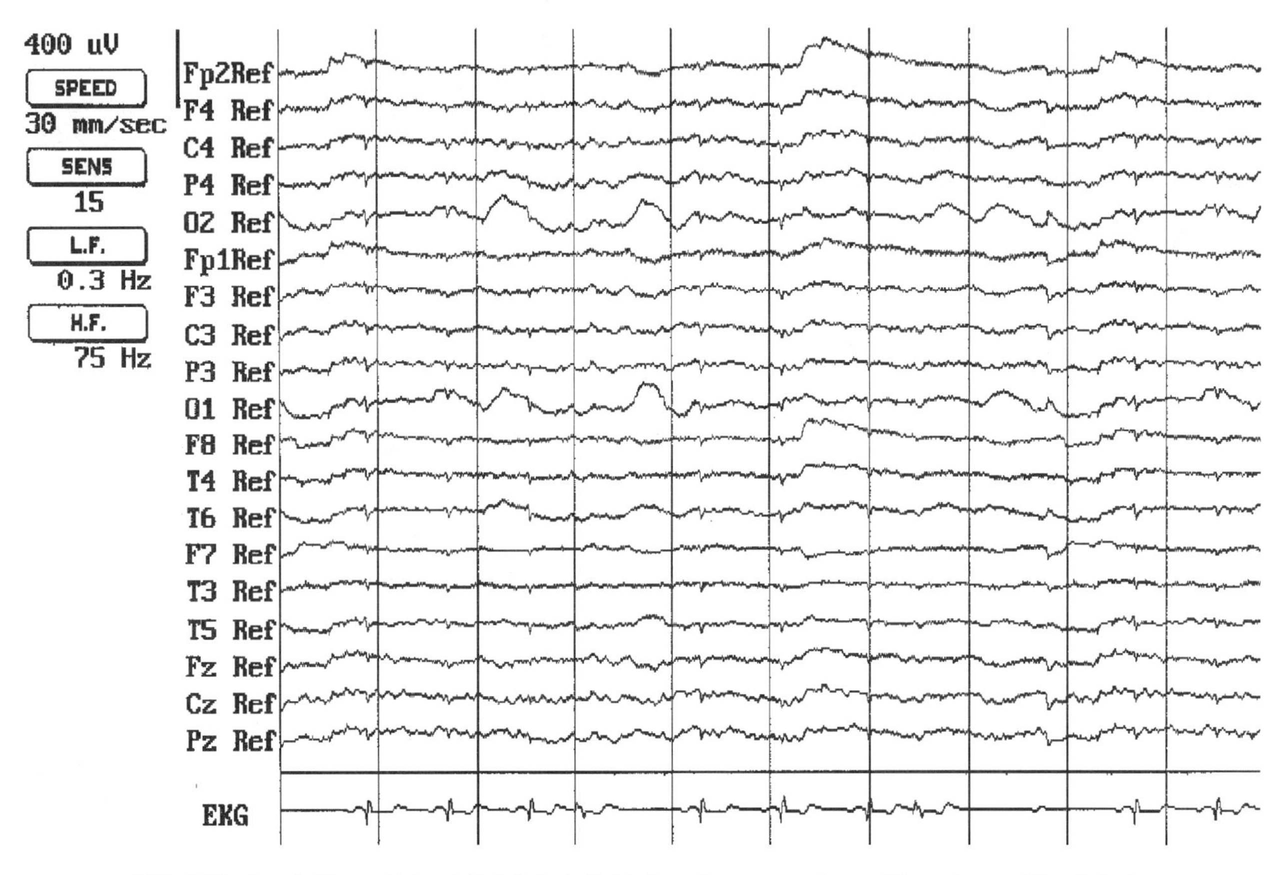

FIG. 4-23a,b,c,d Normal bioccipital delta in light sleep is seen on three different runs. The delta is best seen on run 4 due to the phase reversals. The paper speed of 15 mm/s further enhances the delta. Also of note is the arrhythmic EKG contaminating the reference on run 1 that is eliminated by runs 2 and 3.

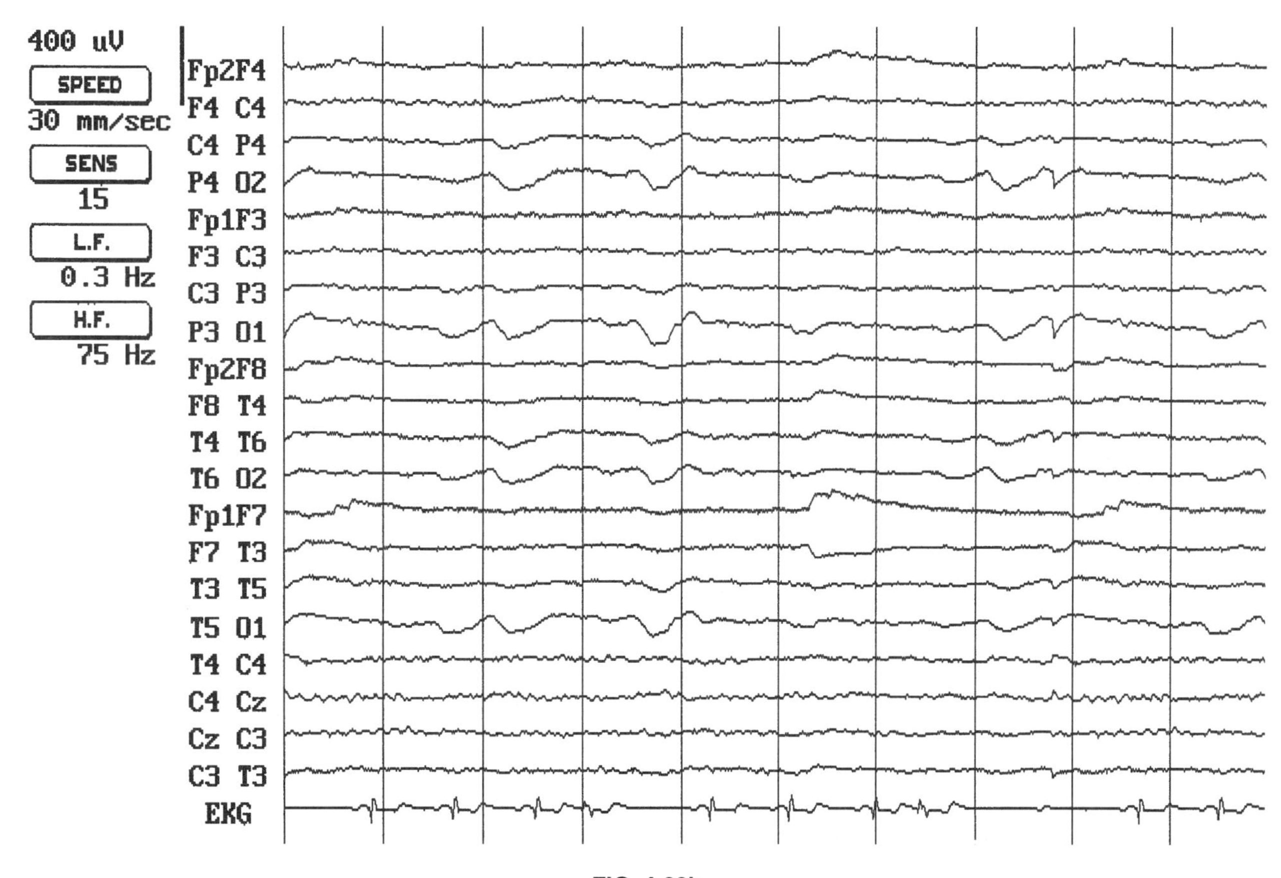
400 uV
SPEED
30 mm/sec
SENS
15
L.F.
0.3 Hz
H.F.
75 Hz
Fp2F4
F4 C4
C4 P4
P4 O2
Fp1F3
F3 C3
C3 P3
P3 O1
Fp2F8
F8 T4
T4 T6
T6 O2
Fp1F7
F7 T3
T3 T5
T5 O1
T4 C4
C4 Cz
Cz C3
C3 T3
EKG

FIG. 4-23b

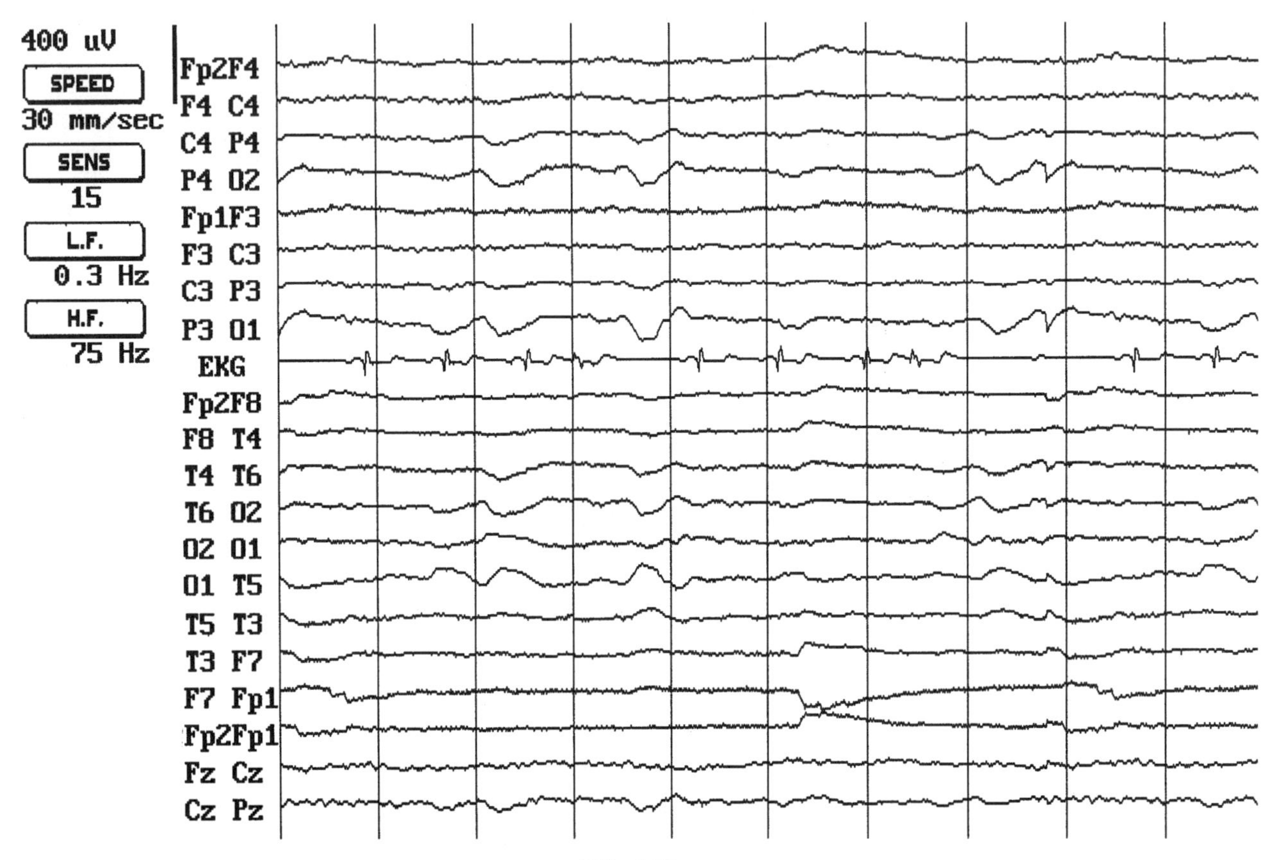
400 uV
SPEED
30 mm/sec
SENS
15
L.F.
0.3 Hz
H.F.
75 Hz
Fp2F4
F4 C4
C4 P4
P4 O2
Fp1F3
F3 C3
C3 P3
P3 O1
EKG
Fp2F8
F8 T4
T4 T6
T6 O2
O2 O1
O1 T5
T5 T3
T3 F7
F7 Fp1
Fp2Fp1
Fz Cz
Cz Pz

FIG. 4-23c

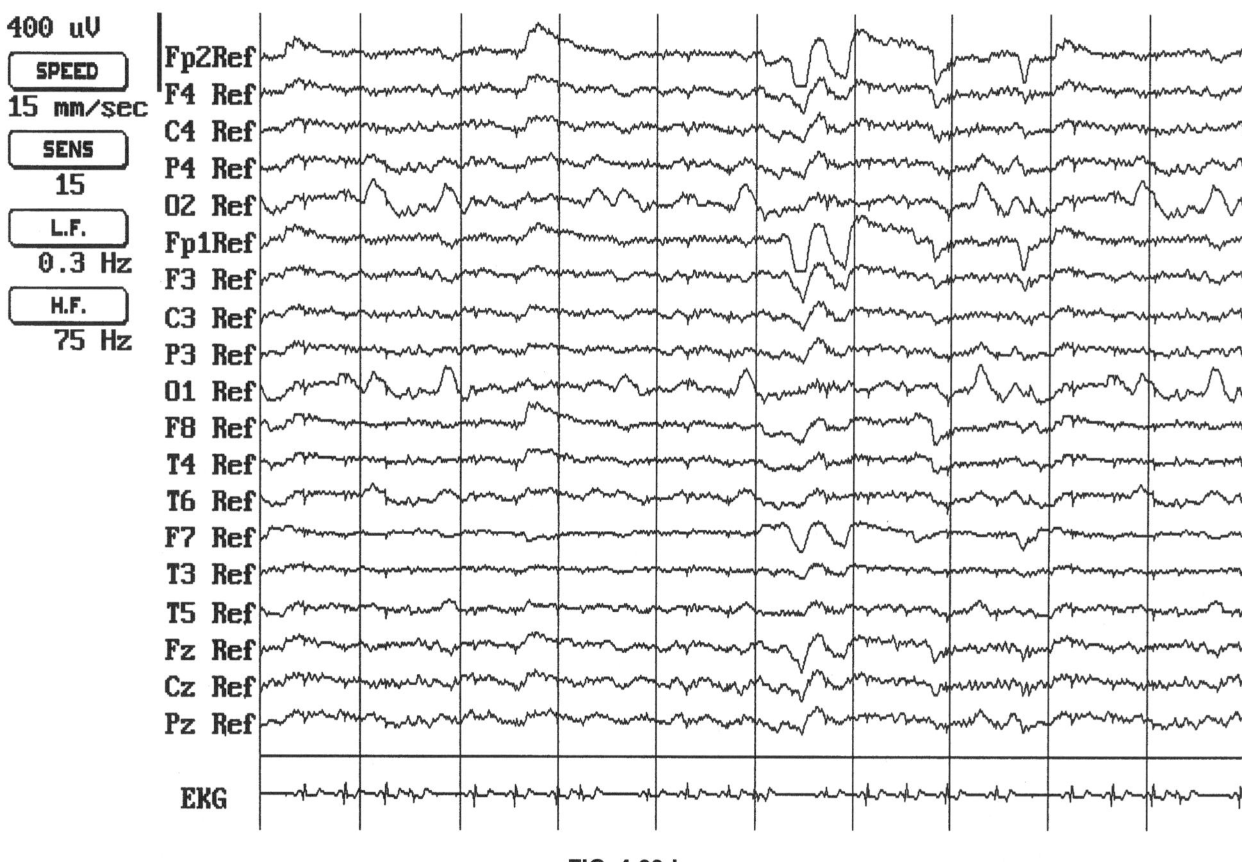
400 uV
SPEED
15 mm/sec
SENS
15
L.F.
0.3 Hz
H.F.
75 Hz
Fp2Ref
F4 Ref
C4 Ref
P4 Ref
O2 Ref
Fp1Ref
F3 Ref
C3 Ref
P3 Ref
O1 Ref
F8 Ref
T4 Ref
T6 Ref
F7 Ref
T3 Ref
T5 Ref
Fz Ref
Cz Ref
Pz Ref
EKG

FIG. 4-23d

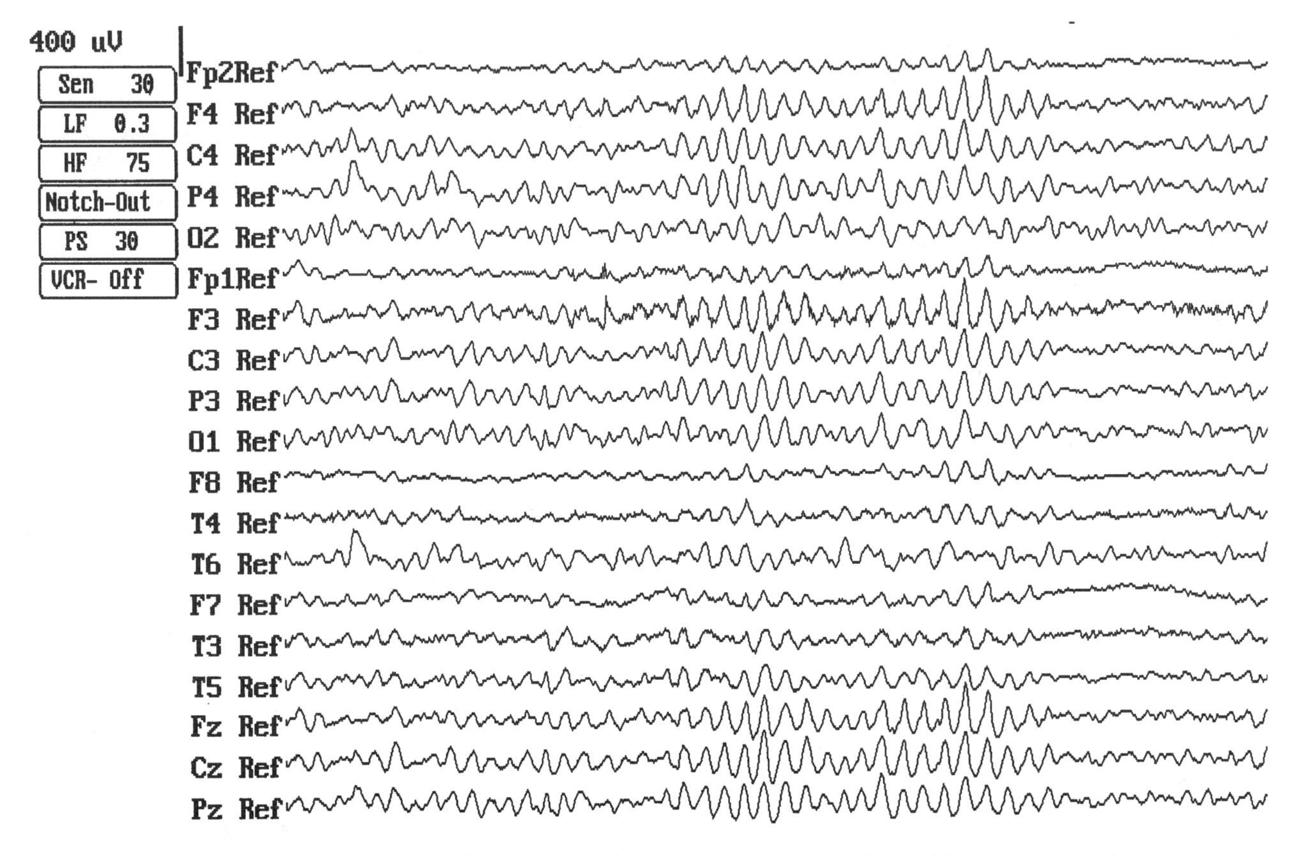

FIG. 4-24a,b,c A well regulated drowsy burst is seen better on run 1 than 2. The paper speed, 15 mm/s, further enhances the rhythmicity of the burst.

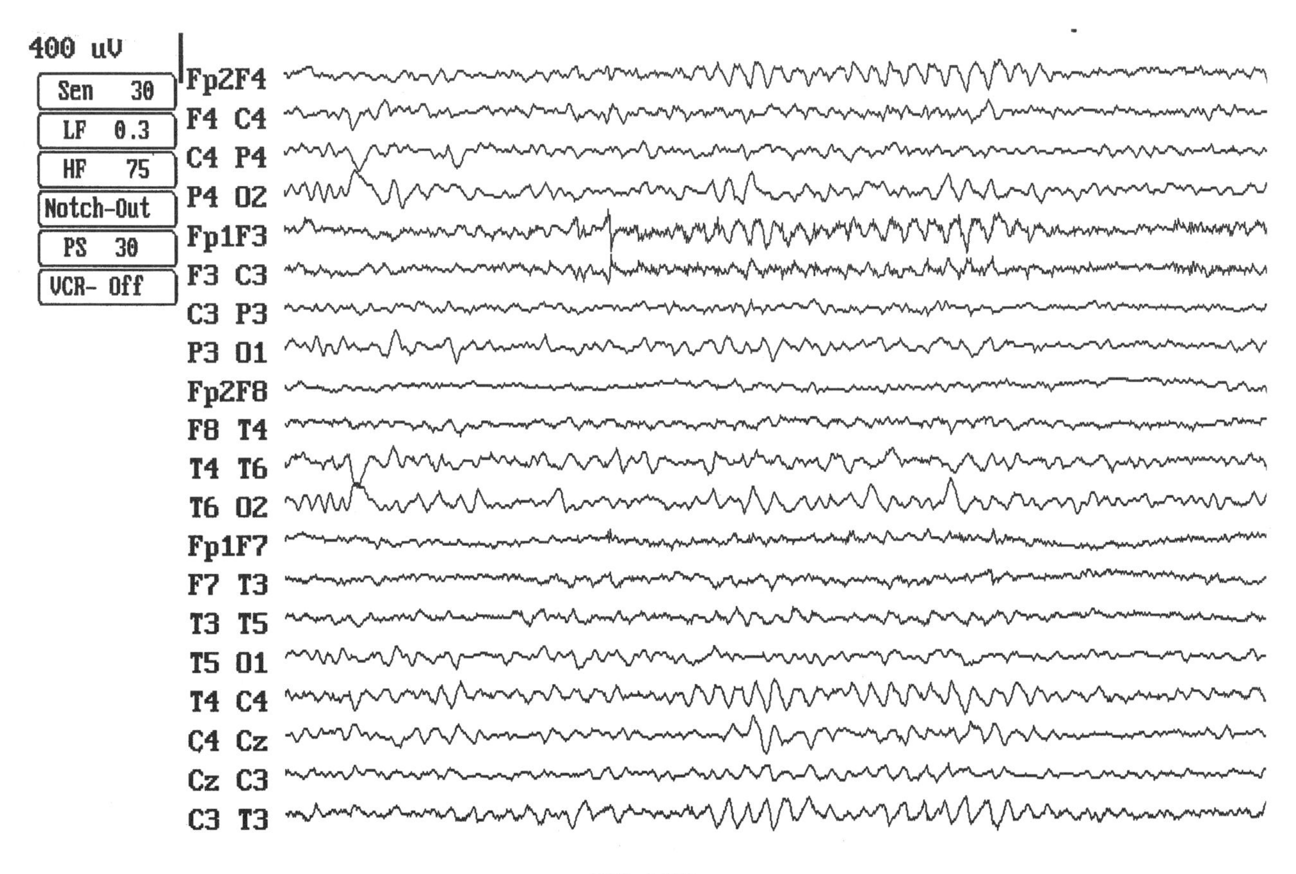
400 uV
Sen 30
LF 0.3
HF 75
Notch-Out
PS 30
VCR- Off
Fp2F4
F4 C4
C4 P4
P4 O2
Fp1F3
F3 C3
C3 P3
P3 O1
Fp2F8
F8 T4
T4 T6
T6 O2
Fp1F7
F7 T3
T3 T5
T5 O1
T4 C4
C4 Cz
Cz C3
C3 T3

FIG. 4-24b

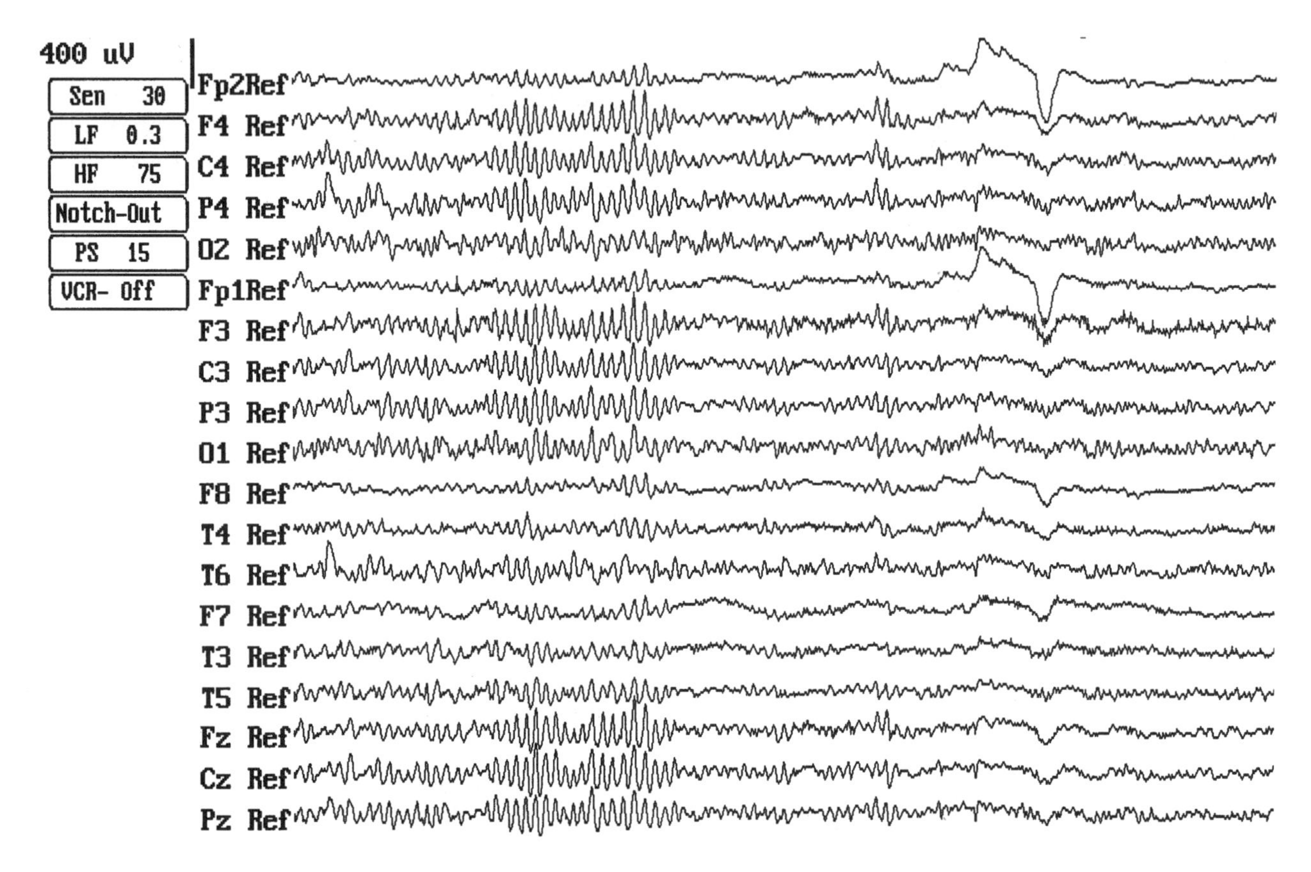
400 uV
Sen 30
LF 0.3
HF 75
Notch-Out
PS 15
VCR- Off
Fp2Ref
F4 Ref
C4 Ref
P4 Ref
O2 Ref
Fp1Ref
F3 Ref
C3 Ref
P3 Ref
O1 Ref
F8 Ref
T4 Ref
T6 Ref
F7 Ref
T3 Ref
T5 Ref
Fz Ref
Cz Ref
Pz Ref

FIG. 4-24c

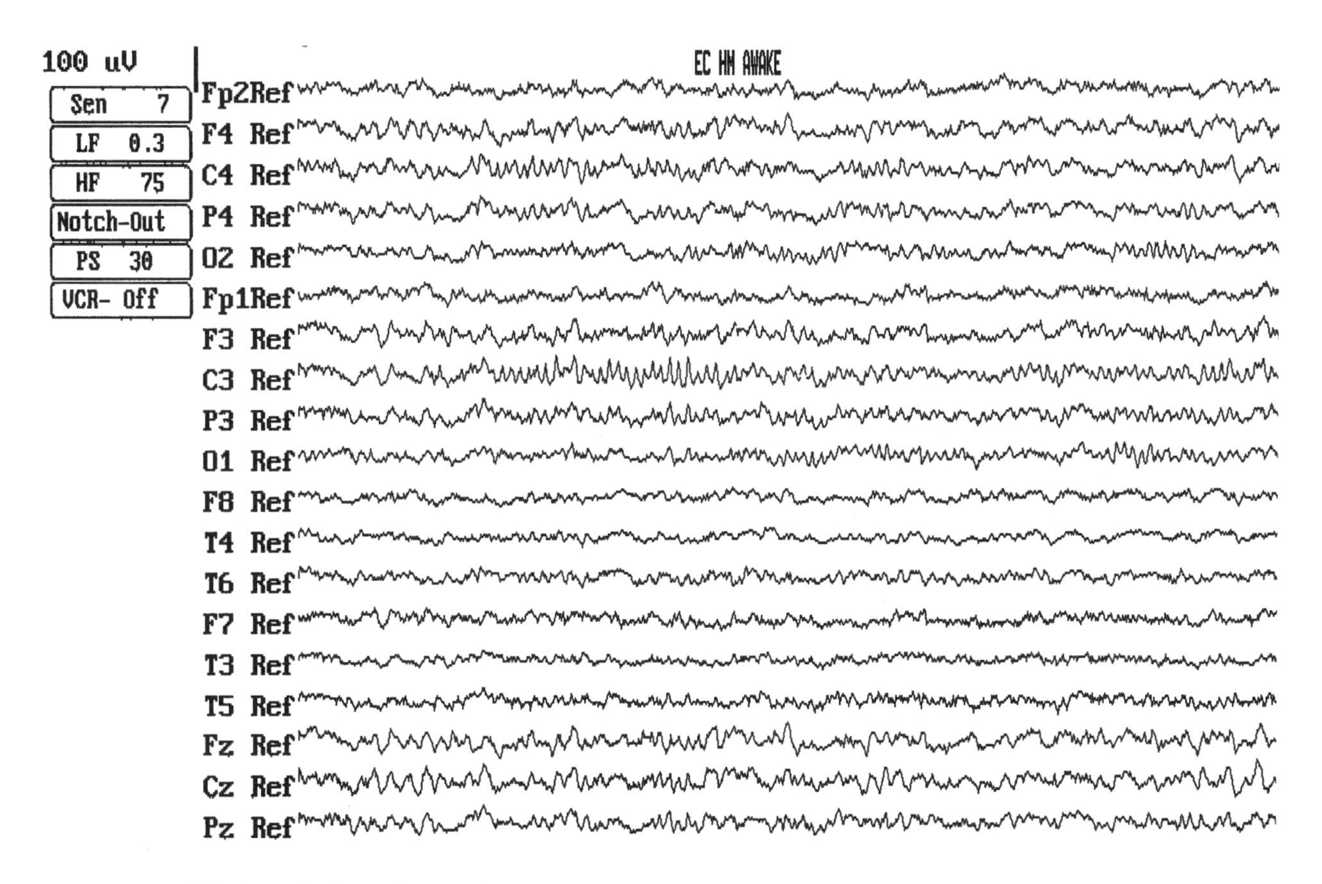

FIG. 4-25a,b Central mu rhythm, which is slightly higher on the left, is seen on runs 1 and 2.

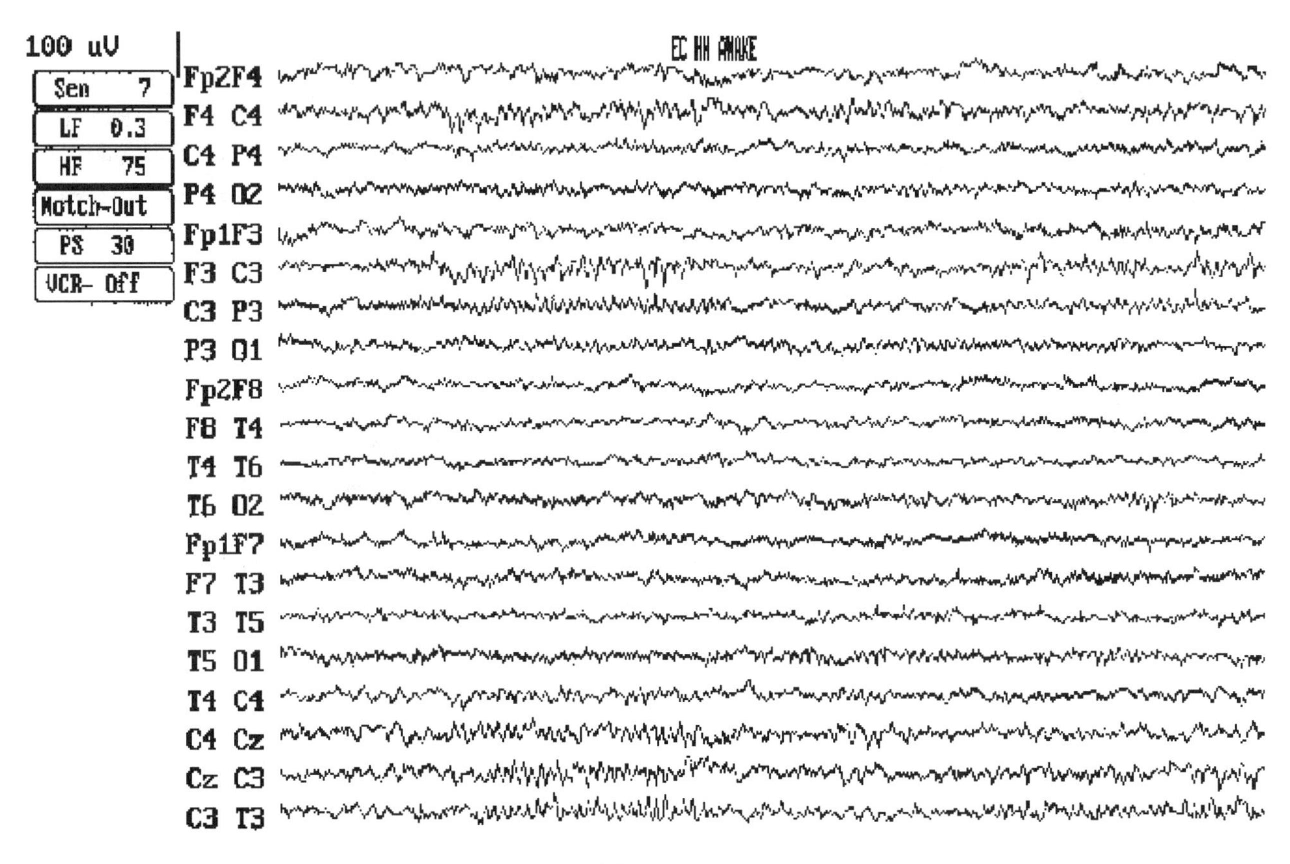

100 uV
Sen 7
LF 0.3
HF 75
Notch-Out
PS 30
VCR- Off
EC HH AWAKE
Fp2F4
F4 C4
C4 P4
P4 O2
Fp1F3
F3 C3
C3 P3
P3 O1
Fp2F8
F8 T4
T4 T6
T6 O2
Fp1F7
F7 T3
T3 T5
T5 O1
T4 C4
C4 Cz
Cz C3
C3 T3

FIG. 4-25b

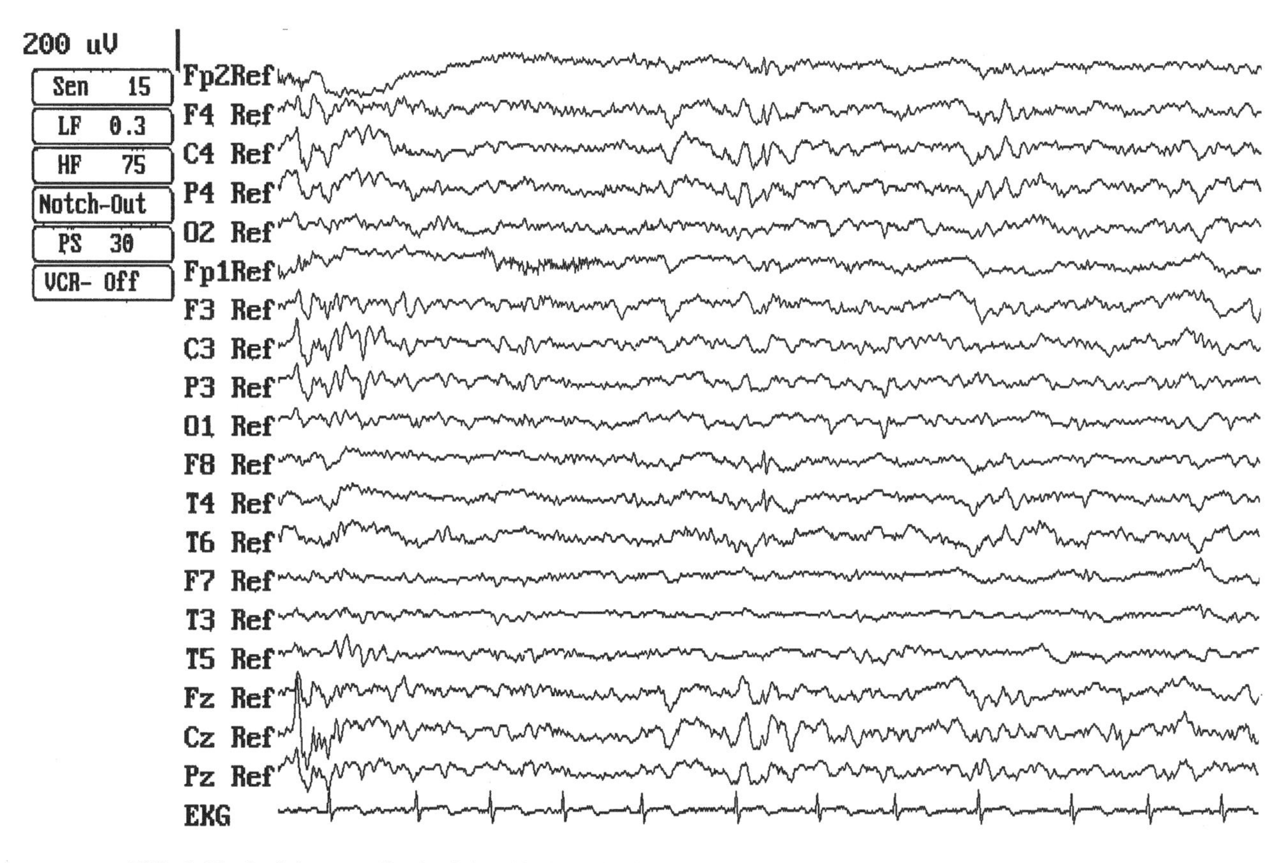

FIG. 4-26a,b A low amplitude right sided small sharp spike is seen clearly on run 1 but disappears on run 2.

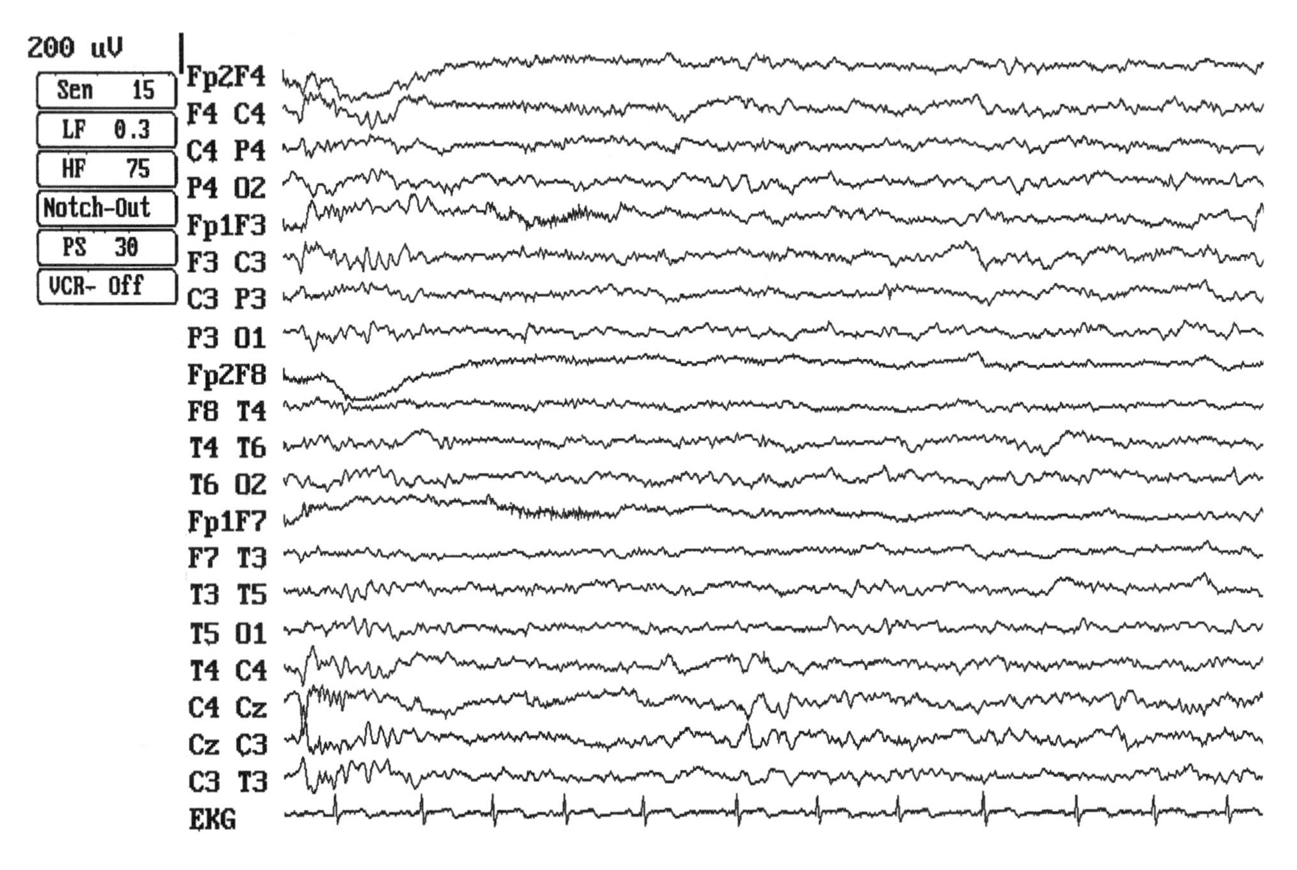
200 uV
Sen 15
LF 0.3
HF 75
Notch-Out
PS 30
VCR- Off
Fp2F4
F4 C4
C4 P4
P4 O2
Fp1F3
F3 C3
C3 P3
P3 O1
Fp2F8
F8 T4
T4 T6
T6 O2
Fp1F7
F7 T3
T3 T5
T5 O1
T4 C4
C4 Cz
Cz C3
C3 T3
EKG

FIG. 4-26b

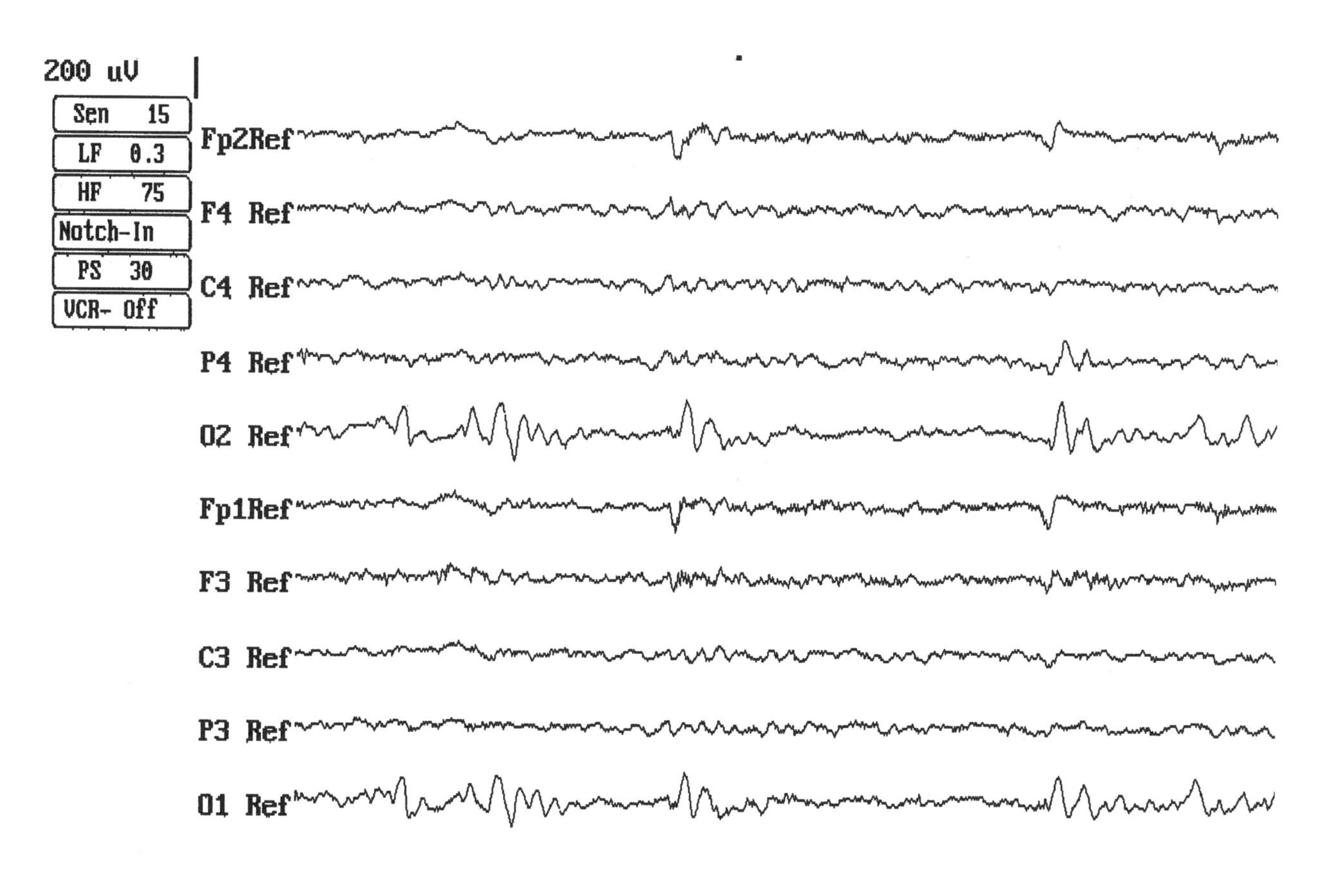

FIG. 4-27a,b High amplitude symmetrical lambda is seen equally well on runs 1 and 2.

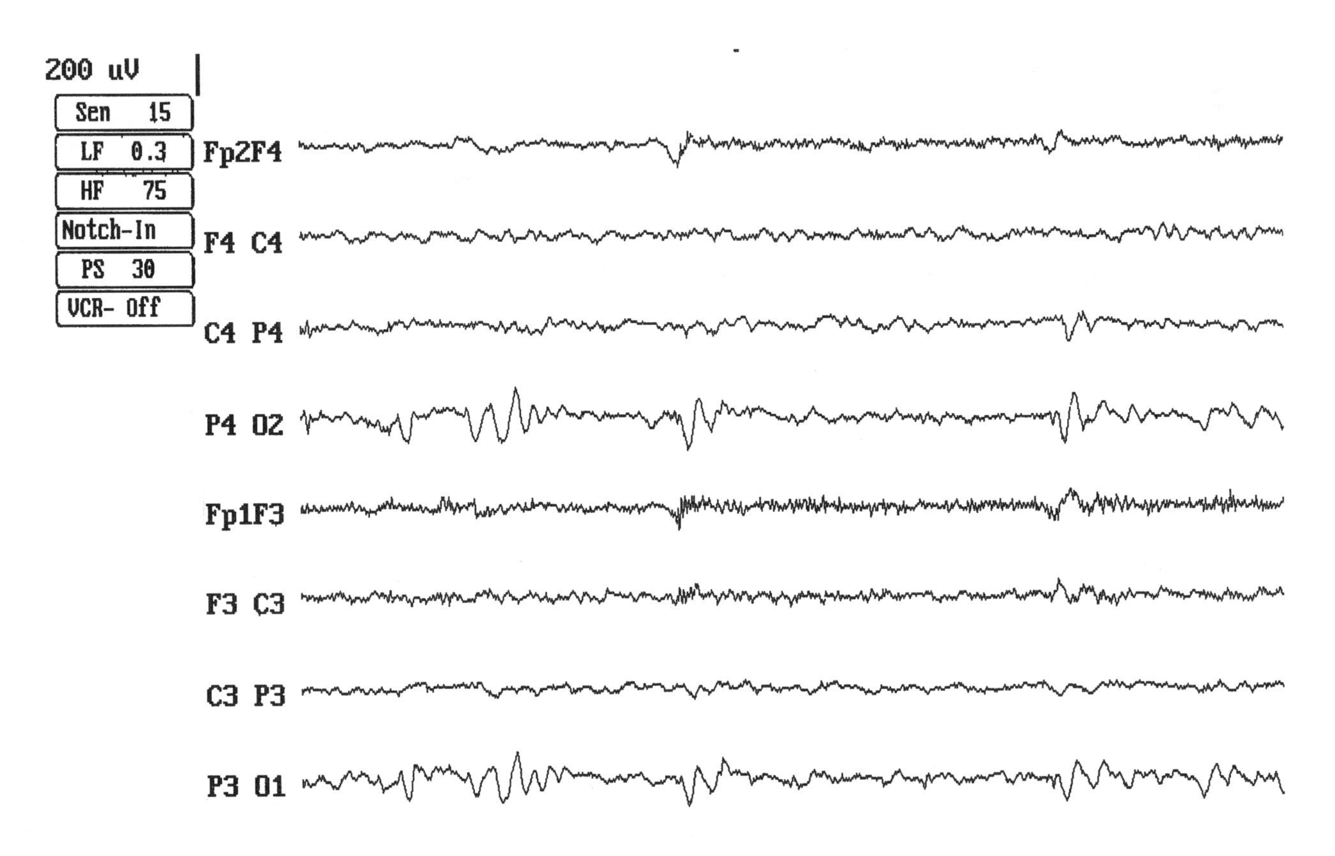
200 uV
Sen 15
LF 0.3
HF 75
Notch-In
PS 30
VCR- Off
Fp2F4
F4 C4
C4 P4
P4 O2
Fp1F3
F3 C3
C3 P3
P3 O1

FIG. 4-27b

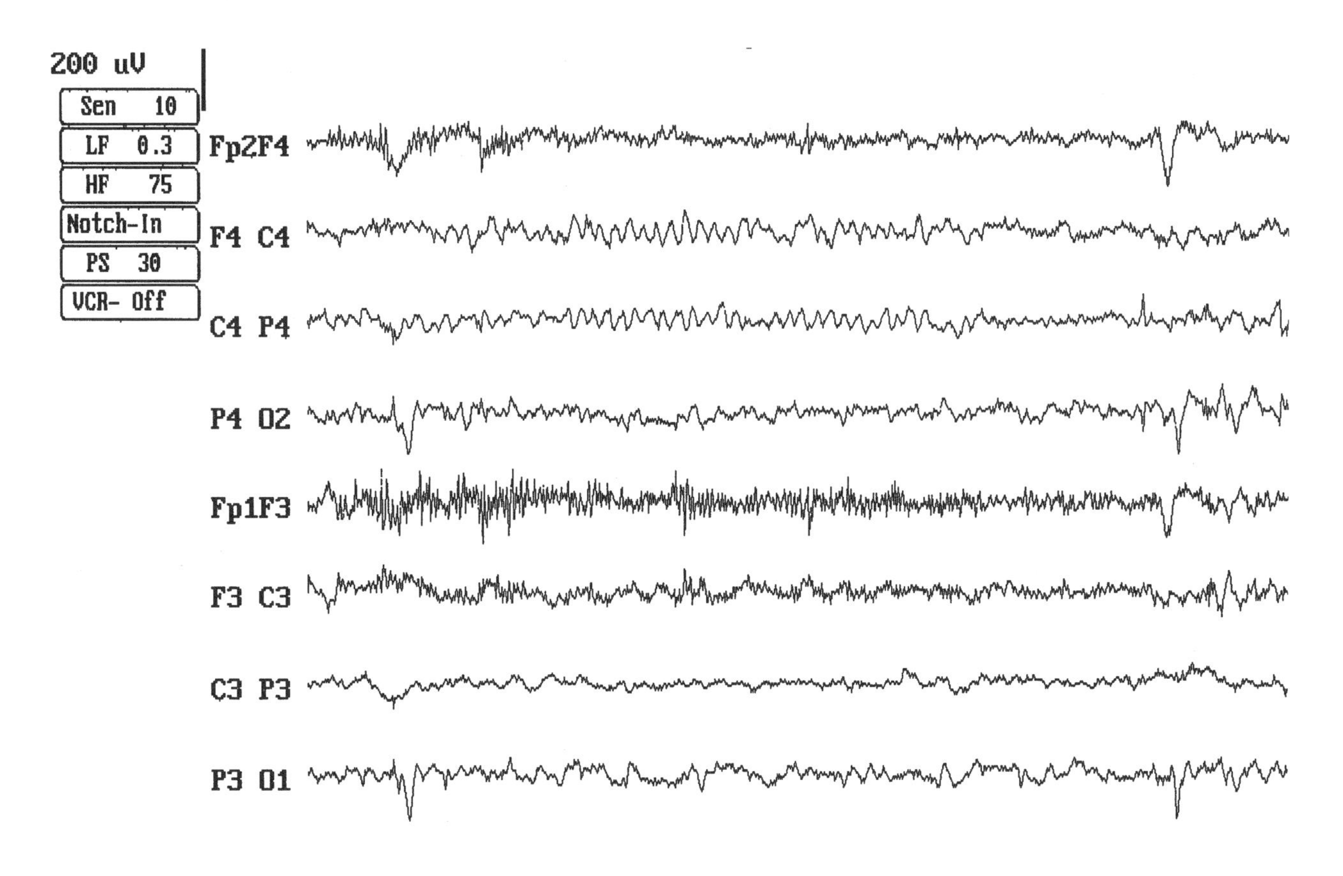

FIG. 4-28a,b Sharp transients are seen with eye closure at the bioccipital area in the first and last second of this sample. This transient is seen well on both runs. Also an asymmetric mu rhythm is seen at the right central.

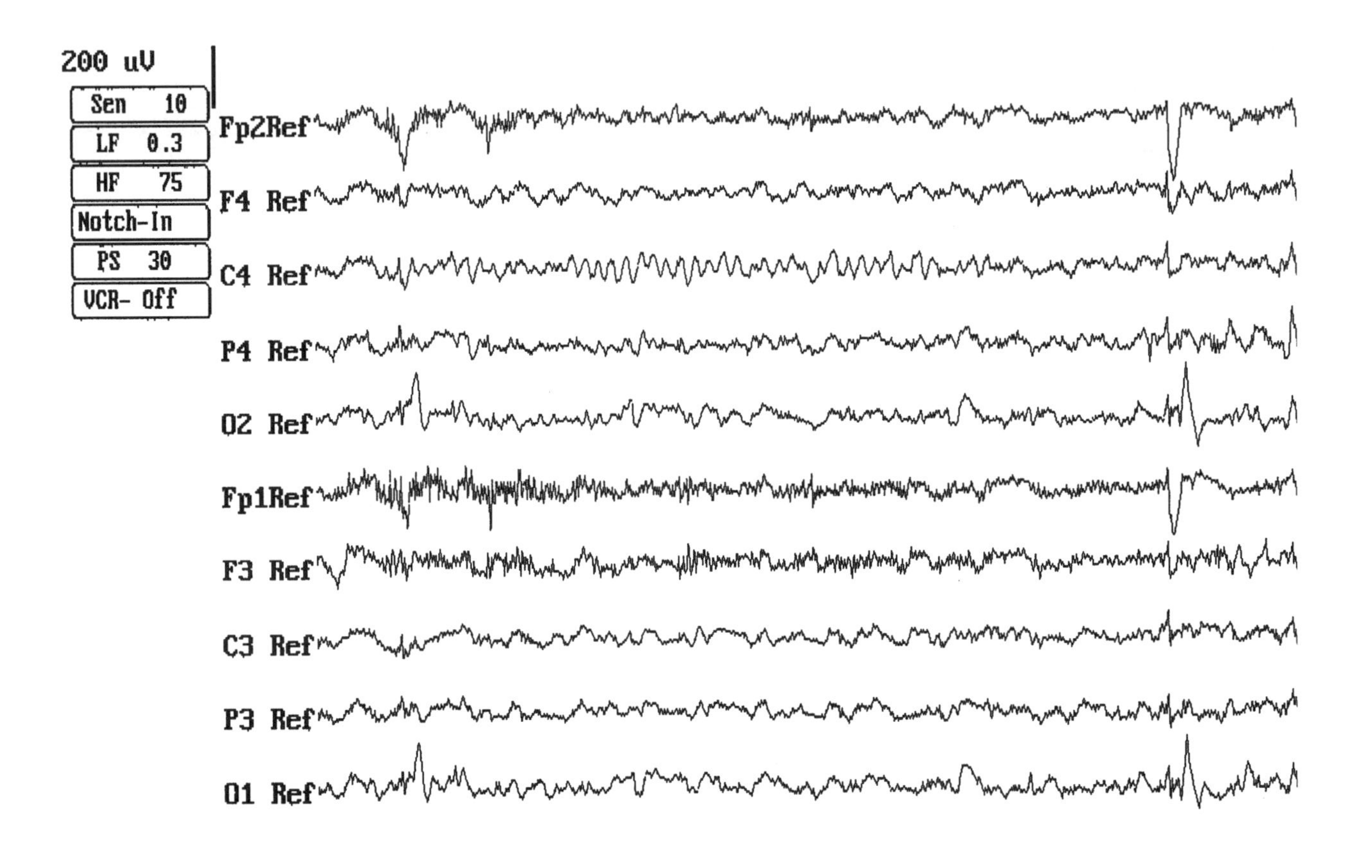
200 uV
Sen 10
LF 0.3
HF 75
Notch-In
PS 30
VCR- Off
Fp2Ref
F4 Ref
C4 Ref
P4 Ref
O2 Ref
Fp1Ref
F3 Ref
C3 Ref
P3 Ref
O1 Ref

FIG. 4-28b

Neonatal Examples

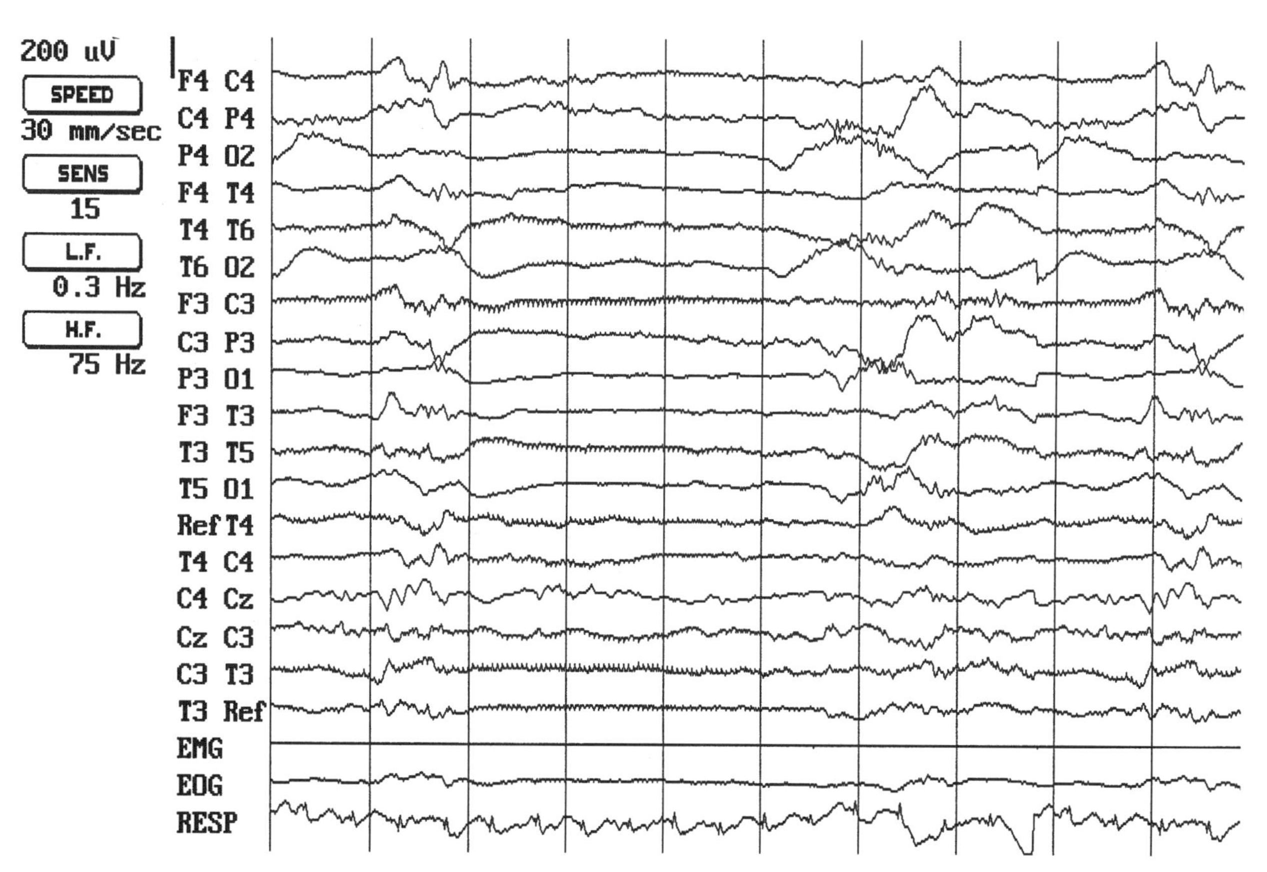

FIG. 4-29a,b This shows a sleep EEG in a neonate 39 weeks conceptional age (CA). The paper speed, 15 mm/s, demonstrates the periodicity of bursts.

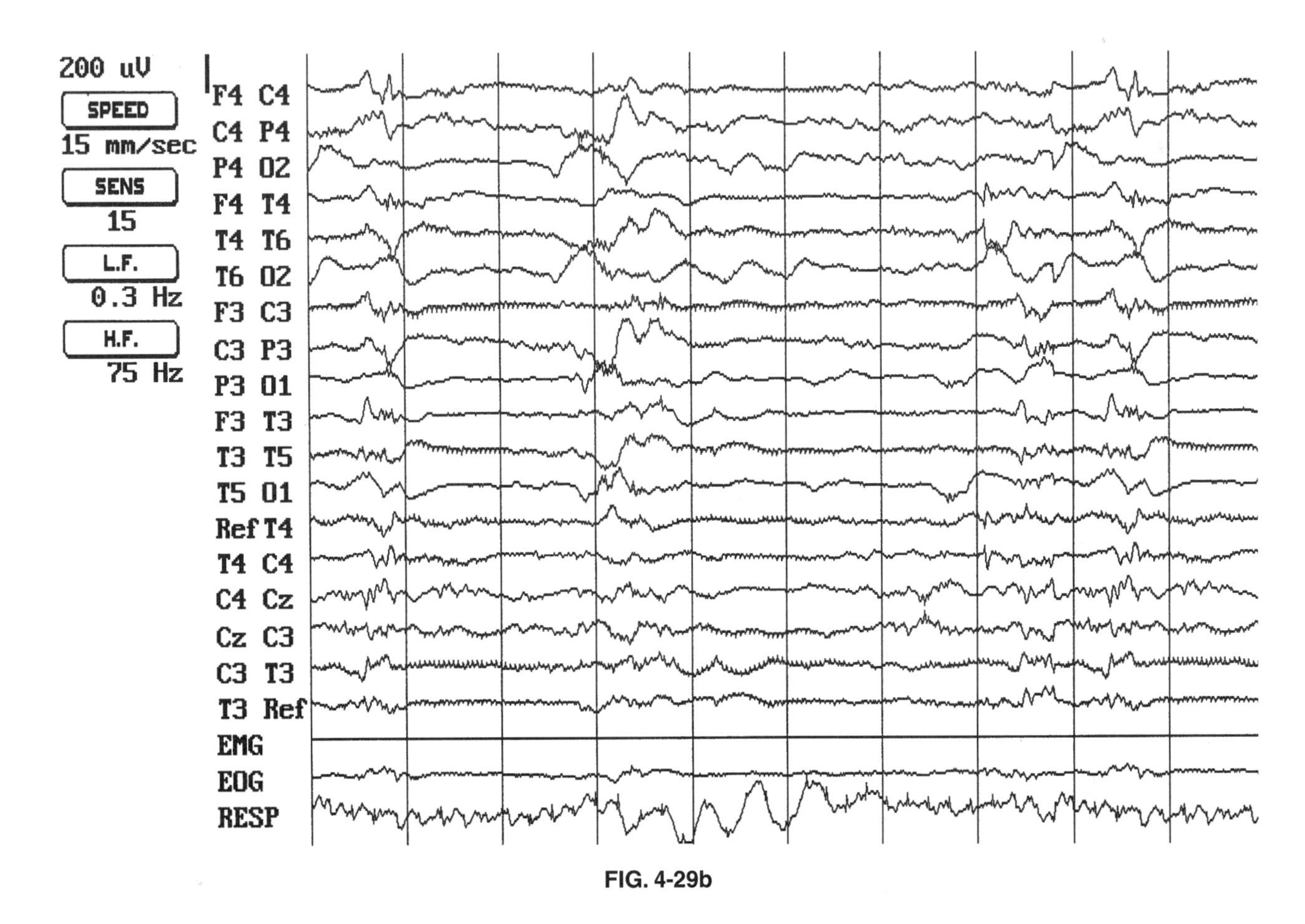
200 uV
SPEED
15 mm/sec
SENS
15
L.F.
0.3 Hz
H.F.
75 Hz
F4 C4
C4 P4
P4 O2
F4 T4
T4 T6
T6 O2
F3 C3
C3 P3
P3 O1
F3 T3
T3 T5
T5 O1
Ref T4
T4 C4
C4 Cz
Cz C3
C3 T3
T3 Ref
EMG
EOG
RESP

FIG. 4-29b

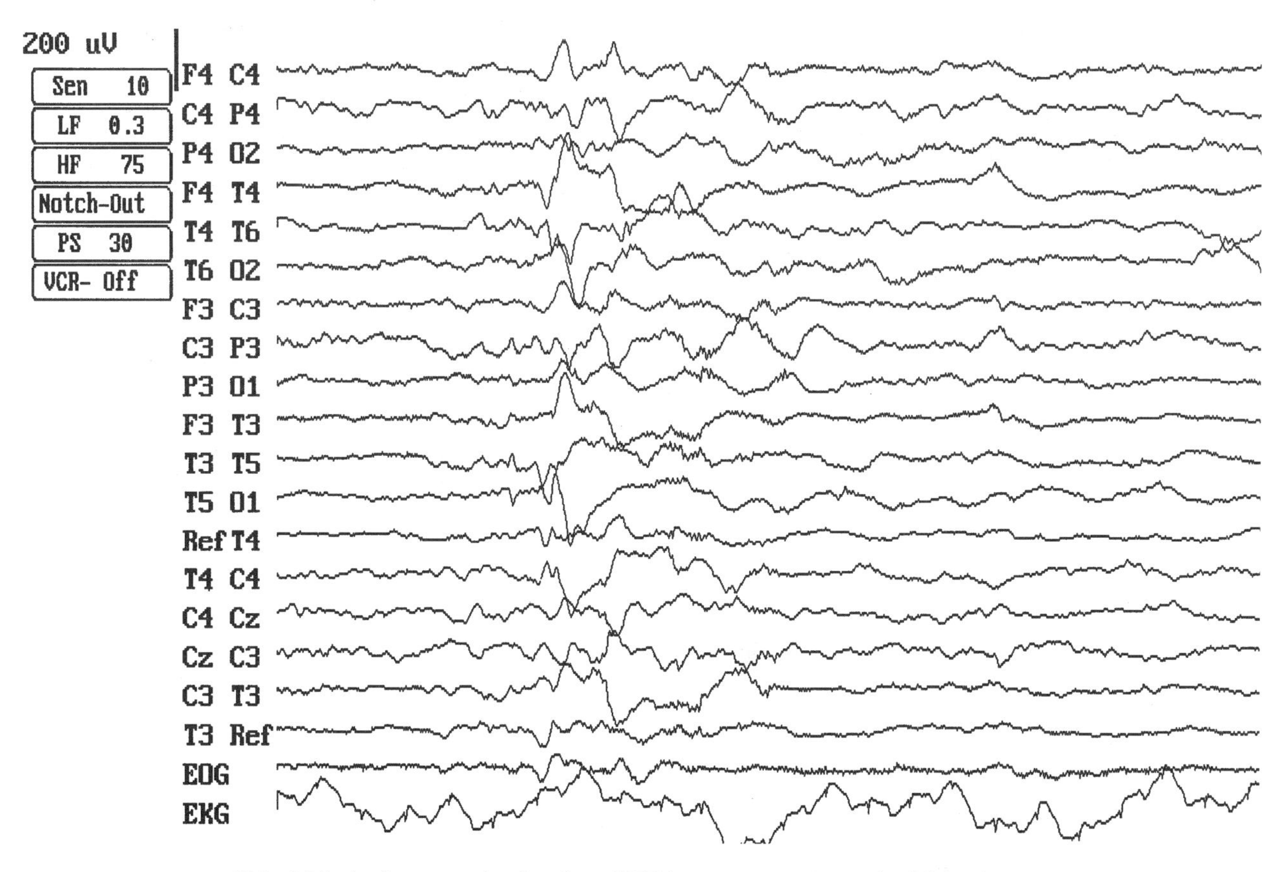

FIG. 4-30a,b An example of a sleep EEG in a neonate 40 weeks CA is shown.

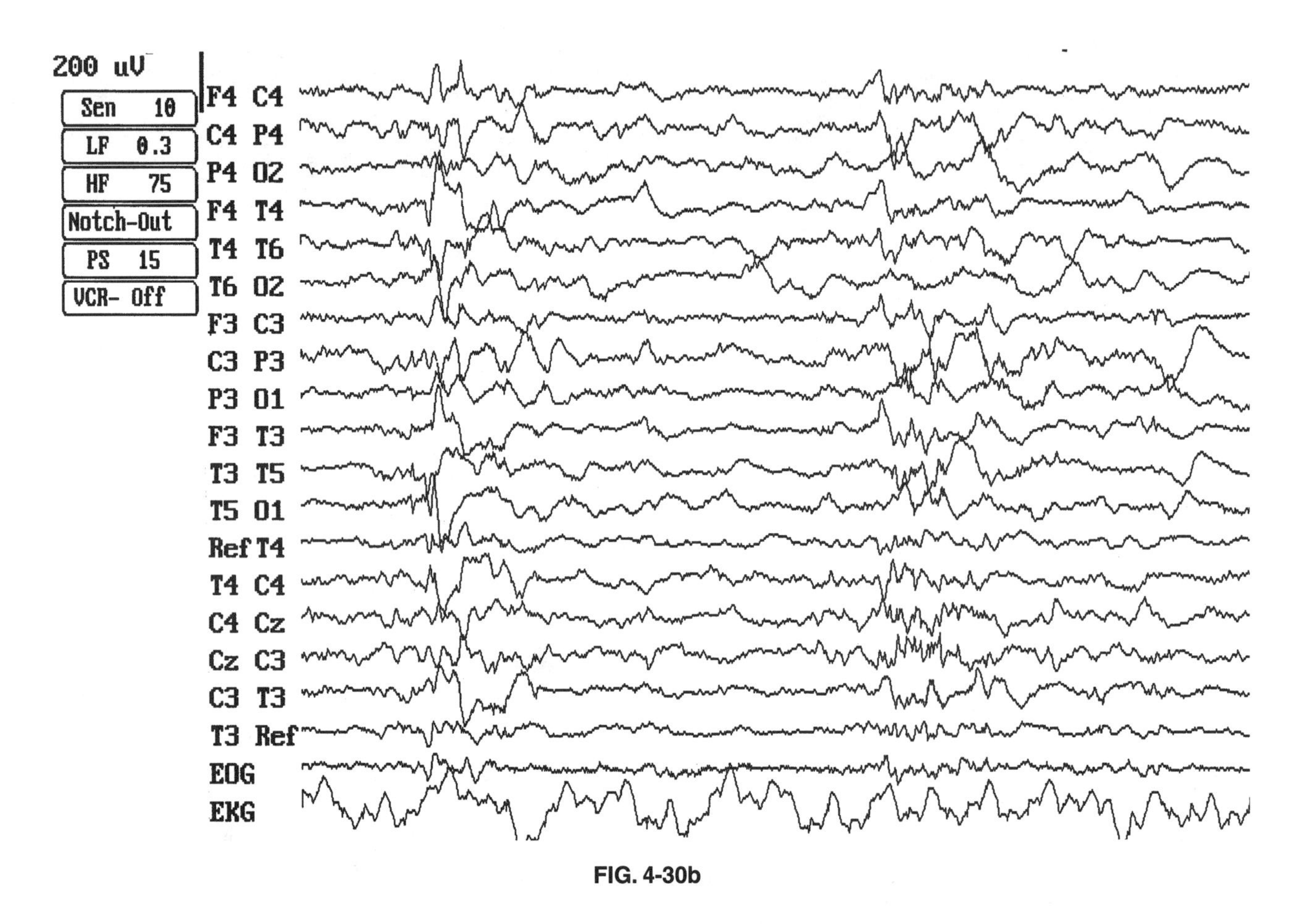
200 uV
Sen 10
LF 0.3
HF 75
Notch-Out
PS 15
VCR- Off
F4 C4
C4 P4
P4 O2
F4 T4
T4 T6
T6 O2
F3 C3
C3 P3
P3 O1
F3 T3
T3 T5
T5 O1
Ref T4
T4 C4
C4 Cz
Cz C3
C3 T3
T3 Ref
EOG
EKG

FIG. 4-30b

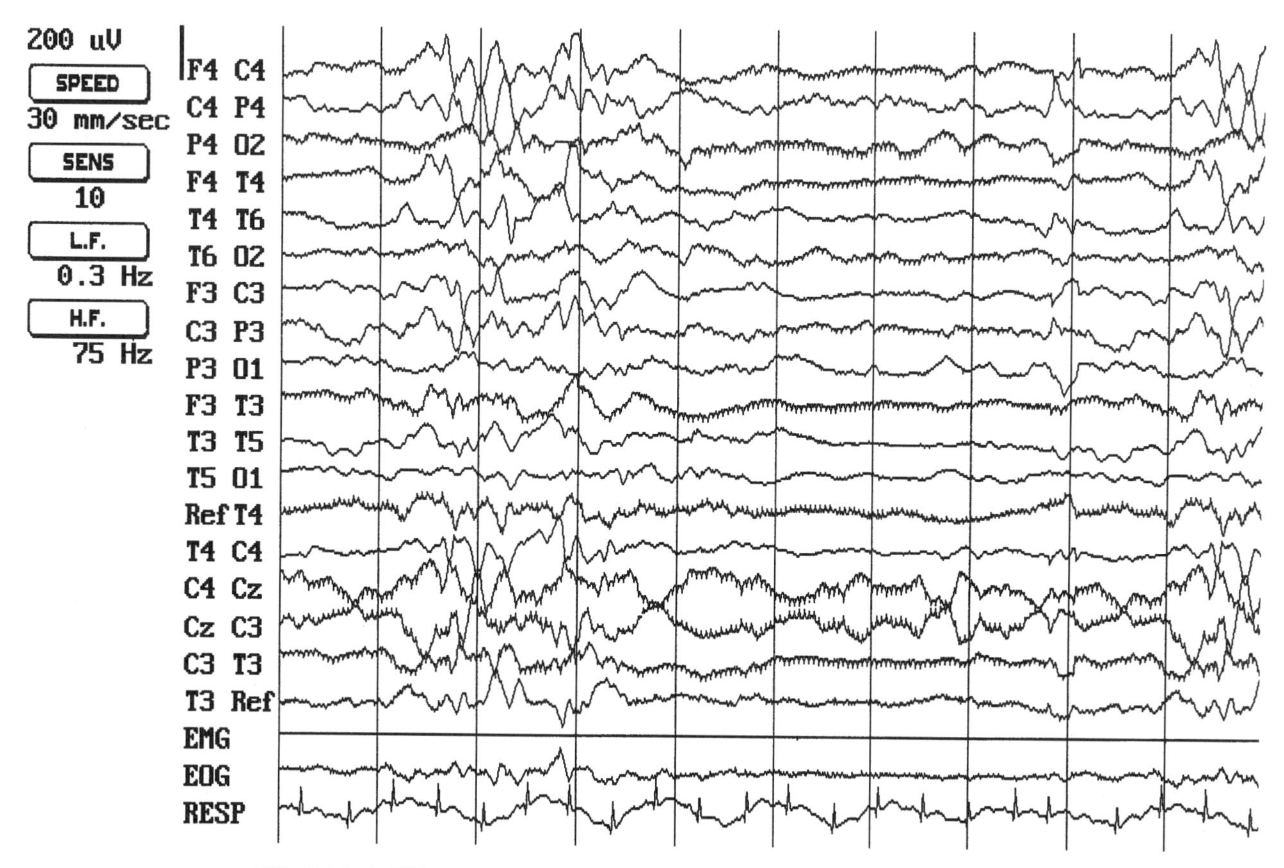

FIG. 4-31a,b This example shows a sleep EEG in a neonate 42 weeks CA.

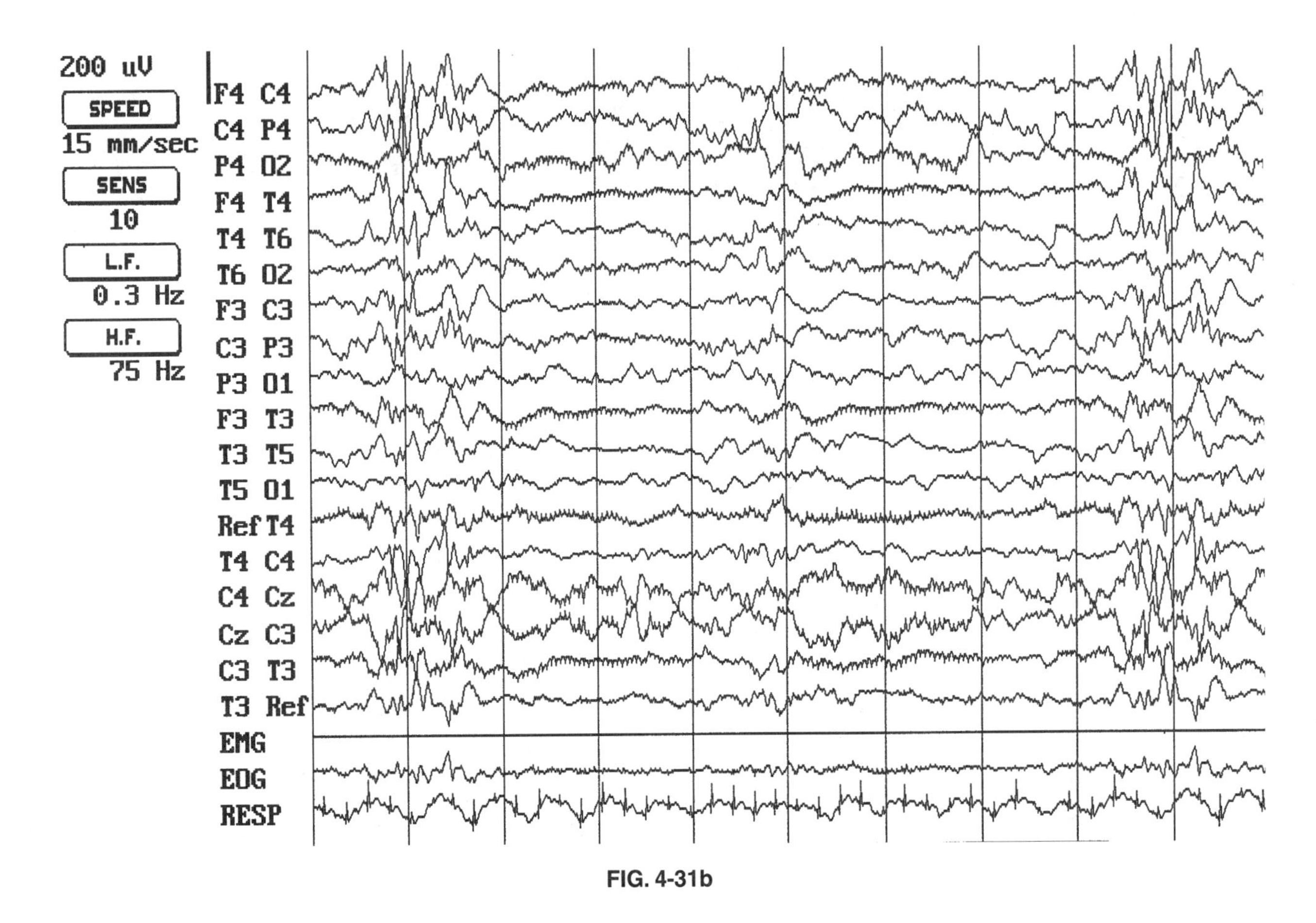
200 uV
SPEED
15 mm/sec
SENS
10
L.F.
0.3 Hz
H.F.
75 Hz
F4 C4
C4 P4
P4 O2
F4 T4
T4 T6
T6 O2
F3 C3
C3 P3
P3 O1
F3 T3
T3 T5
T5 O1
Ref T4
T4 C4
C4 Cz
Cz C3
C3 T3
T3 Ref
EMG
EOG
RESP

FIG. 4-31b

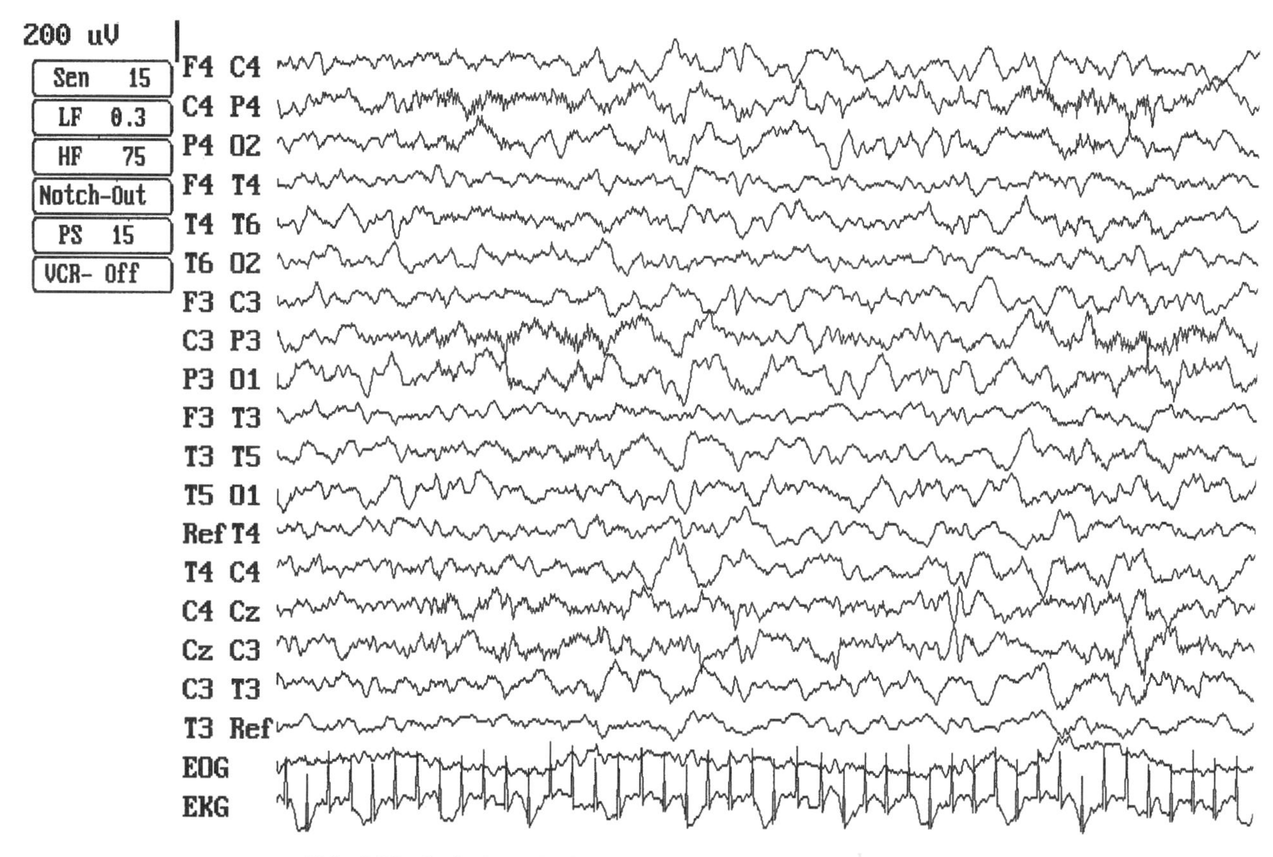

FIG. 4-32a,b A sleep EEG in a neonate 46 weeks CA is shown.

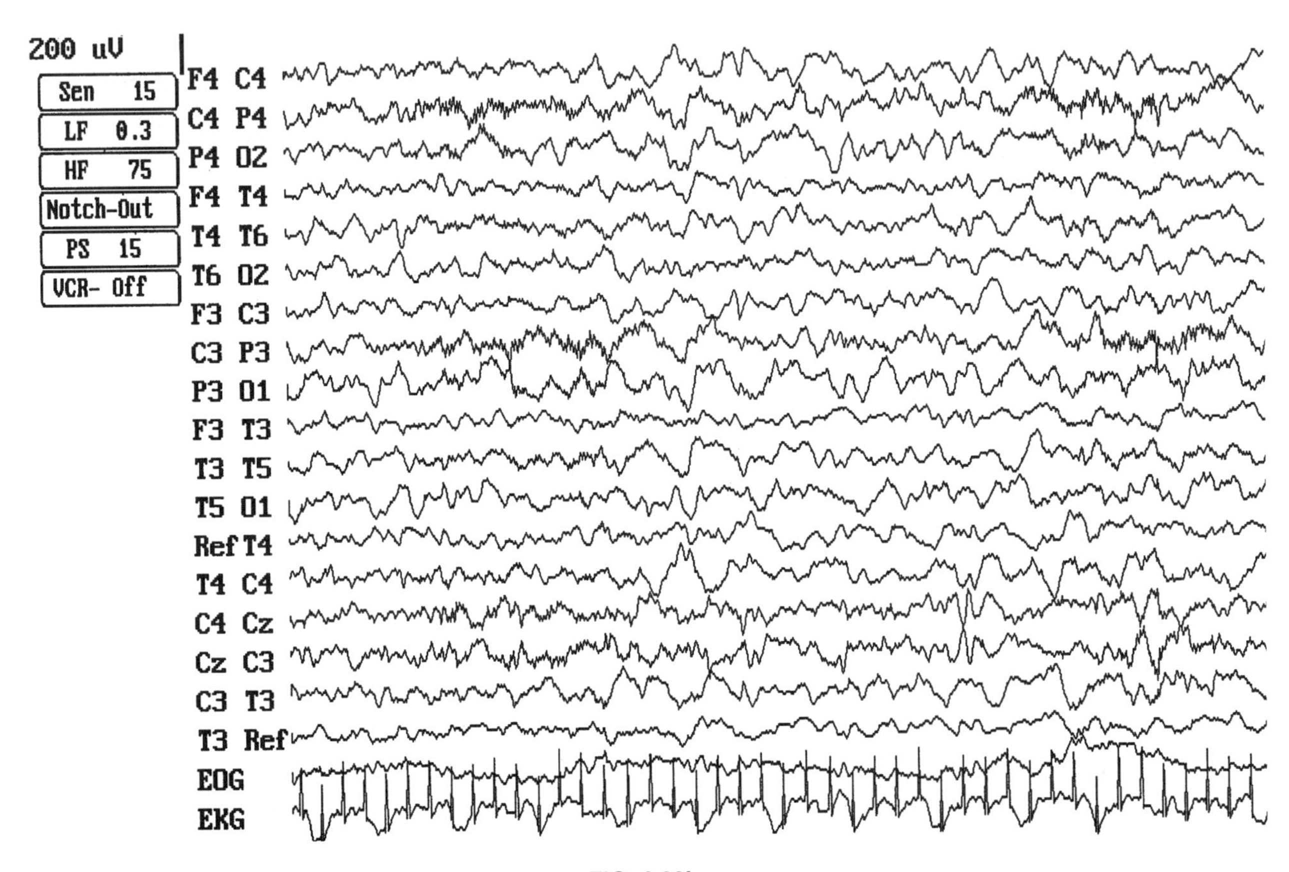
200 uV
Sen 15
LF 0.3
HF 75
Notch-Out
PS 15
VCR- Off
F4 C4
C4 P4
P4 O2
F4 T4
T4 T6
T6 O2
F3 C3
C3 P3
P3 O1
F3 T3
T3 T5
T5 O1
Ref T4
T4 C4
C4 Cz
Cz C3
C3 T3
T3 Ref
EOG
EKG

FIG. 4-32b

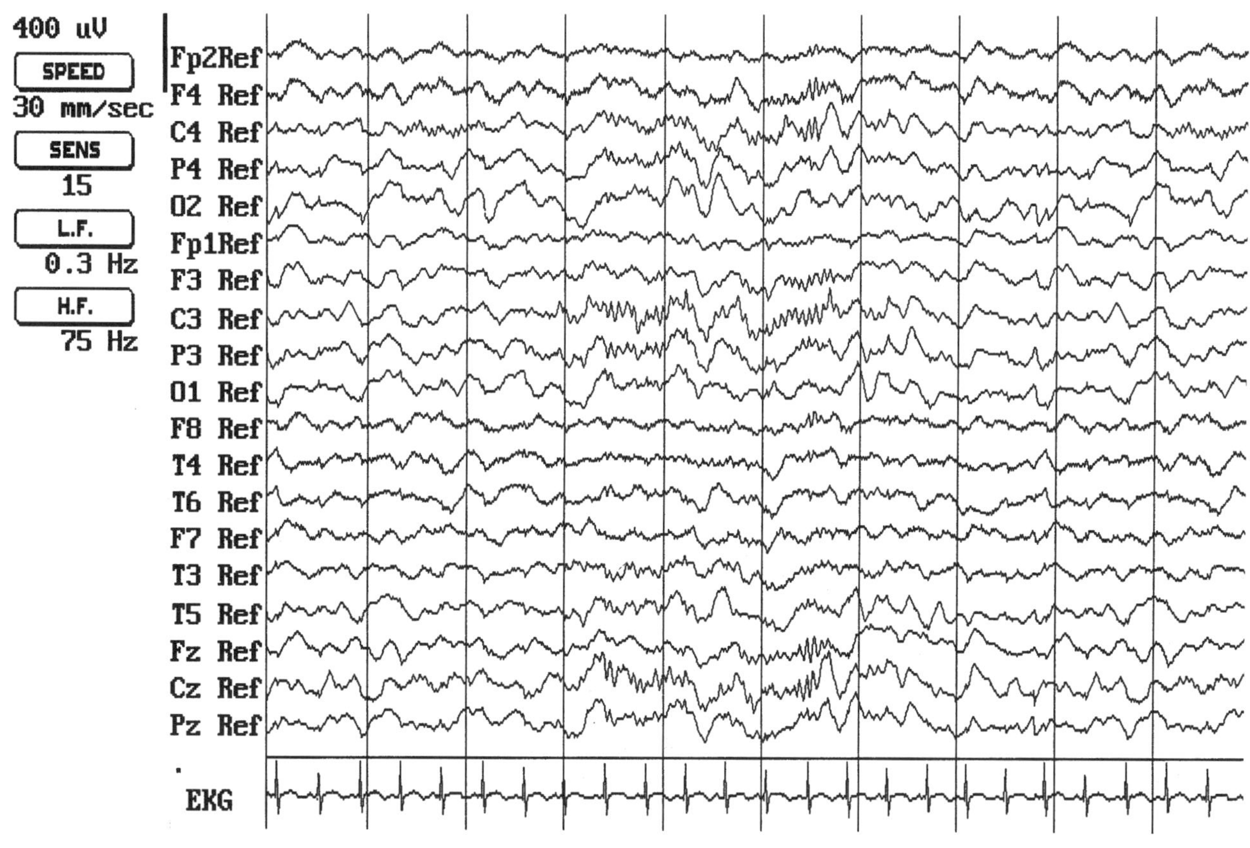

FIG. 4-33a,b,c This sleep EEG in a 3 month old shows Vertex waves and sleep spindles.

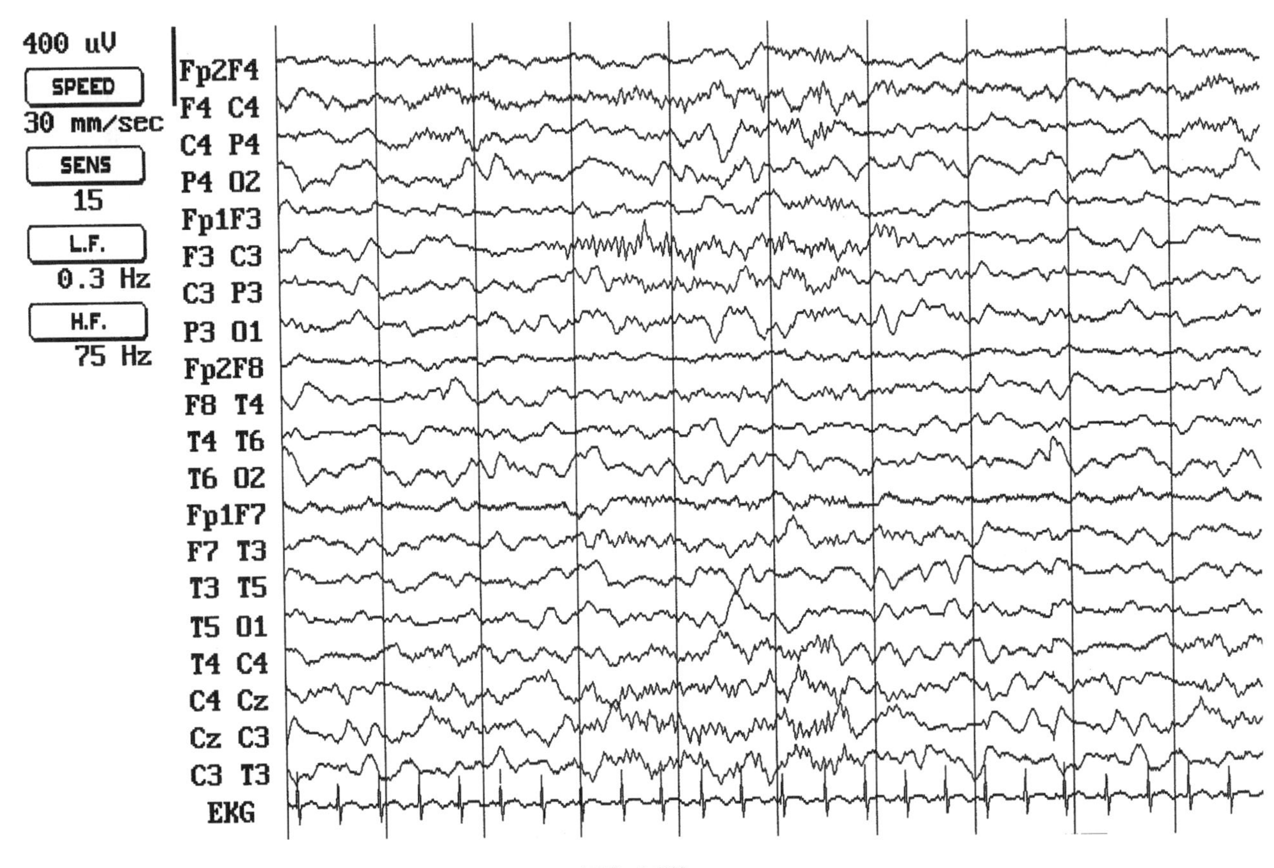
400 uV
SPEED
30 mm/sec
SENS
15
L.F.
0.3 Hz
H.F.
75 Hz
Fp2F4
F4 C4
C4 P4
P4 O2
Fp1F3
F3 C3
C3 P3
P3 O1
Fp2F8
F8 T4
T4 T6
T6 O2
Fp1F7
F7 T3
T3 T5
T5 O1
T4 C4
C4 Cz
Cz C3
C3 T3
EKG

FIG. 4-33b

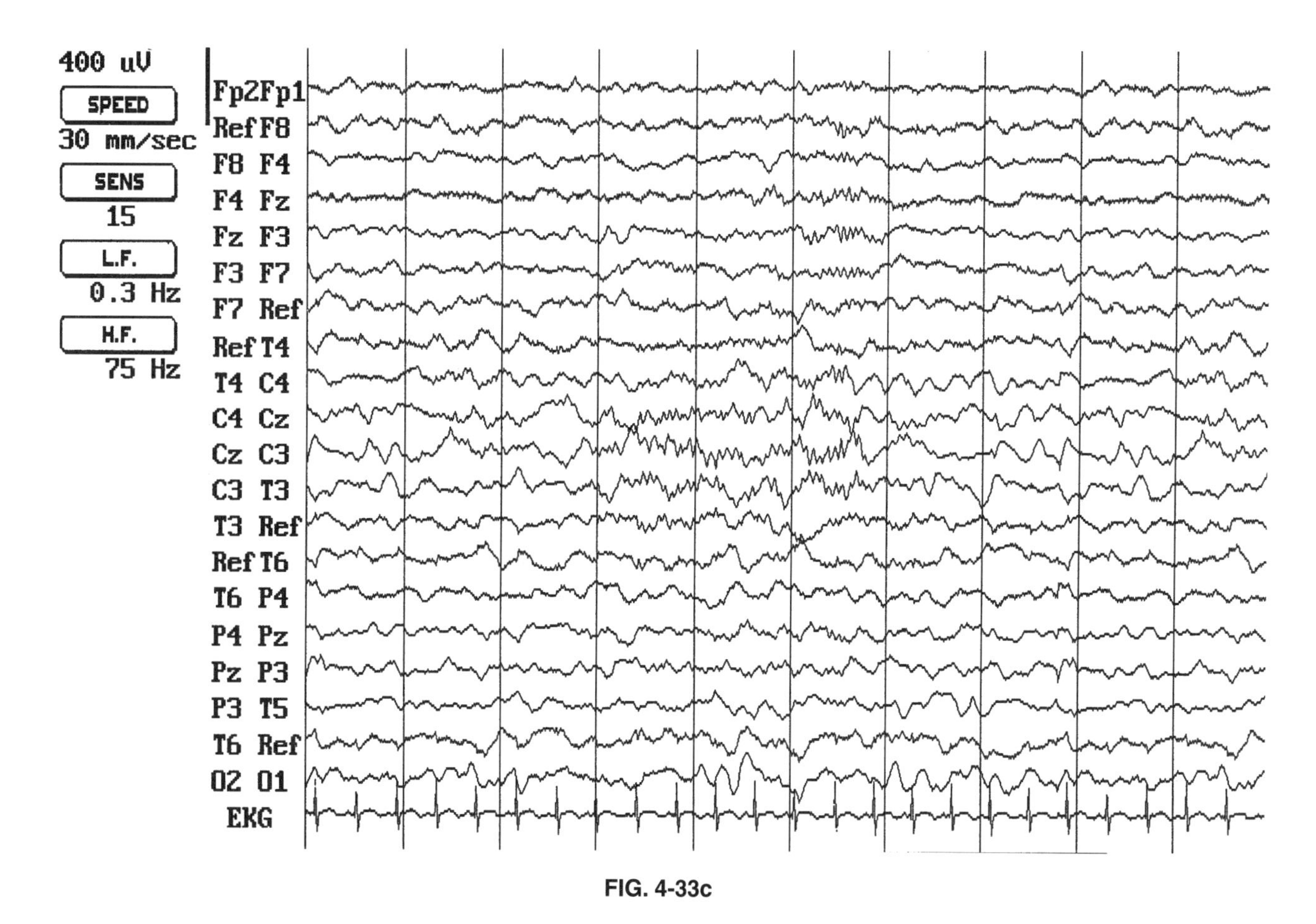
400 uV
SPEED
30 mm/sec
SENS
15
L.F.
0.3 Hz
H.F.
75 Hz
Fp2Fp1
Ref F8
F8 F4
F4 Fz
Fz F3
F3 F7
F7 Ref
Ref T4
T4 C4
C4 Cz
Cz C3
C3 T3
T3 Ref
Ref T6
T6 P4
P4 Pz
Pz P3
P3 T5
T6 Ref
O2 O1
EKG

FIG. 4-33c

Apparent Delta Focus

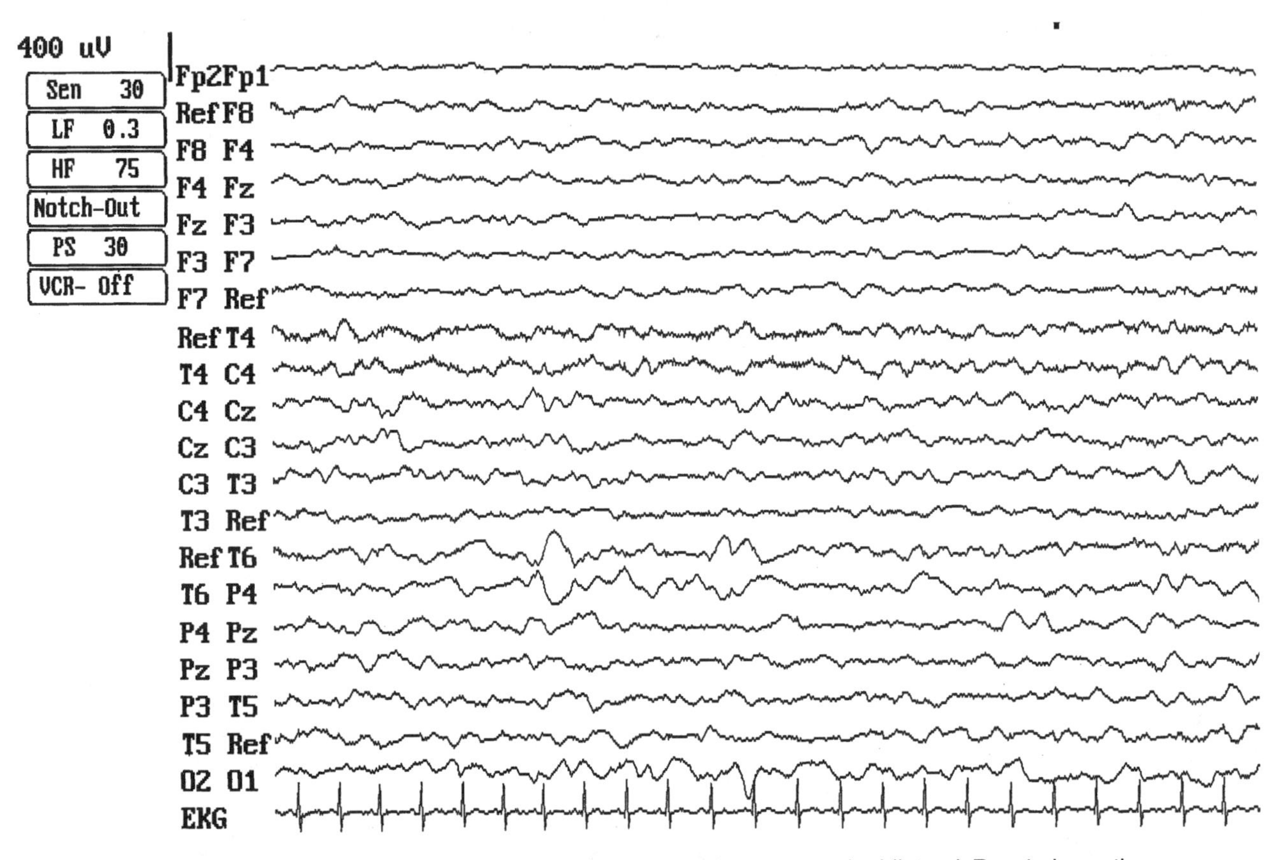

FIG. 4-34a,b,c Run 3 shows a focal delta at T6; on run 2 it appears to be bilateral. Run 1 shows the slow wave to be lower voltage at T5; therefore the apparent focality at T6 is due to the lower amplitude delta at T5. This delta activity has the characteristics of benign posterior slow waves of youth.

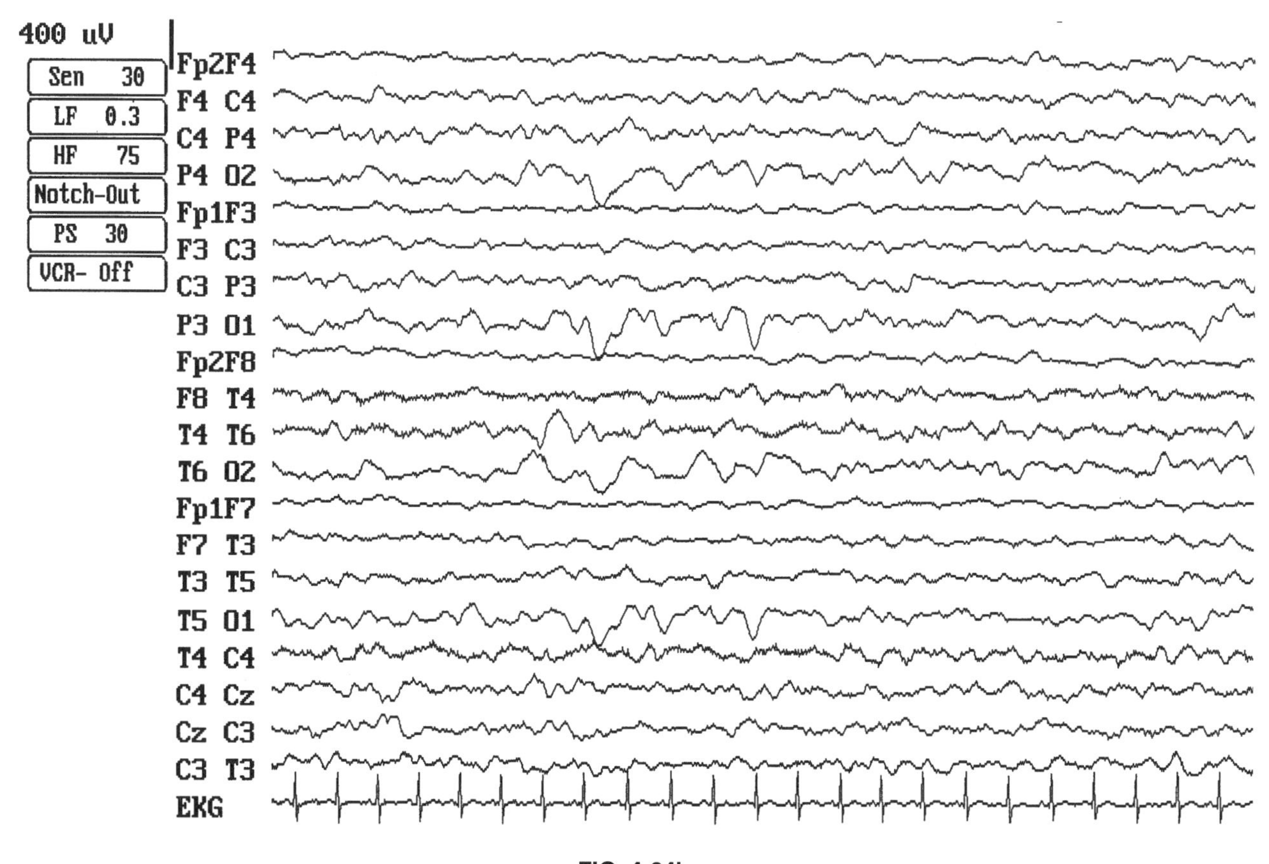
400 uV
Sen 30
LF 0.3
HF 75
Notch-Out
PS 30
VCR- Off
Fp2F4
F4 C4
C4 P4
P4 O2
Fp1F3
F3 C3
C3 P3
P3 O1
Fp2F8
F8 T4
T4 T6
T6 O2
Fp1F7
F7 T3
T3 T5
T5 O1
T4 C4
C4 Cz
Cz C3
C3 T3
EKG

FIG. 4-34b

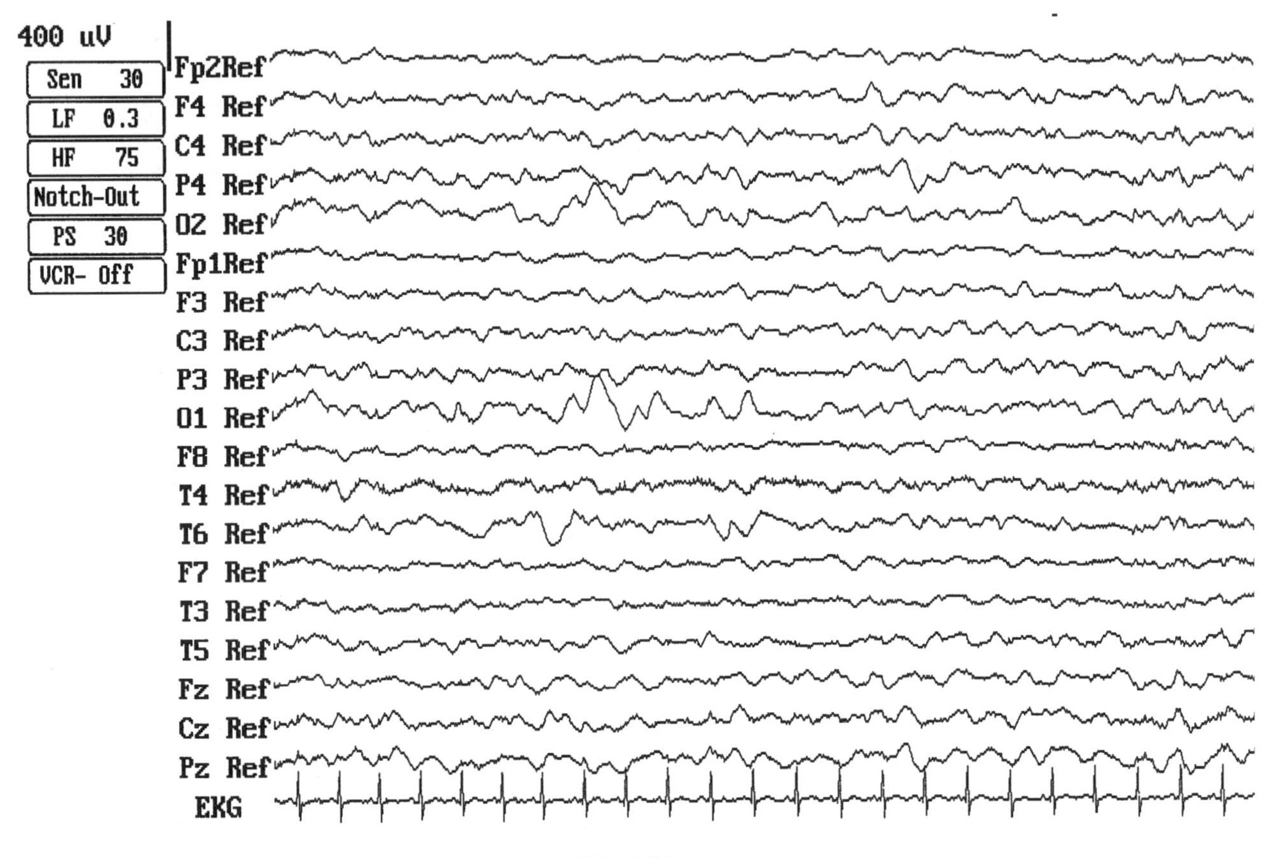
400 uV
Sen 30
LF 0.3
HF 75
Notch-Out
PS 30
VCR- Off
Fp2Ref
F4 Ref
C4 Ref
P4 Ref
O2 Ref
Fp1Ref
F3 Ref
C3 Ref
P3 Ref
O1 Ref
F8 Ref
T4 Ref
T6 Ref
F7 Ref
T3 Ref
T5 Ref
Fz Ref
Cz Ref
Pz Ref
EKG

FIG. 4-34c

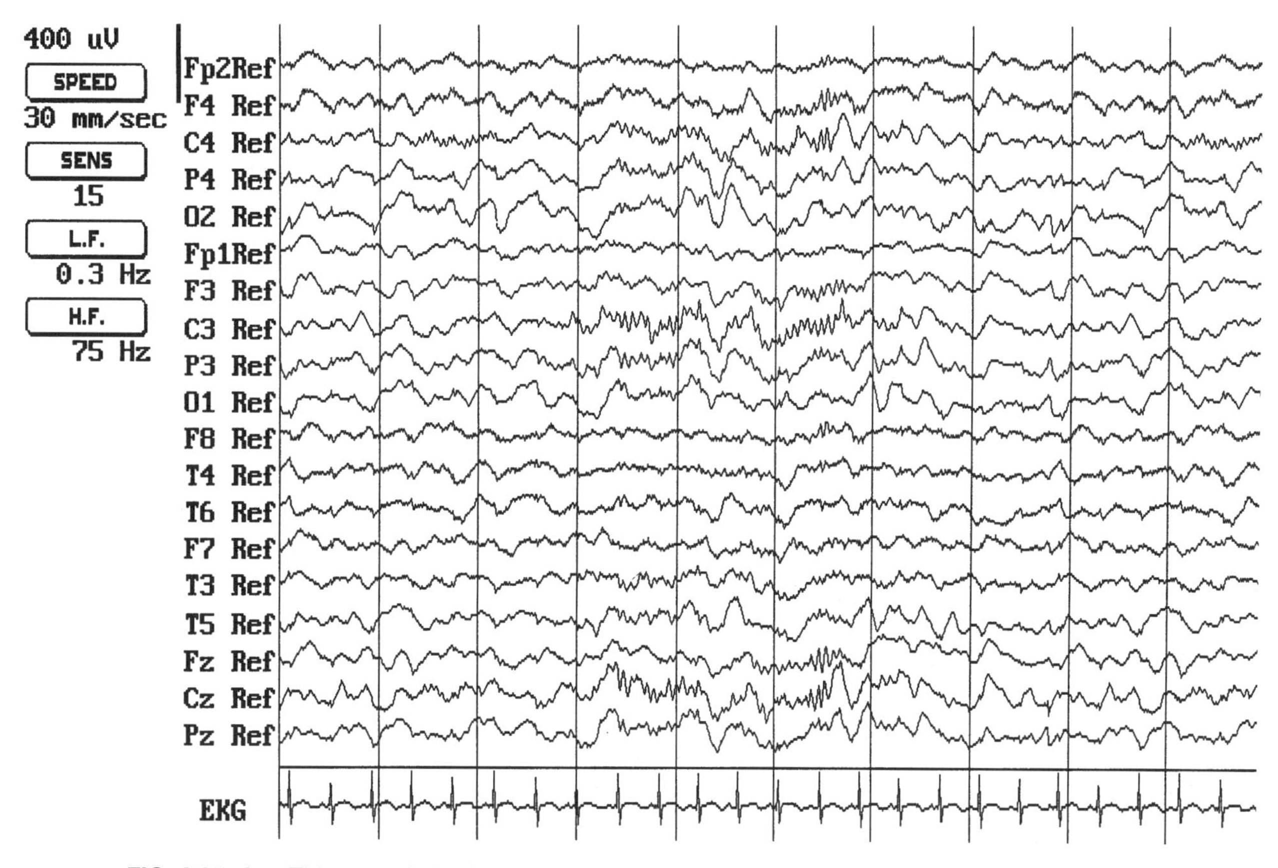

FIG. 4-35a,b,c This example is similar to the previous one but the slowing is of higher frequency (4 to 5 Hz).

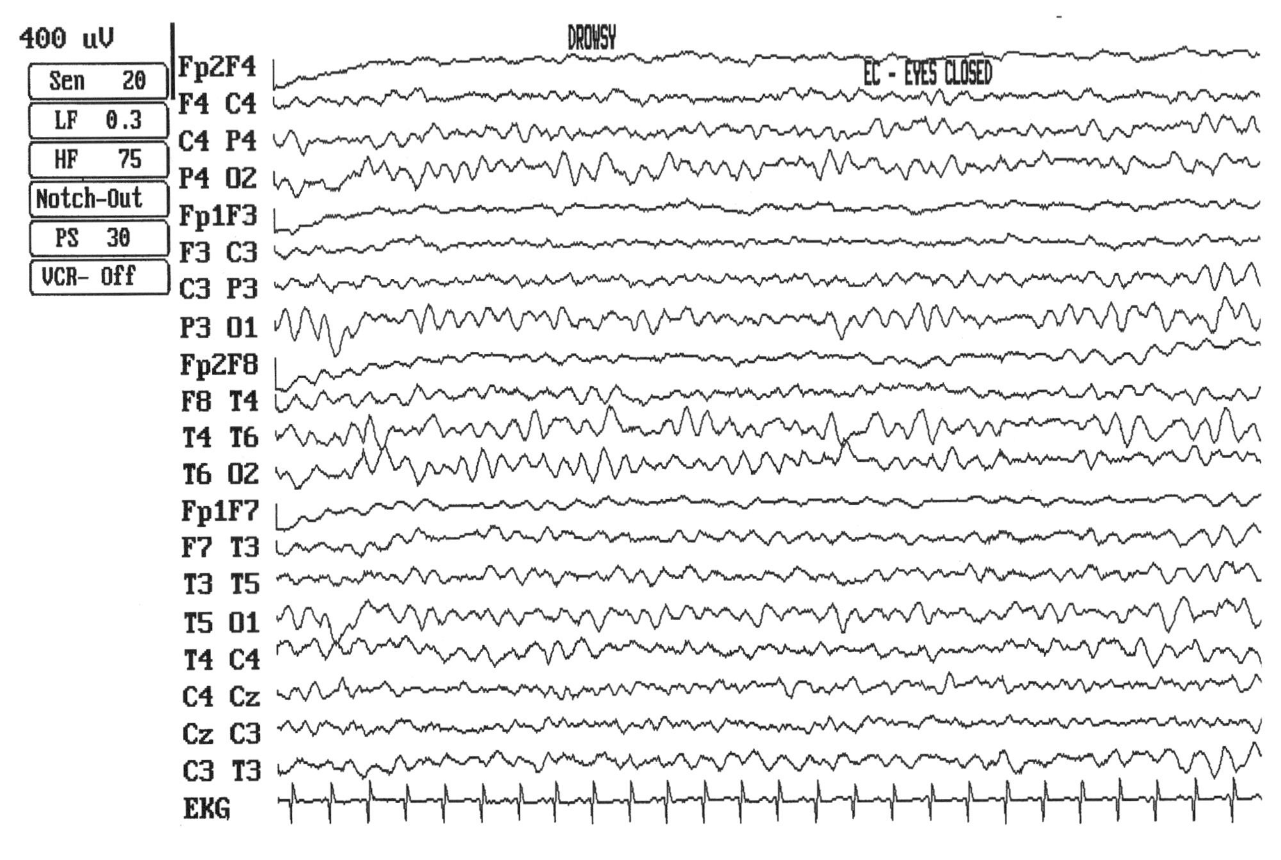
400 uV
Sen 20
LF 0.3
HF 75
Notch-Out
PS 30
VCR- Off
DROWSY
EC - EYES CLOSED
Fp2F4
F4 C4
C4 P4
P4 O2
Fp1F3
F3 C3
C3 P3
P3 O1
Fp2F8
F8 T4
T4 T6
T6 O2
Fp1F7
F7 T3
T3 T5
T5 O1
T4 C4
C4 Cz
Cz C3
C3 T3
EKG

FIG. 4-35b

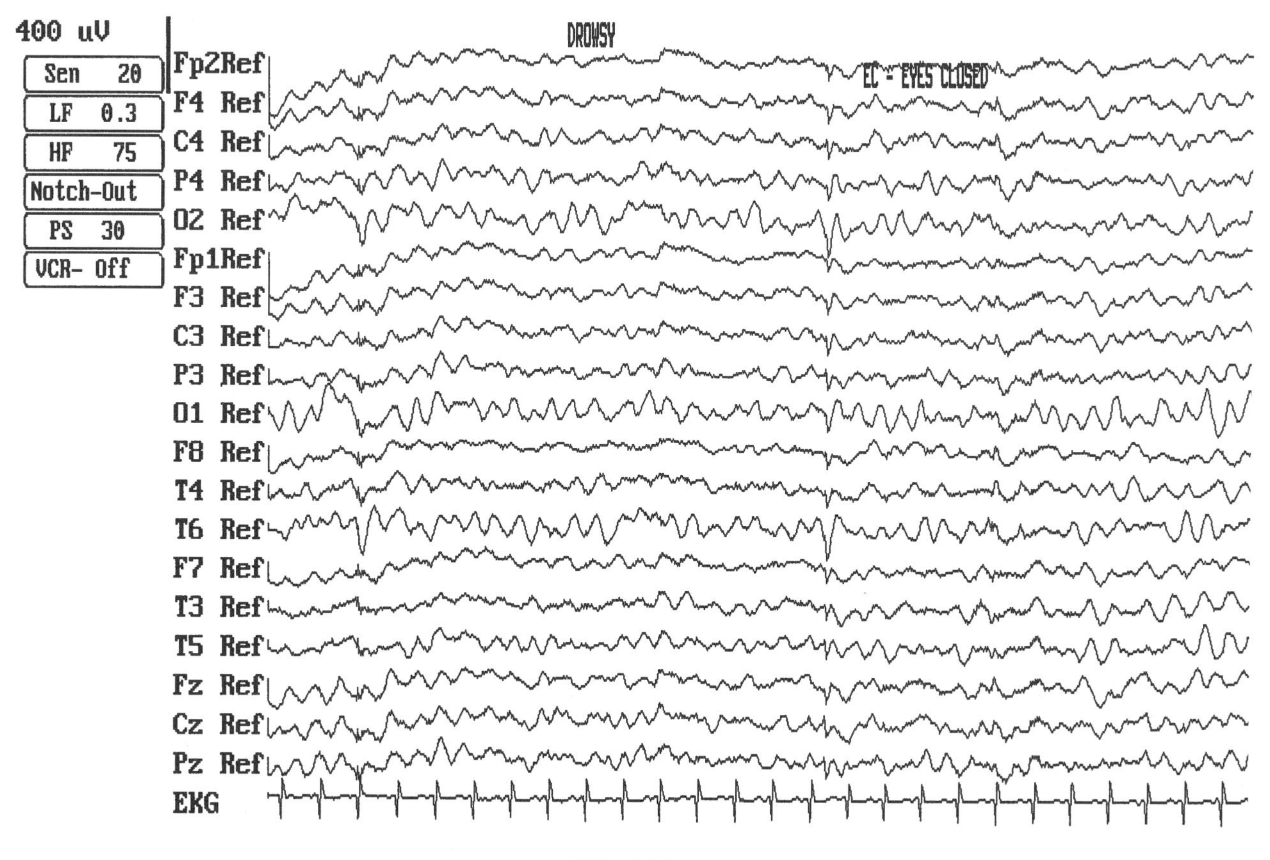
400 uV
Sen 20
LF 0.3
HF 75
Notch-Out
PS 30
VCR- Off
DROWSY
EC = EYES CLOSED
Fp2Ref
F4 Ref
C4 Ref
P4 Ref
O2 Ref
Fp1Ref
F3 Ref
C3 Ref
P3 Ref
O1 Ref
F8 Ref
T4 Ref
T6 Ref
F7 Ref
T3 Ref
T5 Ref
Fz Ref
Cz Ref
Pz Ref
EKG

FIG. 4-35c

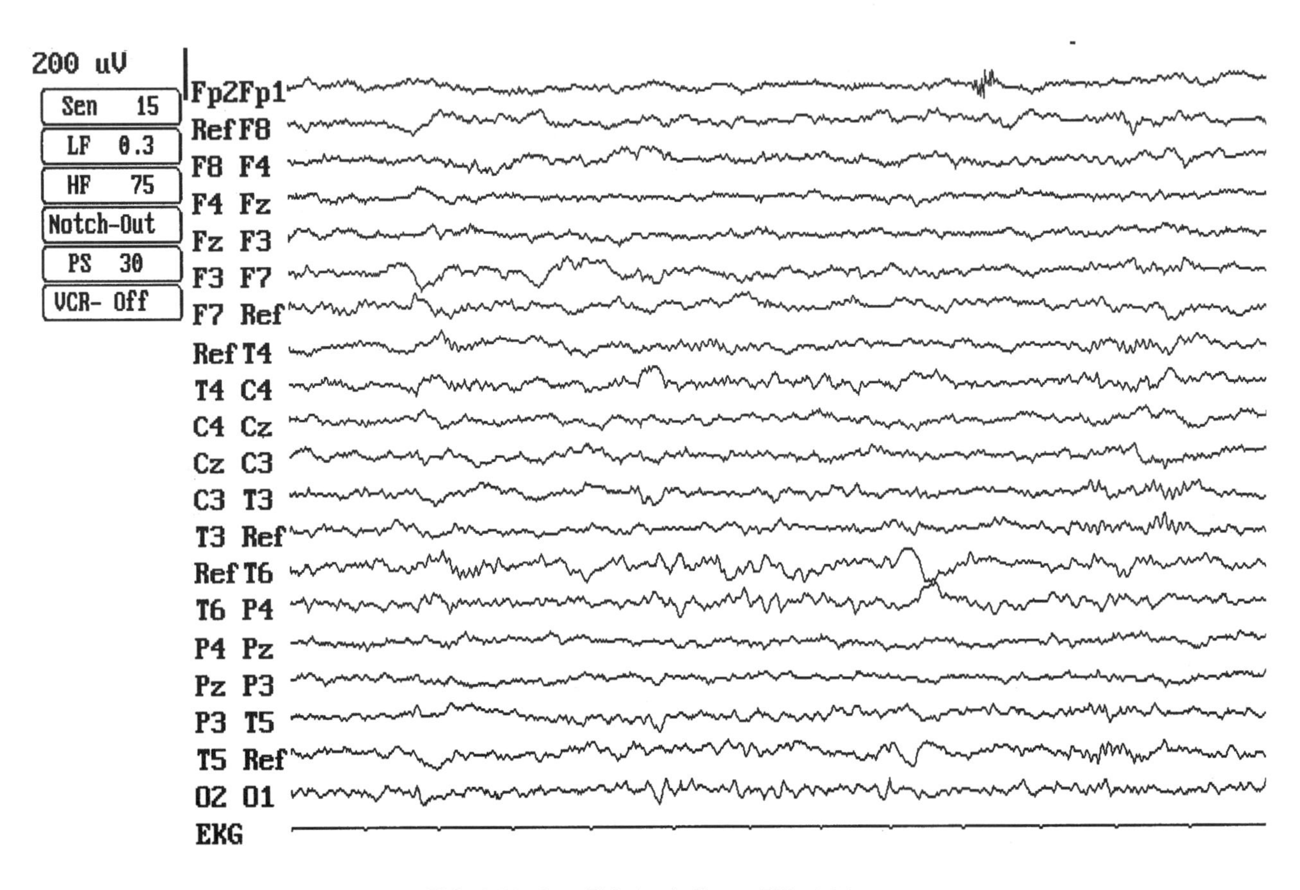

FIG. 4-36a,b,c This is similar to FIG. 4-34.

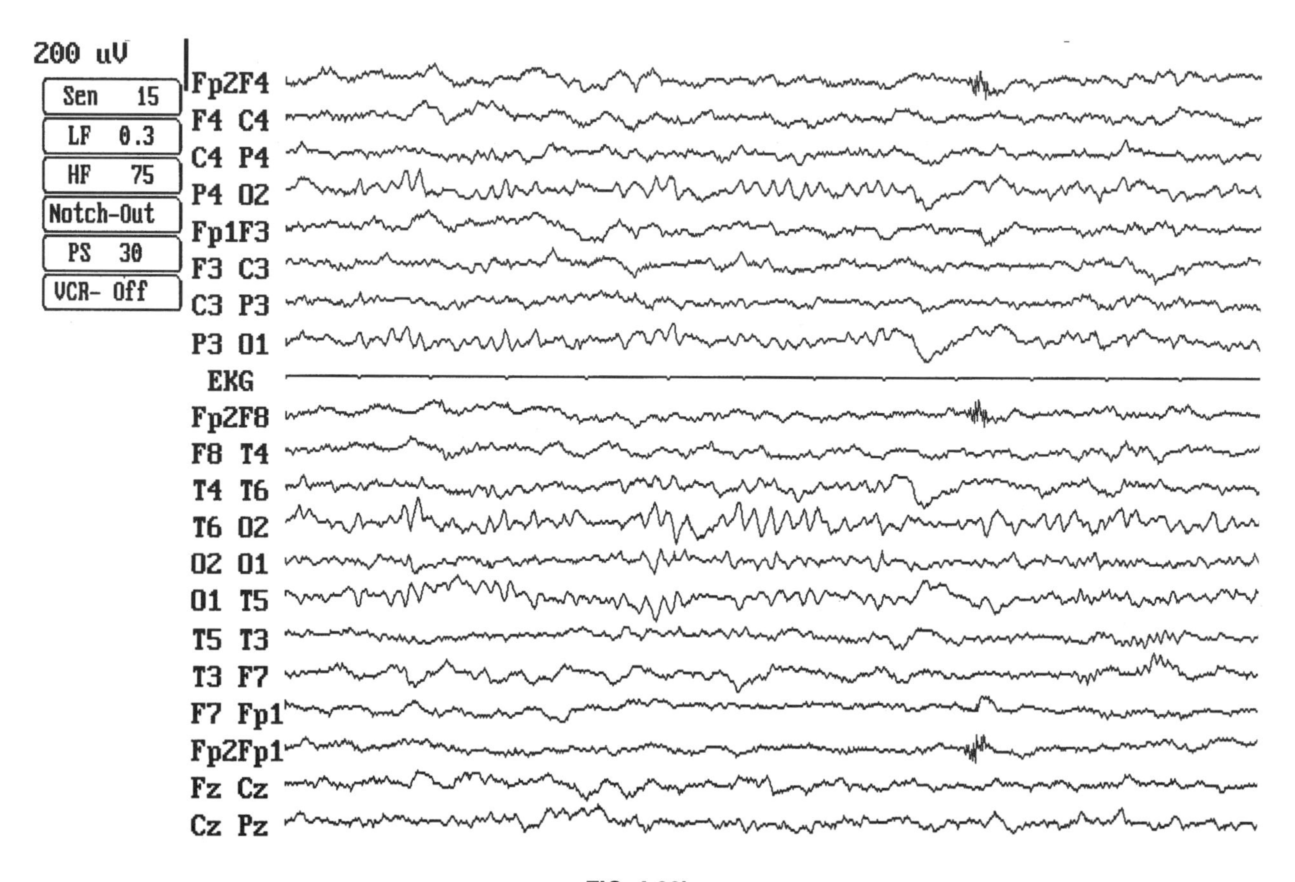
200 uV
Sen 15
LF 0.3
HF 75
Notch-Out
PS 30
VCR- Off
Fp2F4
F4 C4
C4 P4
P4 O2
Fp1F3
F3 C3
C3 P3
P3 O1
EKG
Fp2F8
F8 T4
T4 T6
T6 O2
O2 O1
O1 T5
T5 T3
T3 F7
F7 Fp1
Fp2Fp1
Fz Cz
Cz Pz

FIG. 4-36b

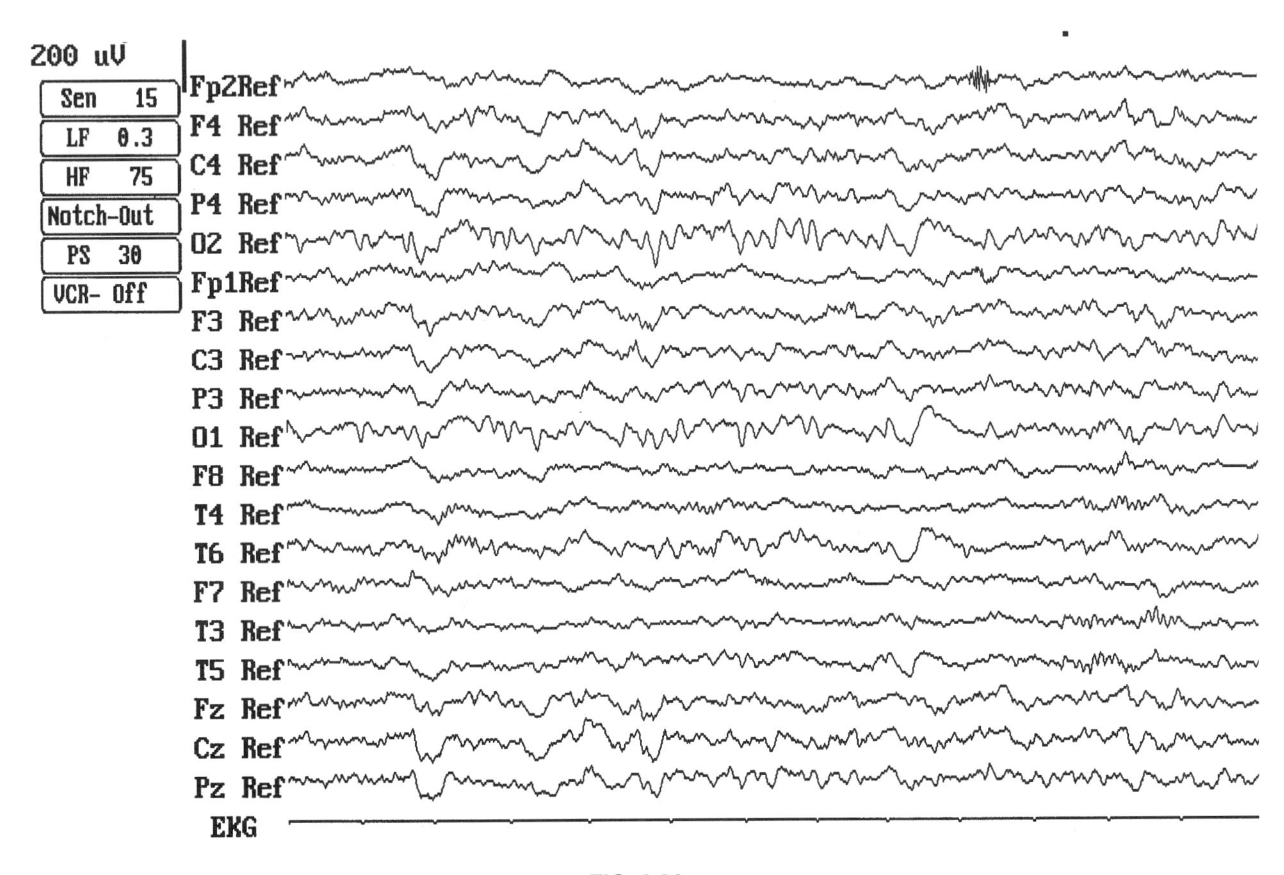
200 uV
Sen 15
LF 0.3
HF 75
Notch-Out
PS 30
VCR- Off
Fp2Ref
F4 Ref
C4 Ref
P4 Ref
O2 Ref
Fp1Ref
F3 Ref
C3 Ref
P3 Ref
O1 Ref
F8 Ref
T4 Ref
T6 Ref
F7 Ref
T3 Ref
T5 Ref
Fz Ref
Cz Ref
Pz Ref
EKG

FIG. 4-36c

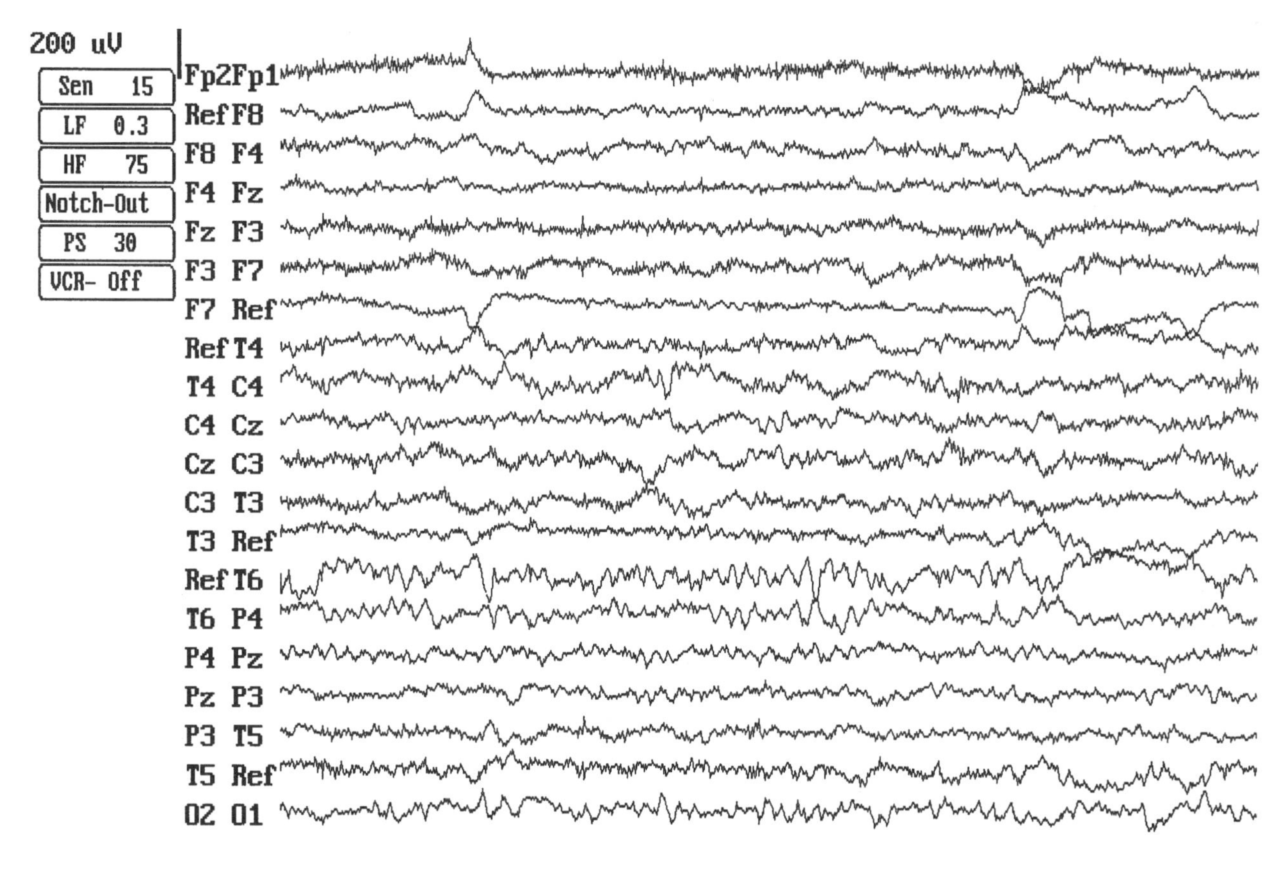

FIG. 4-37a,b,c This example is similar to FIG. 4-34 except that the slowing is at theta frequency.

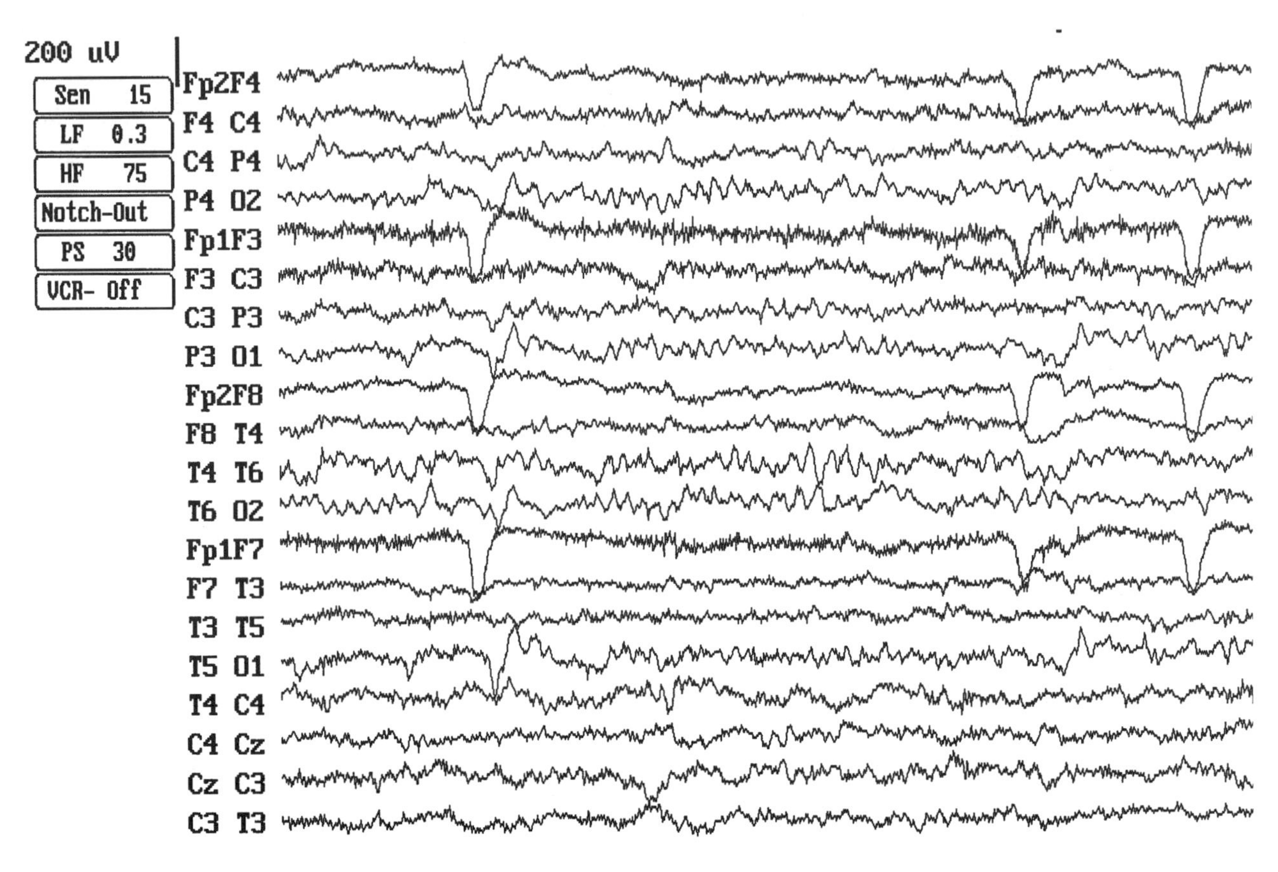
200 uV
Sen 15
LF 0.3
HF 75
Notch-Out
PS 30
VCR- Off
Fp2F4
F4 C4
C4 P4
P4 O2
Fp1F3
F3 C3
C3 P3
P3 O1
Fp2F8
F8 T4
T4 T6
T6 O2
Fp1F7
F7 T3
T3 T5
T5 O1
T4 C4
C4 Cz
Cz C3
C3 T3

FIG. 4-37b

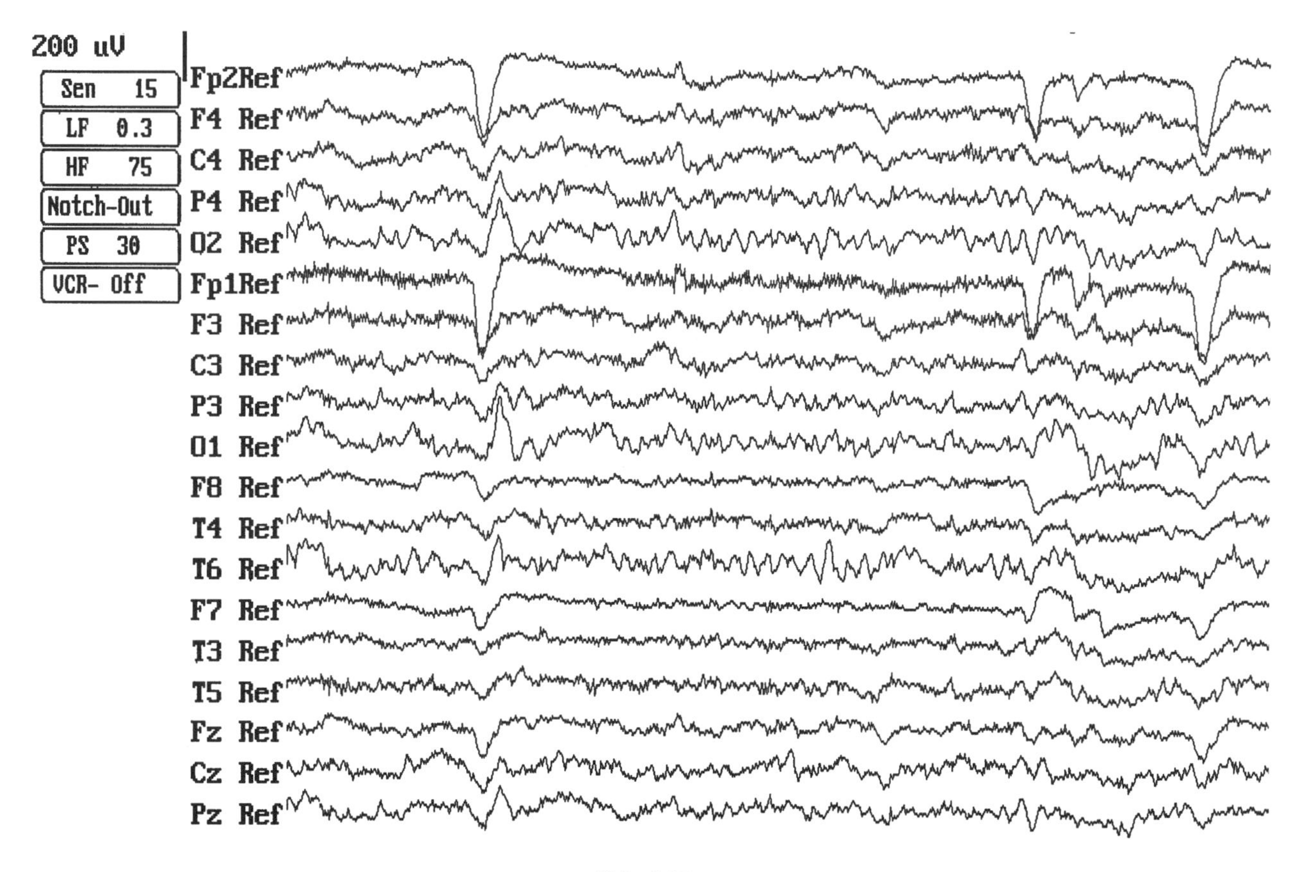
200 uV
Sen 15
LF 0.3
HF 75
Notch-Out
PS 30
VCR- Off
Fp2Ref
F4 Ref
C4 Ref
P4 Ref
O2 Ref
Fp1Ref
F3 Ref
C3 Ref
P3 Ref
O1 Ref
F8 Ref
T4 Ref
T6 Ref
F7 Ref
T3 Ref
T5 Ref
Fz Ref
Cz Ref
Pz Ref

FIG. 4-37c

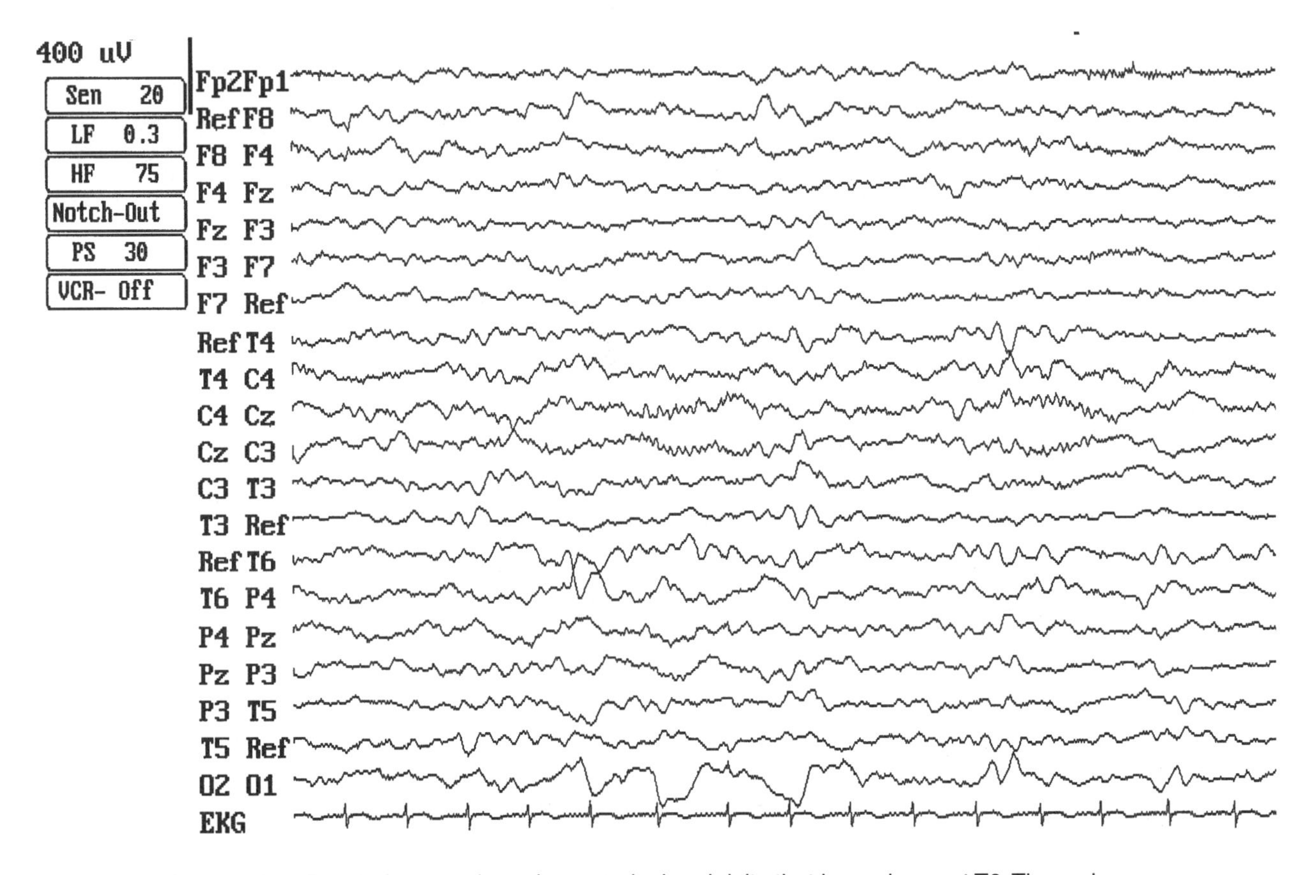

FIG. 4-38a,b,c Run 3 shows an irregular posterior head delta that is maximum at T6. There also appears to be a sharp wave at T6. Run 2 shows the bilateral nature of the slowing. Run 1 further clarifies that indeed there is a posterior head delta, but that it is not focal to T6. It is lower amplitude at T5. Also the appearance of the "sharp wave" at T6 was merely a random occurrence from subtracting two relatively large slow waves.

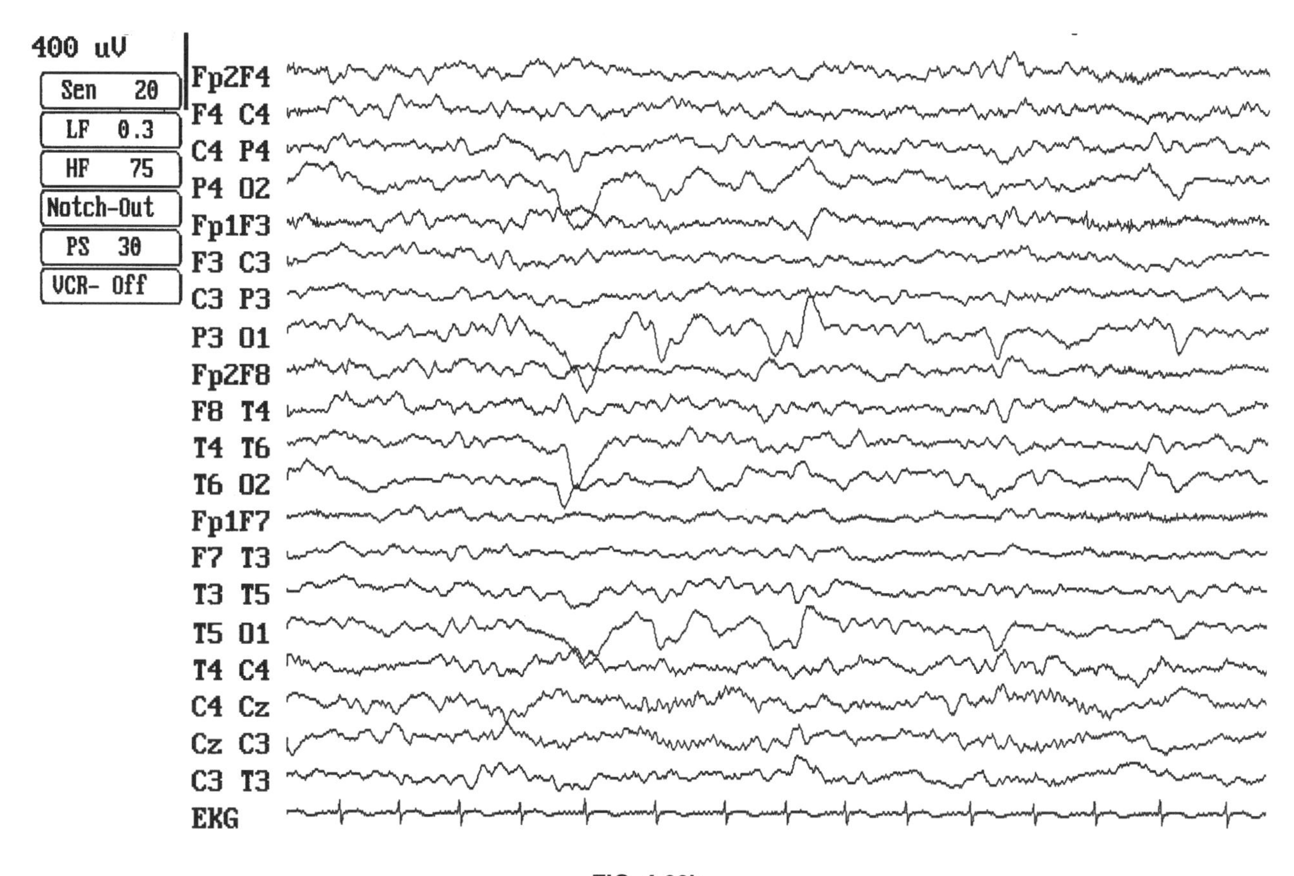
400 uV
Sen 20
LF 0.3
HF 75
Notch-Out
PS 30
VCR- Off
Fp2F4
F4 C4
C4 P4
P4 O2
Fp1F3
F3 C3
C3 P3
P3 O1
Fp2F8
F8 T4
T4 T6
T6 O2
Fp1F7
F7 T3
T3 T5
T5 O1
T4 C4
C4 Cz
Cz C3
C3 T3
EKG

FIG. 4-38b

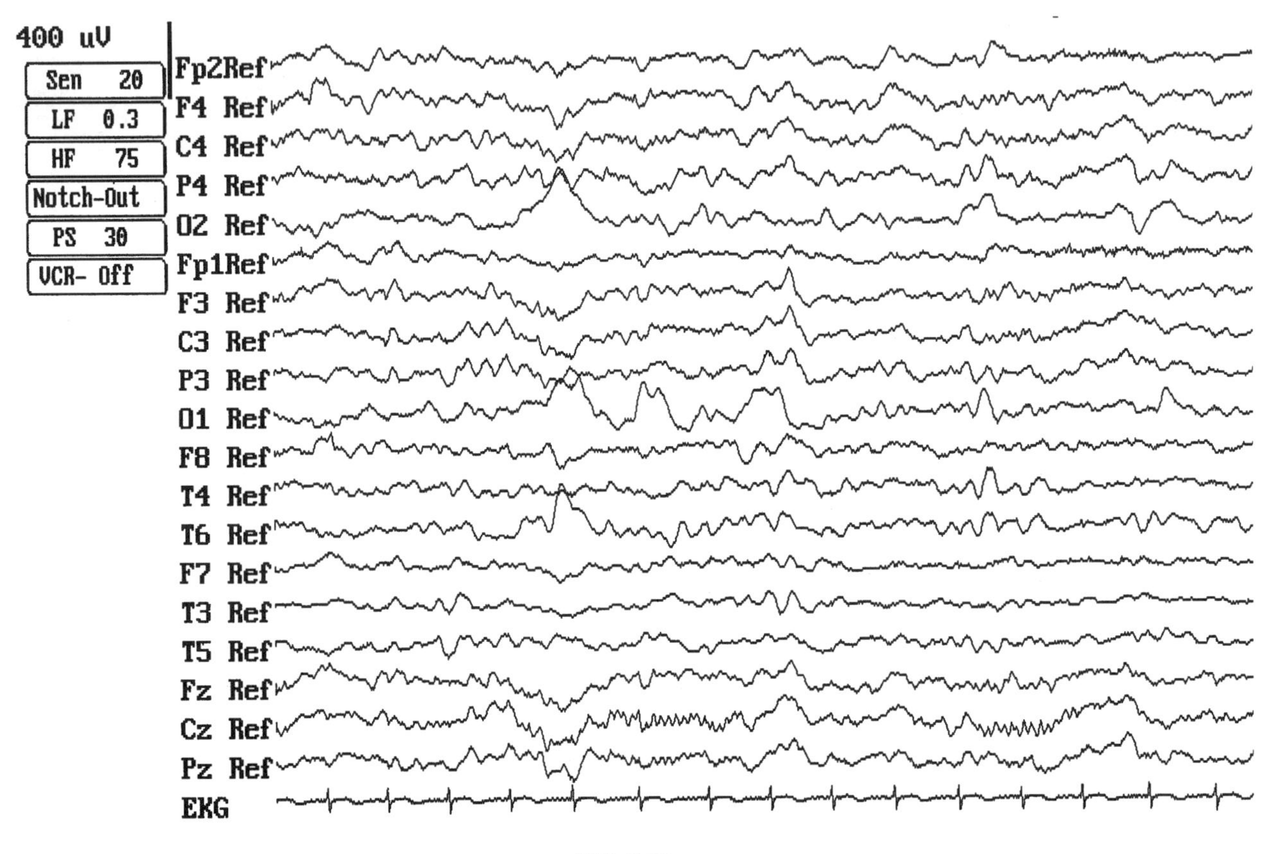
400 uV
Sen 20
LF 0.3
HF 75
Notch-Out
PS 30
VCR- Off
Fp2Ref
F4 Ref
C4 Ref
P4 Ref
O2 Ref
Fp1Ref
F3 Ref
C3 Ref
P3 Ref
O1 Ref
F8 Ref
T4 Ref
T6 Ref
F7 Ref
T3 Ref
T5 Ref
Fz Ref
Cz Ref
Pz Ref
EKG

FIG. 4-38c

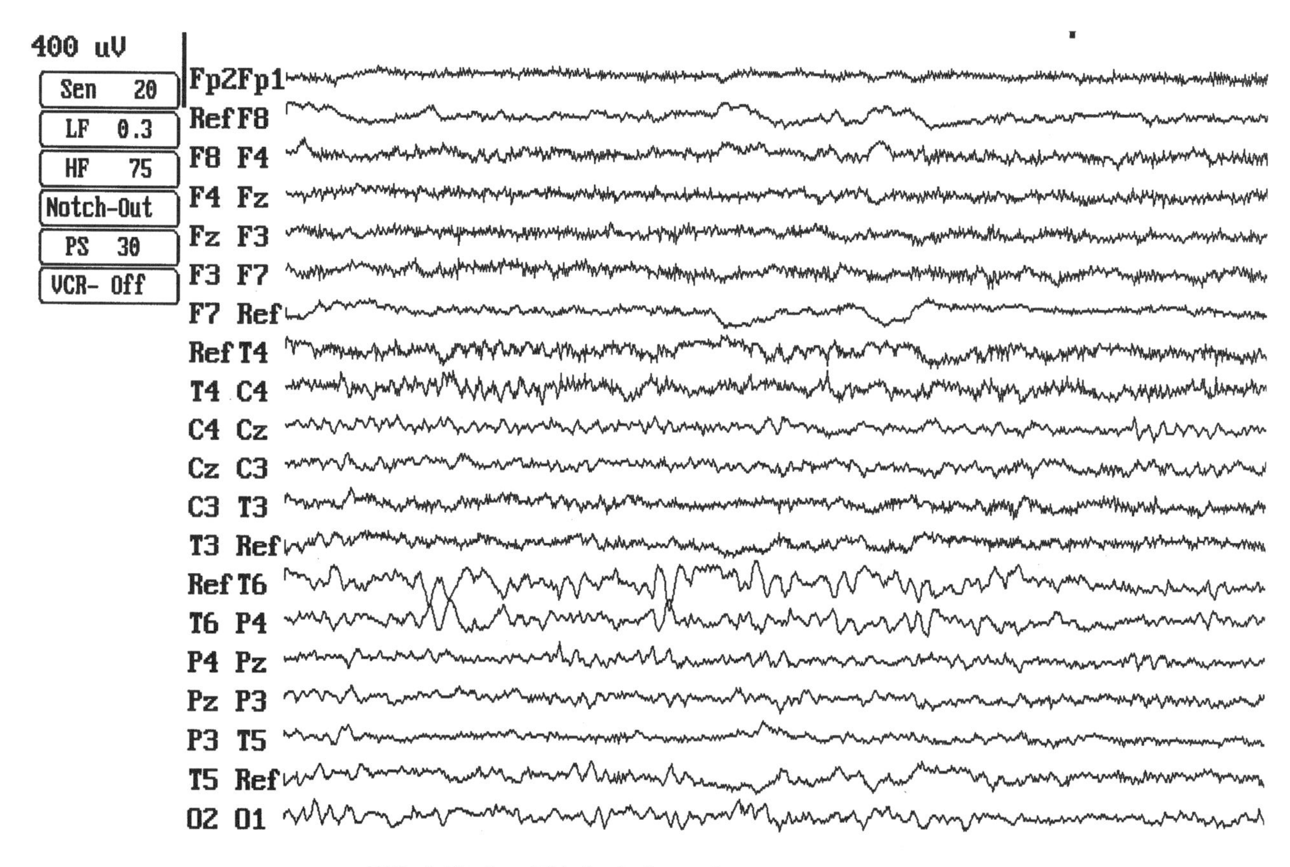

FIG. 4-39a,b,c This is similar to the previous sample.

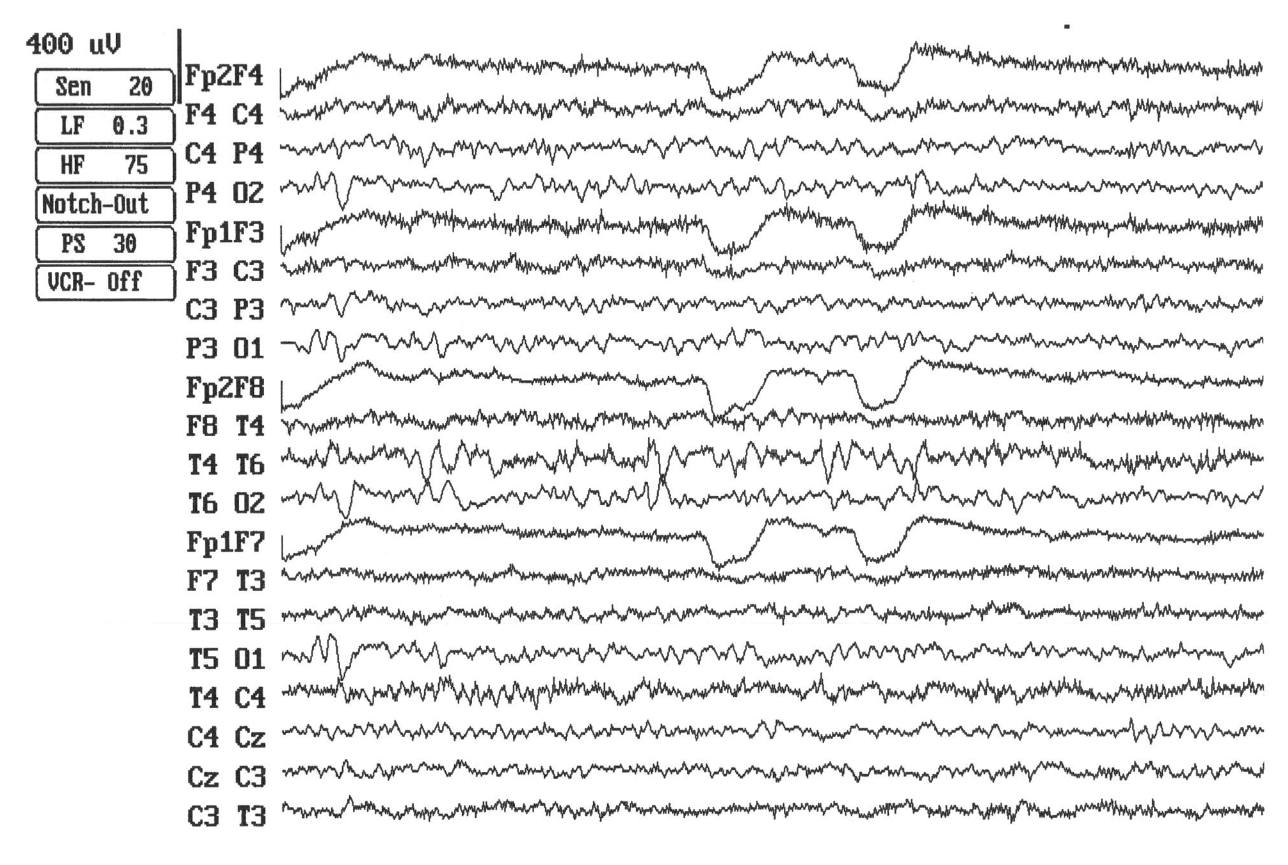
400 uV
Sen 20
LF 0.3
HF 75
Notch-Out
PS 30
VCR- Off
Fp2F4
F4 C4
C4 P4
P4 O2
Fp1F3
F3 C3
C3 P3
P3 O1
Fp2F8
F8 T4
T4 T6
T6 O2
Fp1F7
F7 T3
T3 T5
T5 O1
T4 C4
C4 Cz
Cz C3
C3 T3

FIG. 4-39b

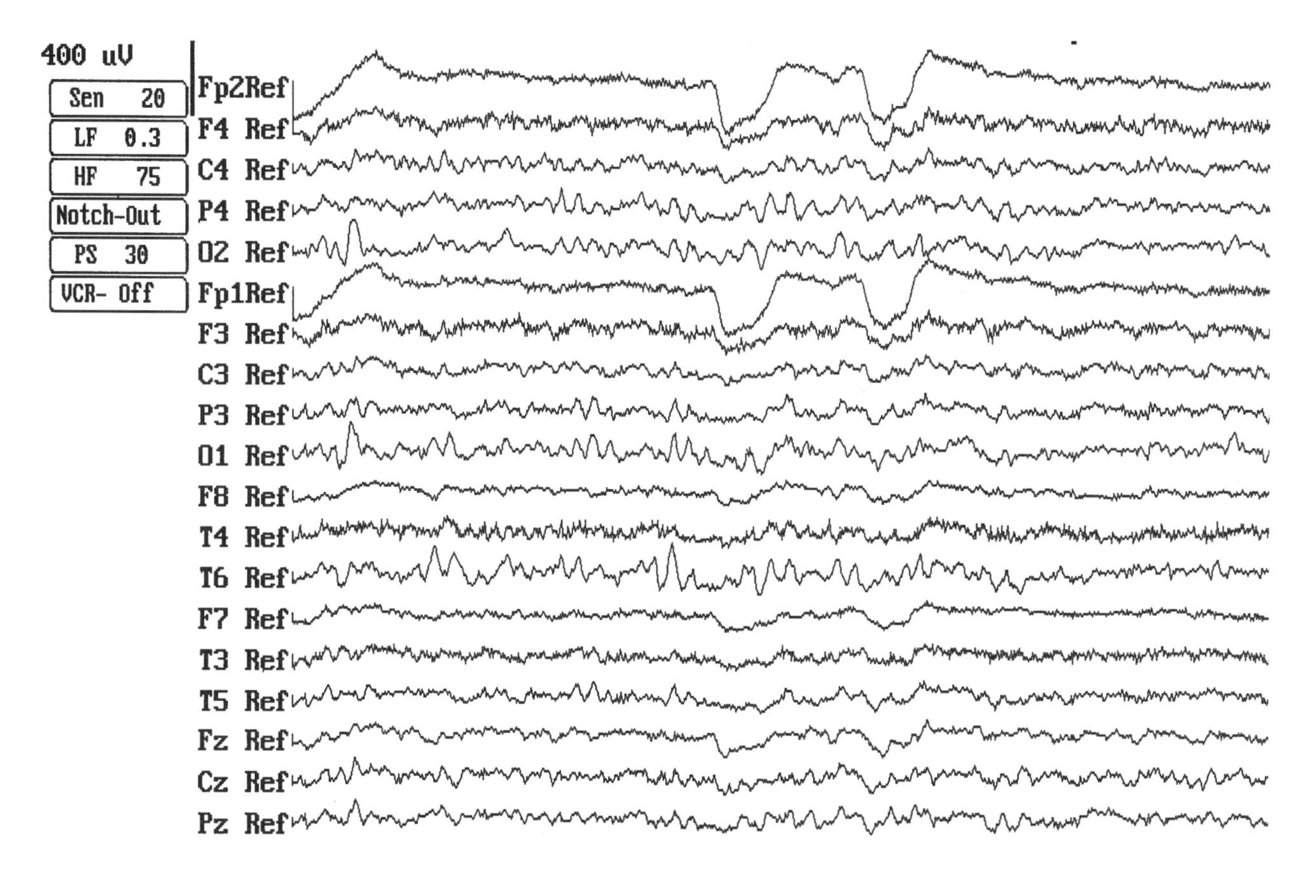
400 uV
Sen 20
LF 0.3
HF 75
Notch-Out
PS 30
VCR- Off
Fp2Ref
F4 Ref
C4 Ref
P4 Ref
O2 Ref
Fp1Ref
F3 Ref
C3 Ref
P3 Ref
O1 Ref
F8 Ref
T4 Ref
T6 Ref
F7 Ref
T3 Ref
T5 Ref
Fz Ref
Cz Ref
Pz Ref

FIG. 4-39c

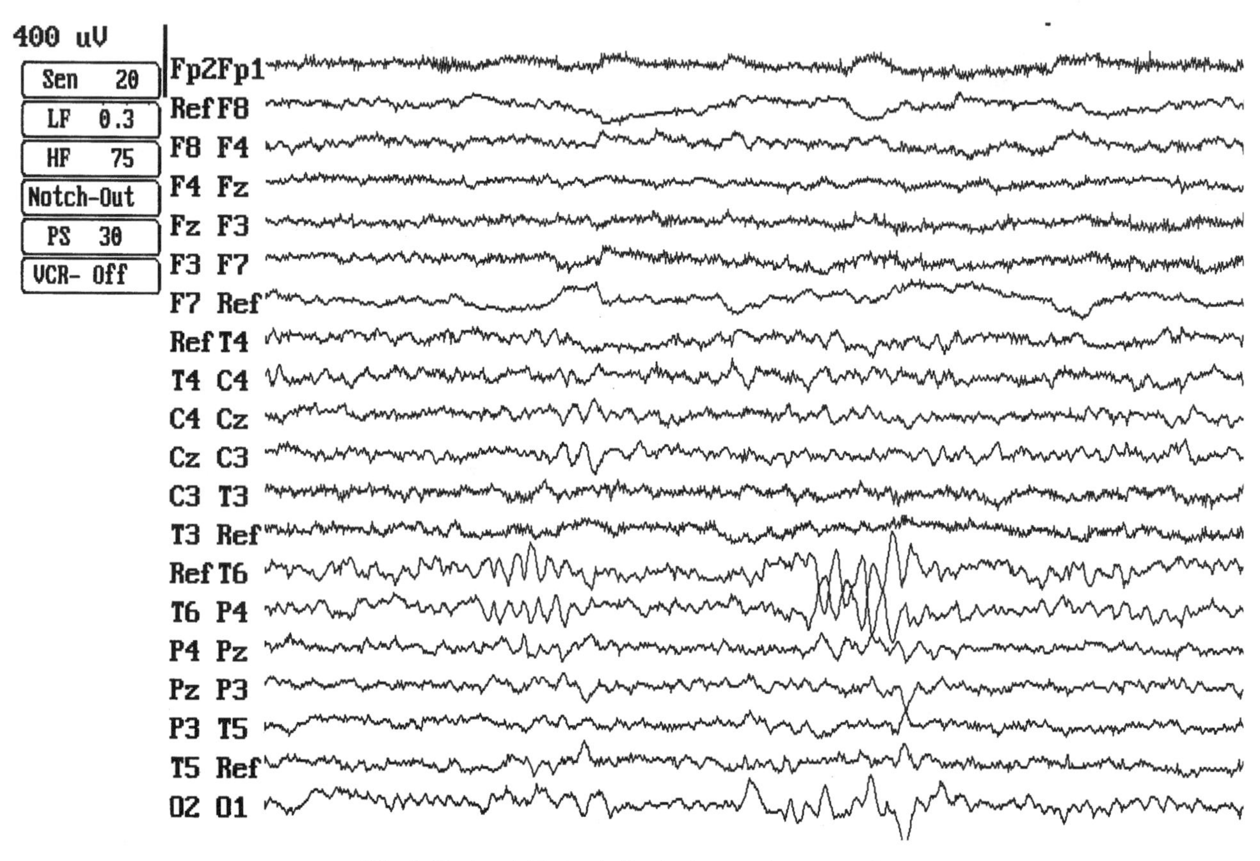

FIG. 4-40a,b,c This is similar to the previous sample.

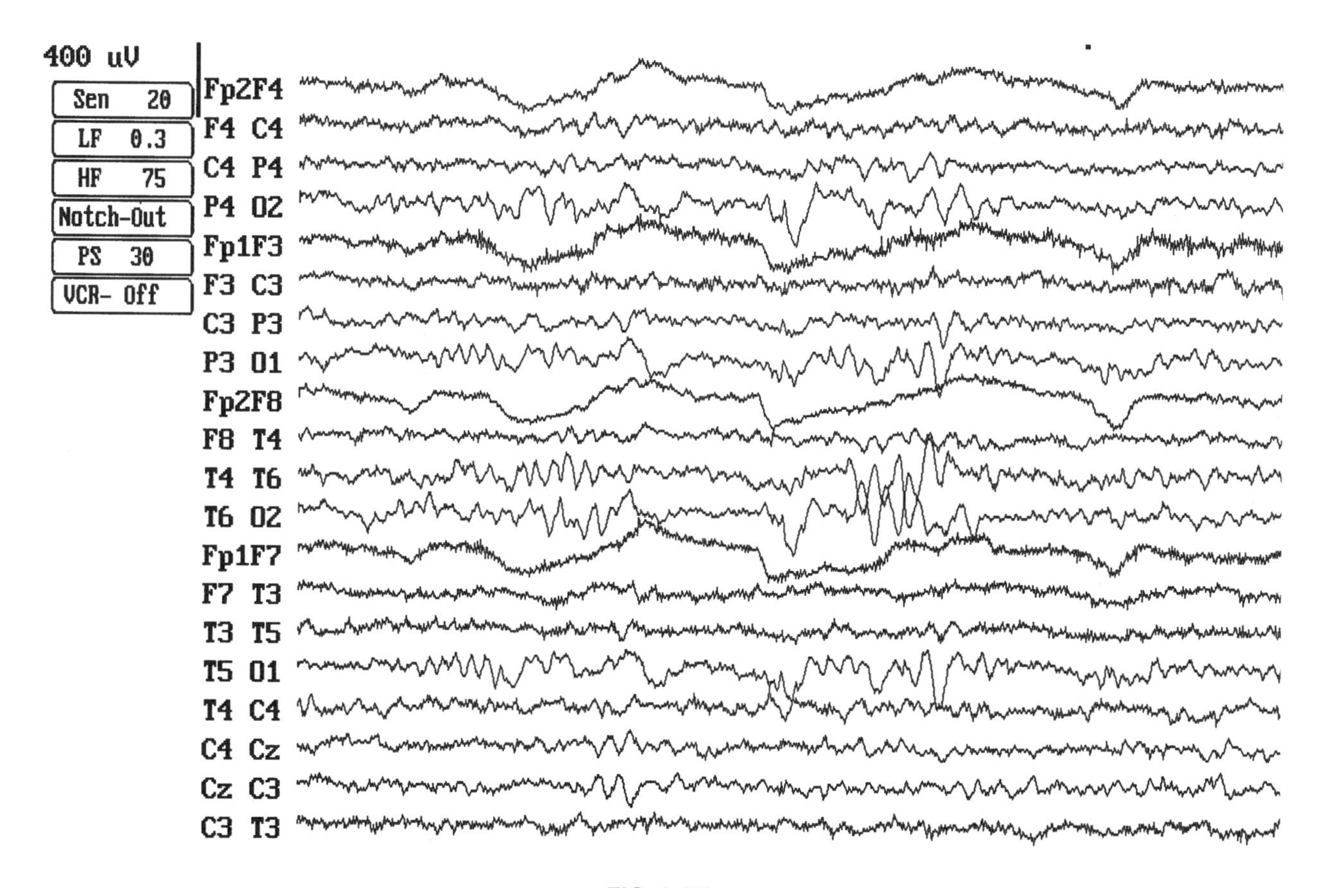
400 uV
Sen 20
LF 0.3
HF 75
Notch-Out
PS 30
VCR- Off
Fp2F4
F4 C4
C4 P4
P4 O2
Fp1F3
F3 C3
C3 P3
P3 O1
Fp2F8
F8 T4
T4 T6
T6 O2
Fp1F7
F7 T3
T3 T5
T5 O1
T4 C4
C4 Cz
Cz C3
C3 T3

FIG. 4-40b

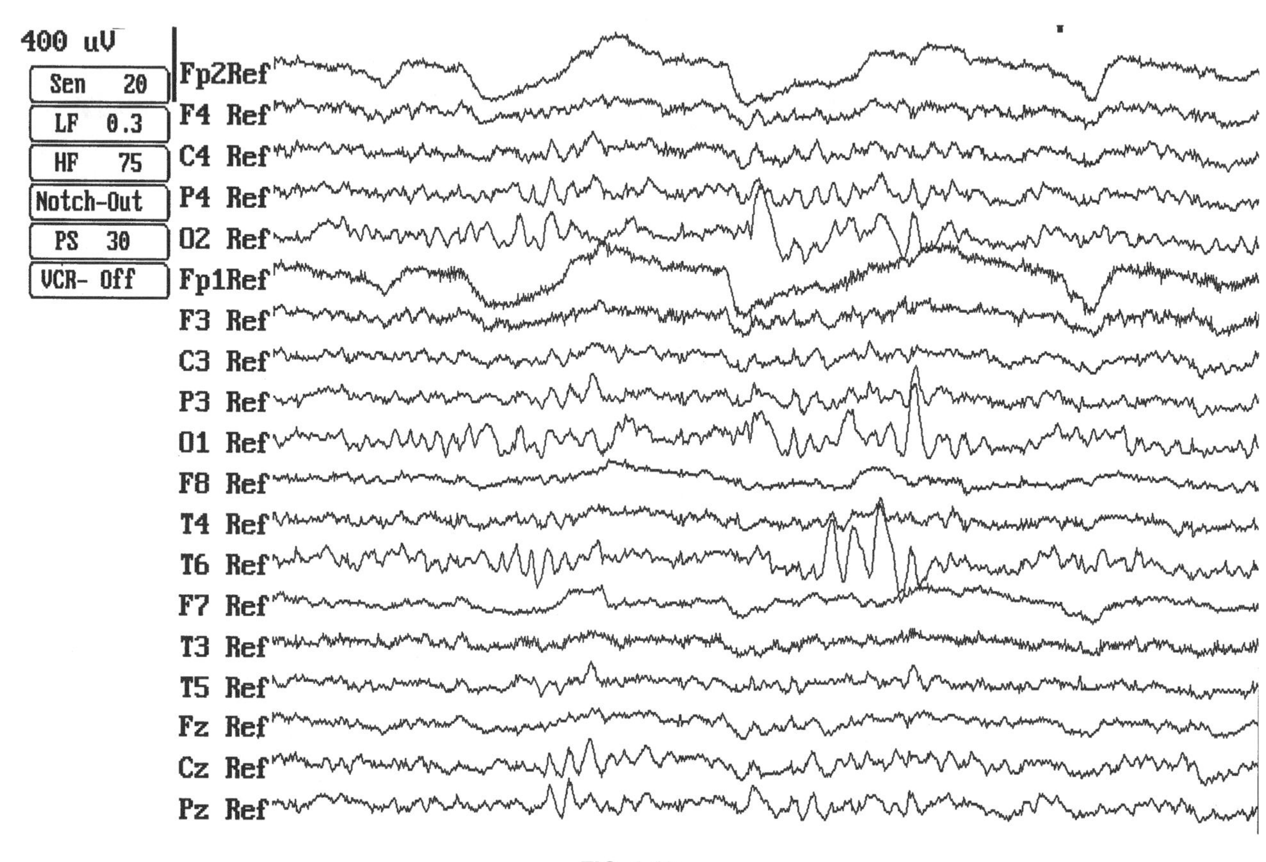
400 uV
Sen 20
LF 0.3
HF 75
Notch-Out
PS 30
VCR- Off
Fp2Ref
F4 Ref
C4 Ref
P4 Ref
O2 Ref
Fp1Ref
F3 Ref
C3 Ref
P3 Ref
O1 Ref
F8 Ref
T4 Ref
T6 Ref
F7 Ref
T3 Ref
T5 Ref
Fz Ref
Cz Ref
Pz Ref

FIG. 4-40c

ABNORMAL EXAMPLES

Suppressions

FIG. 4-41a,b A focal right central parietal suppression is seen on run 2. Run 1 shows the presence of intermixed theta and delta over the same area though with a shallow gradient, thus accounting for the cancellation on run 2.
FIG. 4-42a,b This is similar to the previous sample except that suppression is over the bilateral posterior head, maximum over the right.

Beta

FIG. 4-43a,b Focal paroxysmal beta at T4 is seen on runs 1 and 2.
FIG. 4-44a,b,c Generalized beta in sleep is seen on runs 1 and 3. The paper speed of 60 mm/sec shows morphology of beta.
FIG. 4-45a,b,c,d Bianterior beta is seen on runs 1,2, and 3 and with a paper speed of 60 mm/s.

Theta

FIG. 4-46a,b,c Normal drowsiness showing diffuse theta maximum at right central parietal is seen on run 1. On run 2 there appears to be a right hemispheric dysrhythmia, while run 3 shows a right central temporal dysrhythmia. If the interpretation was limited to a particular montage, different localizations would result from the same data.
FIG. 4-47a,b,c,d,e Persistent rhythmic 4 to 5 Hz biposterior head theta is seen on runs 1,2,3, and 4. Run 1 with a slow paper speed enhances theta. Run 3 gives the worst localization.

Delta

FIG. 4-48a,b,c This example shows a focal bianterior delta, more persistent and rhythmic on the left, more paroxysmal on the right, as seen on run 1 at 30 and 15 mm/s; run 4 is shown for comparison.
FIG. 4-49a,b,c A paroxysmal biposterior delta maximal at Pz is clearly seen on run 1 and is only seen on 1 channel (Cz-Pz) on run 4. There are misleading theta phase reversals at Pz on run 3.
FIG. 4-50a,b,c,d This shows a poorly defined right sided delta on run 1 (better with slow PS). Run 3 shows a suggestion of two distinct delta frequencies, though run 2 shows them best: rhythmic fast delta at F8, and a slower delta maximal at C4.
FIG. 4-51a,b,c Right frontal slowing is seen on run 1. Note the artifact at the 8th second. Faster delta phase reversals are seen at F8 and some slower delta at C4 are seen on run 2. These are most clear with PS for 15 mm/s.

Seizures

FIG. 4-52a,b,c,d A right hemispheric seizure is seen on run 2. Sensitivity = 15 is too high to see the seizure, but is good for seeing the preictal background. At sensitivity = 50, the ictal activity is seen better.
FIG. 4-53a,b,c,d This shows a right parietal temporal seizure (P4,T6) spreading to right central (C4) then to right temporal, later to the left hemisphere, ending with a strong ictal pattern at the left temporal area (run 2 throughout).
FIG. 4-54a,b,c This shows a right anterior temporal seizure vaguely seen at F8 on run 1. On run 2 the ictal onset is seen much better. The development of the ictal pattern is shown 10 s later.
FIG. 4-55a,b,c,d,e This example shows a generalized seizure consisting of diffuse theta then delta. Run 2 shows the eye movements obscuring the ictal onset, whereas run 1 shows the onset better. Subsequent ictal development

continues on run 2 without problems with the ictus ending at P3.

FIG. 4-56a,b,c,d,e This is a generalized tonic clonic seizure showing the use of different sensitivities during the entire seizure (all run 1). First, the ictal onset was recorded at sensitivity = 20, and then increasing the sensitivity to 30 and 50 to accommodate the higher amplitude activity. At ictal offset, sensitivity = 30 is used to see the offset background clearly.

FIG. 4-57a,b,c,d,e,f,g,h In this generalized tonic clonic seizure the ictal onset is seen at sensitivity = 20 and 50. Note the slightly earlier right sided onset. The development of ictus required sensitivity = 100 to avoid clipping. Despite sensitivity = 100 (e) there was some amplifier saturation seen at C4 (flat top and bottom of large waveforms). To appreciate the markedly suppressed offset background, sensitivity = 20 is required.

FIG. 4-58 A generalized 3/s spike and wave was recorded at 8 bits with too high sensitivity. Note the amplifier clipped waves that cannot be corrected by changing the display sensitivity.

FIG. 4-59a,b,c,d A generalized 3/s spike and wave was recorded at 11 bits, then displayed at sensitivities of 20 and 50 to show the absence of clipping. The same data is shown on run 2 for comparison.

FIG. 4-60a,b High amplitude photoconvulsive response is seen on run 1, with PS of 30 and 60 mm/s.

FIG. 4-61a,b A bioccipital seizure is seen on run 1, and is seen better on run 4 as a posterior halo.

FIG. 4-62a,b,c,d,e,f A right posterior temporal seizure is seen on run 1, but run 2 shows nicely how the posterior temporal-parietal seizure involved the central region.

FIG. 4-63a,b,c,d A left temporal seizure with ear contamination is seen. Run 1 with A1+A2 reference shows diffuse slowing, maximal on the right. Run 2 clarifies a left temporal-central discharge, which is optimally displayed using O2 reference, while PS = 15 provides another perspective of the same data as in (c).

Suppressions

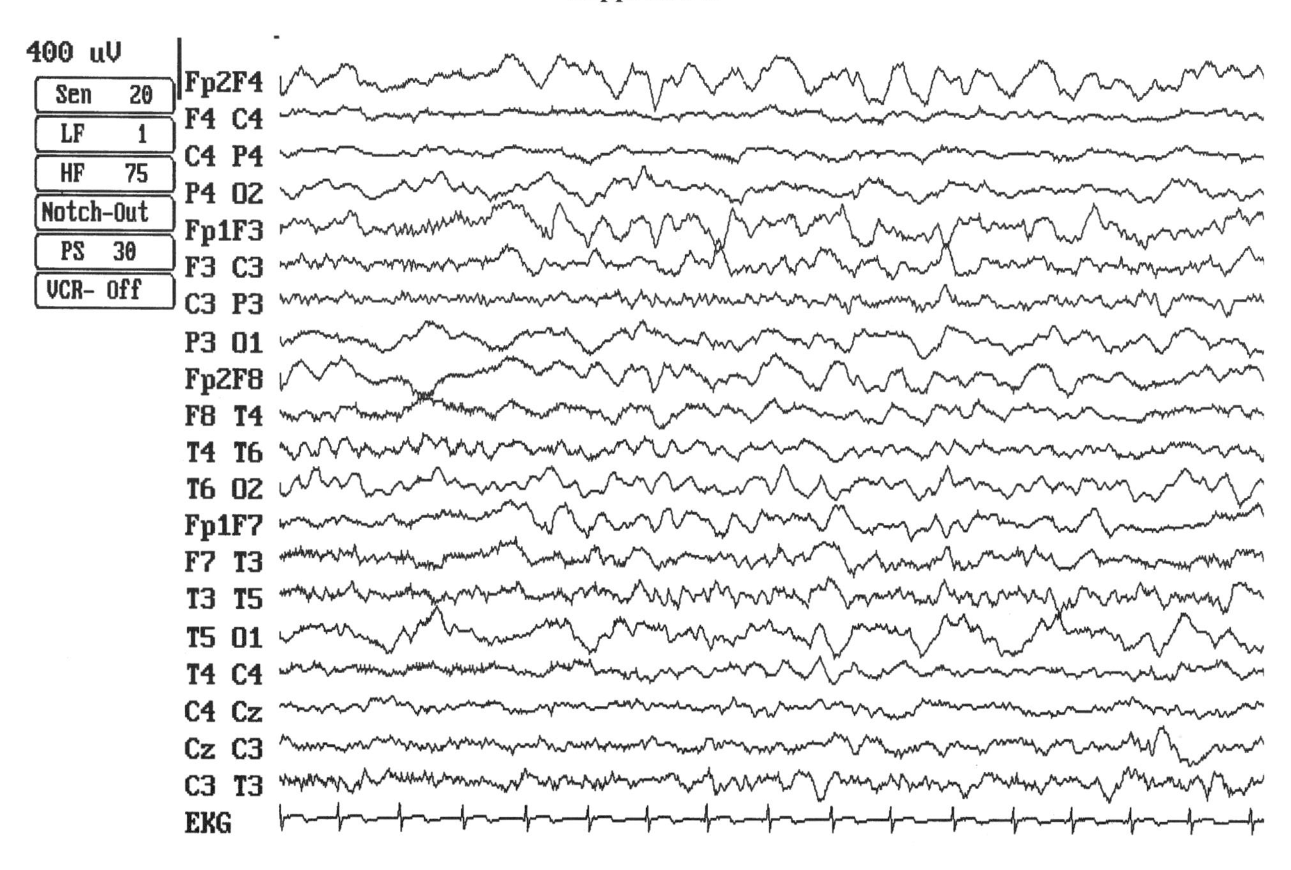

FIG. 4-41a,b A focal right central parietal suppression is seen on run 2. Run 1 shows the presence of intermixed theta and delta over the same area though with a shallow gradient, thus accounting for the cancellation on run 2.

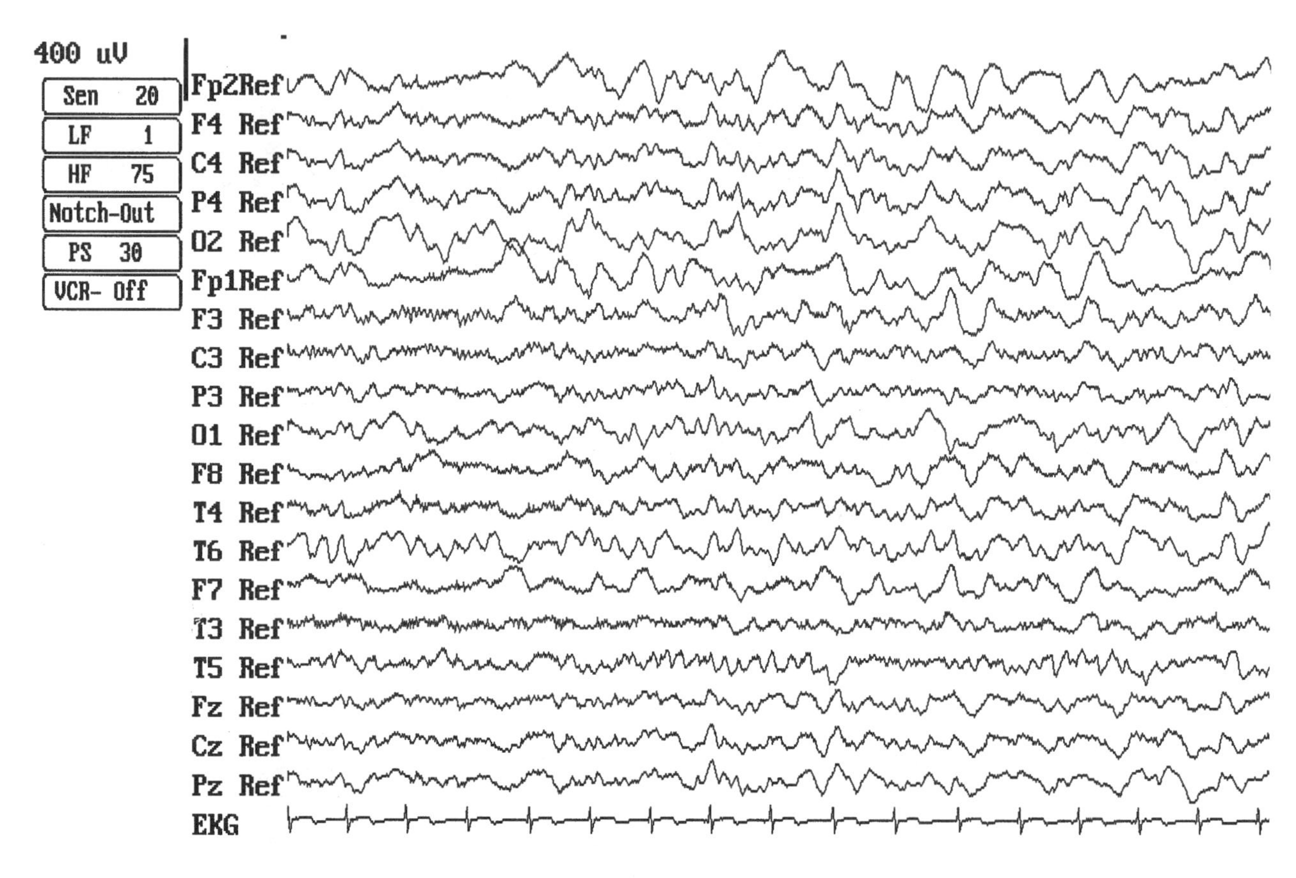
400 uV
Sen 20
LF 1
HF 75
Notch-Out
PS 30
VCR- Off
Fp2Ref
F4 Ref
C4 Ref
P4 Ref
O2 Ref
Fp1Ref
F3 Ref
C3 Ref
P3 Ref
O1 Ref
F8 Ref
T4 Ref
T6 Ref
F7 Ref
T3 Ref
T5 Ref
Fz Ref
Cz Ref
Pz Ref
EKG

FIG. 4-41b

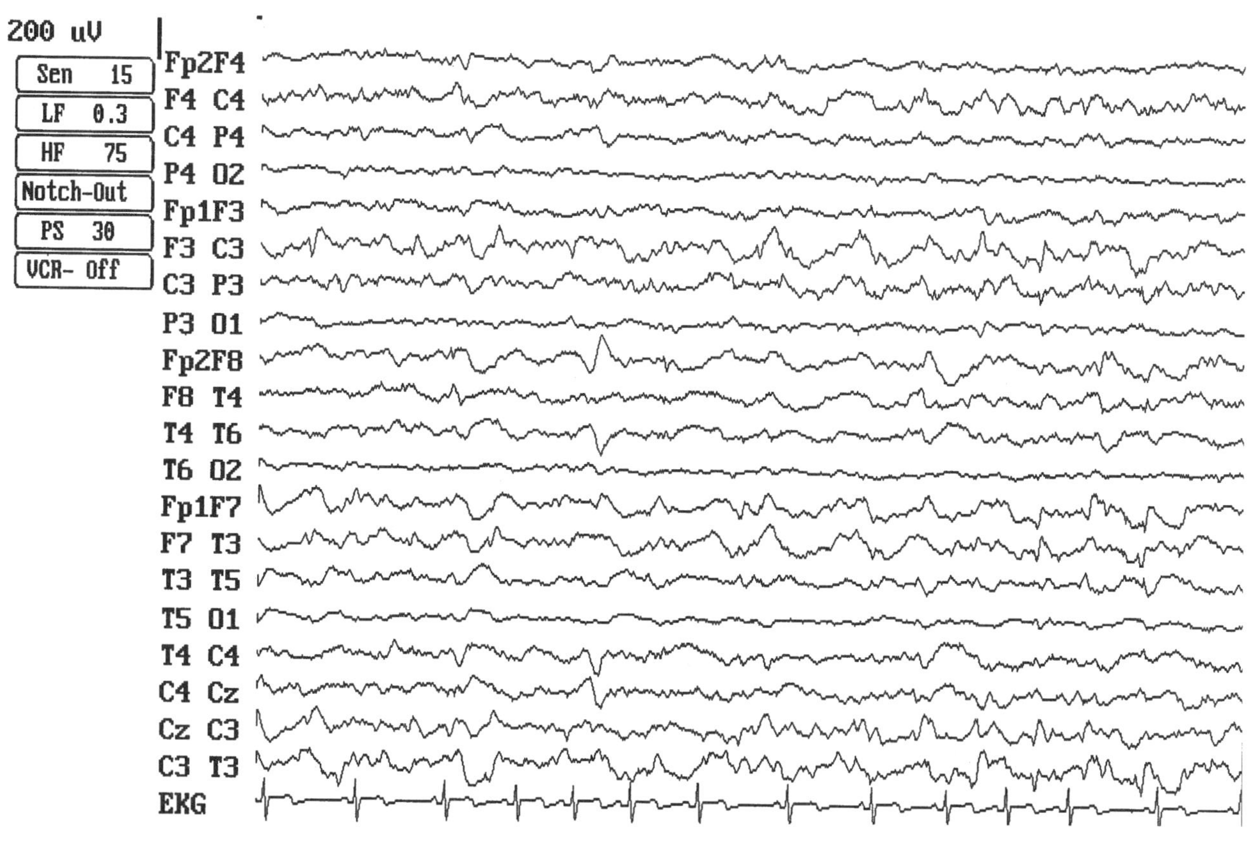

FIG. 4-42a,b This is similar to the previous sample except that suppression is over the bilateral posterior head, maximum over the right.

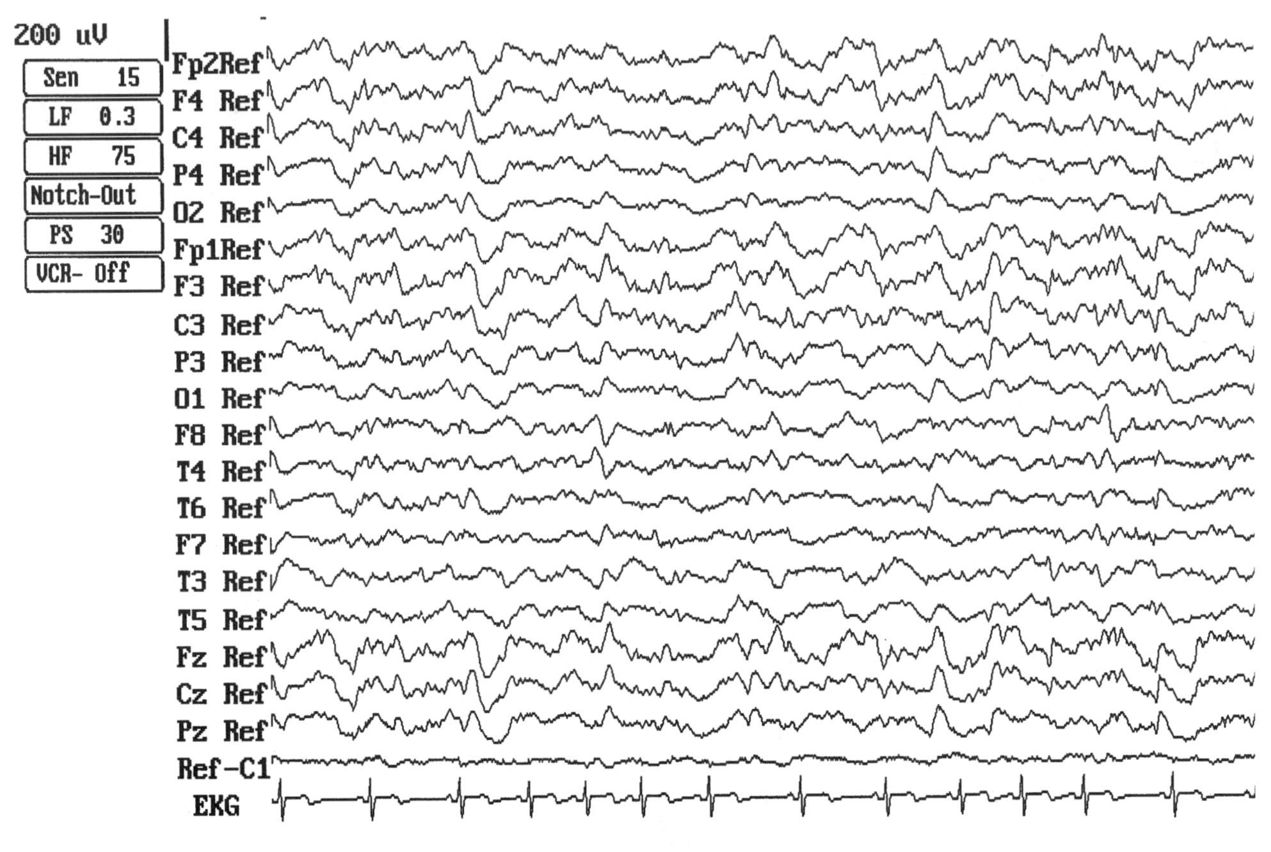
200 uV
Sen 15
LF 0.3
HF 75
Notch-Out
PS 30
VCR- Off
Fp2Ref
F4 Ref
C4 Ref
P4 Ref
O2 Ref
Fp1Ref
F3 Ref
C3 Ref
P3 Ref
O1 Ref
F8 Ref
T4 Ref
T6 Ref
F7 Ref
T3 Ref
T5 Ref
Fz Ref
Cz Ref
Pz Ref
Ref-C1
EKG

FIG. 4-42b

Beta

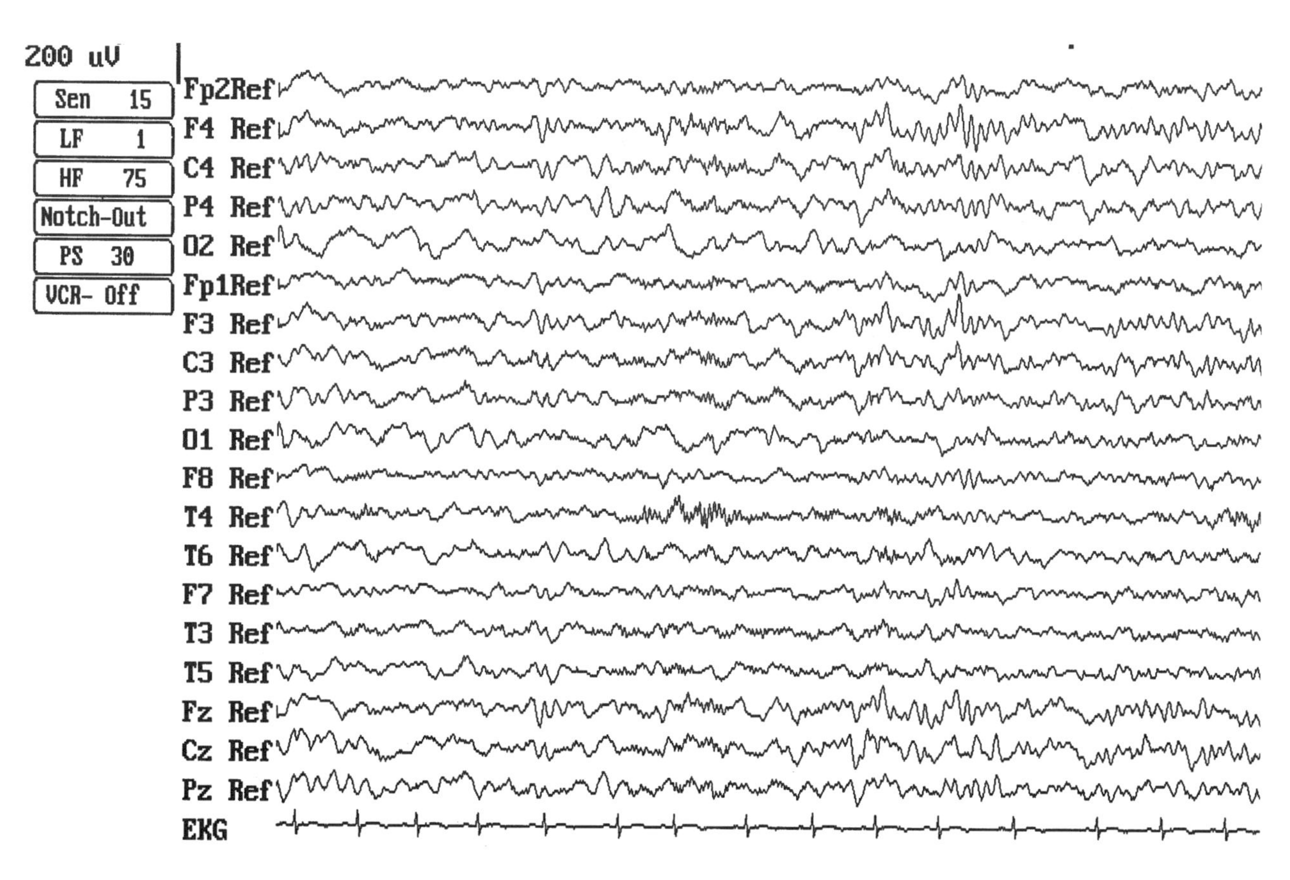

FIG. 4-43a,b Focal paroxysmal beta at T4 is seen on runs 1 and 2.

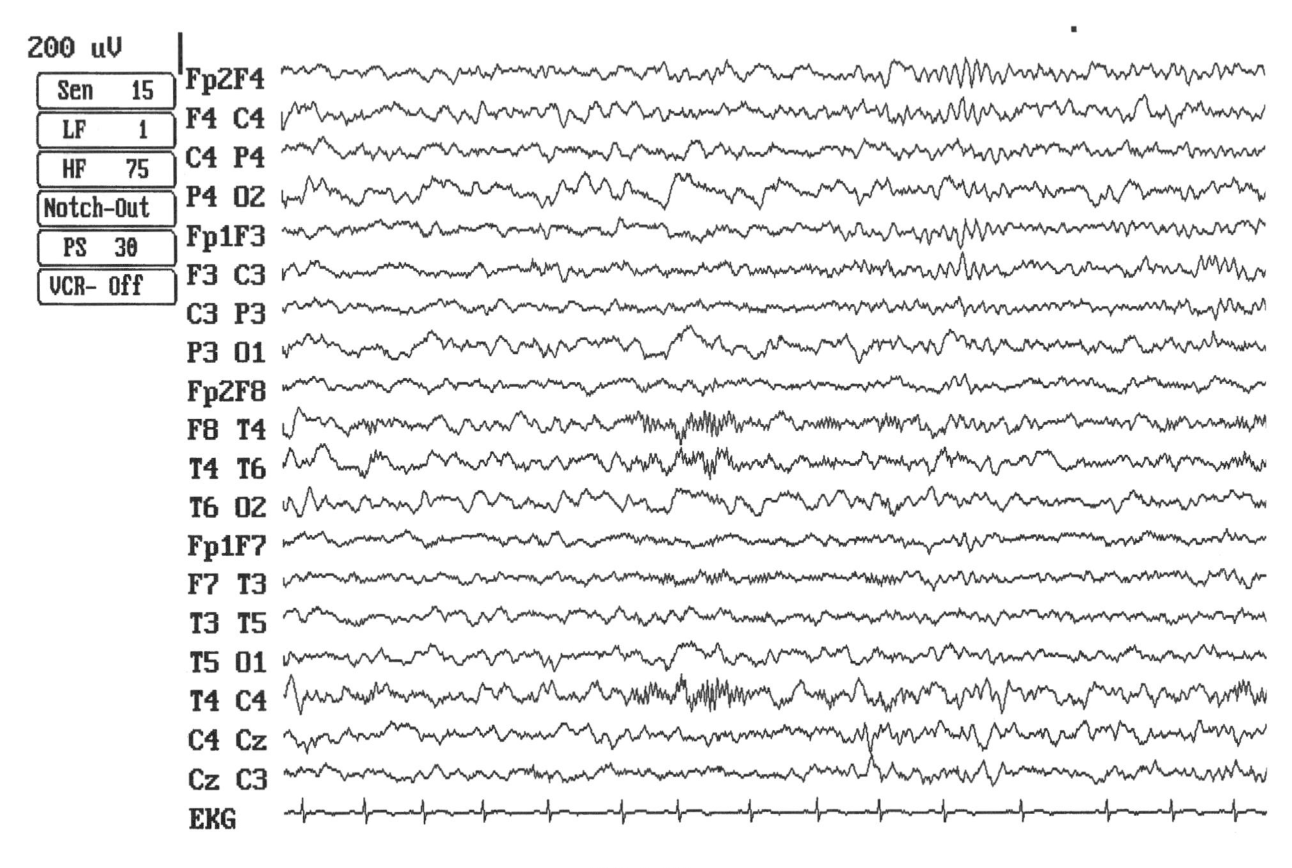
200 uV
Sen 15
LF 1
HF 75
Notch-Out
PS 30
VCR- Off
Fp2F4
F4 C4
C4 P4
P4 O2
Fp1F3
F3 C3
C3 P3
P3 O1
Fp2F8
F8 T4
T4 T6
T6 O2
Fp1F7
F7 T3
T3 T5
T5 O1
T4 C4
C4 Cz
Cz C3
EKG

FIG. 4-43b

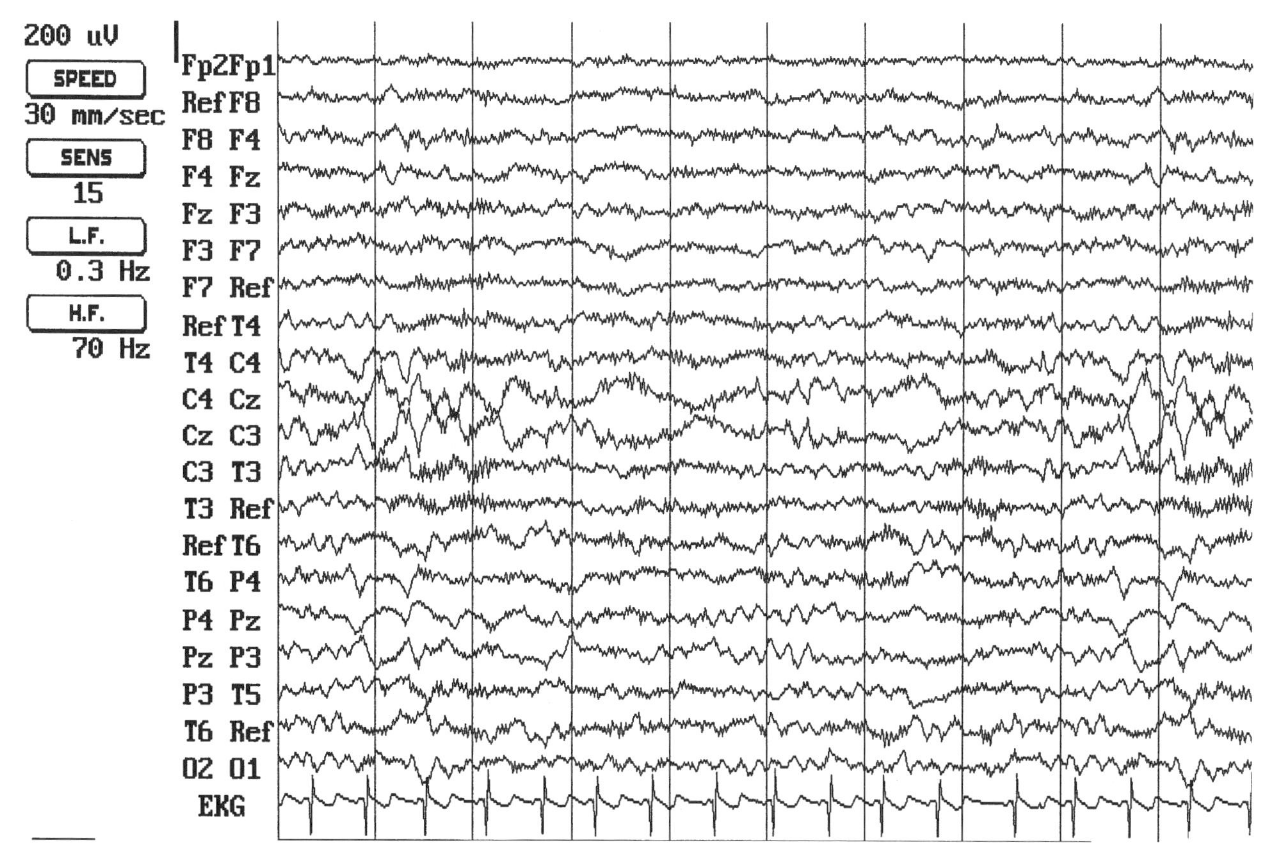

FIG. 4-44a,b,c Generalized beta in sleep is seen on runs 1 and 3. The paper speed of 60 mm/sec shows morphology of beta.

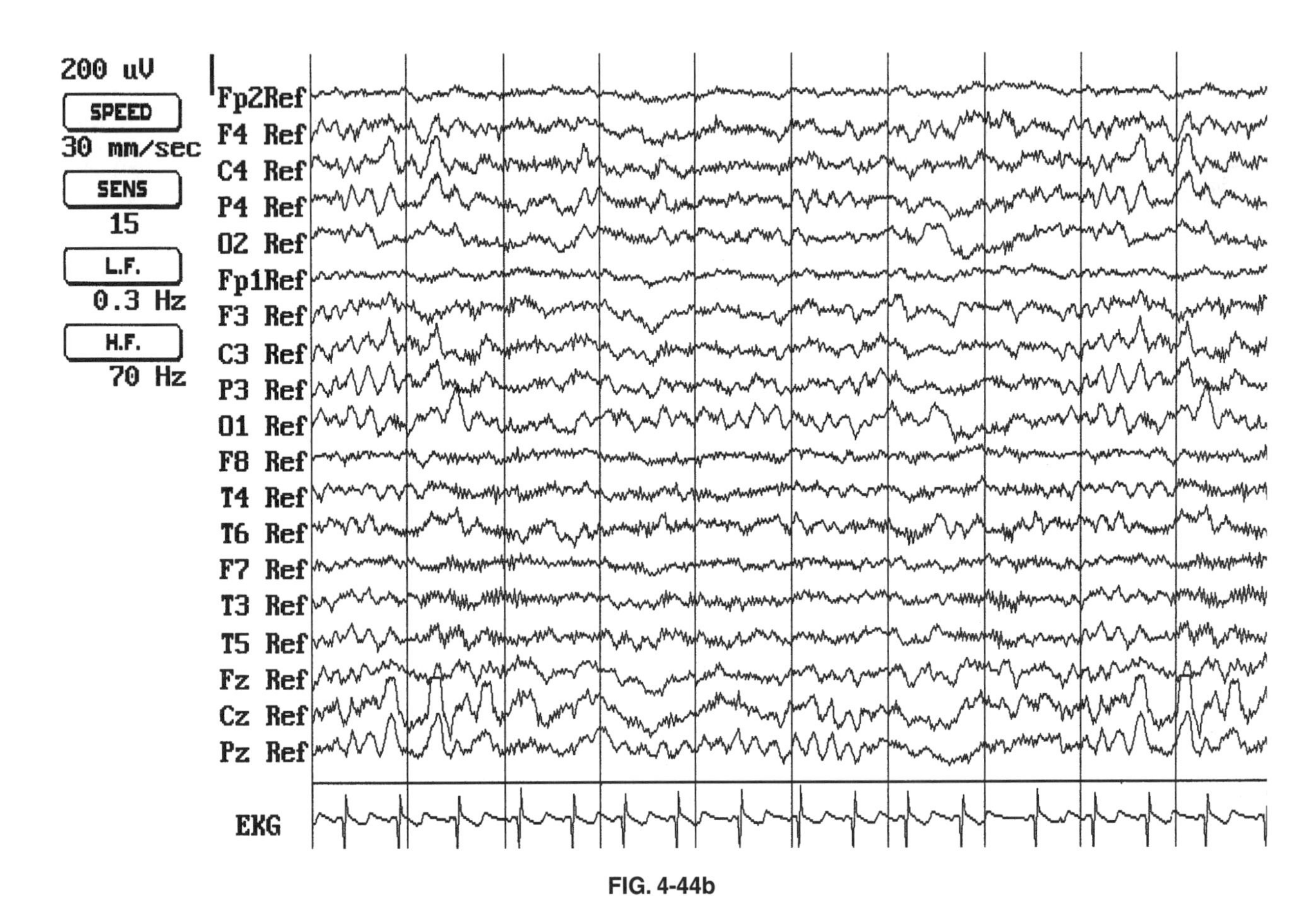
200 uV
SPEED
30 mm/sec
SENS
15
L.F.
0.3 Hz
H.F.
70 Hz
Fp2Ref
F4 Ref
C4 Ref
P4 Ref
O2 Ref
Fp1Ref
F3 Ref
C3 Ref
P3 Ref
O1 Ref
F8 Ref
T4 Ref
T6 Ref
F7 Ref
T3 Ref
T5 Ref
Fz Ref
Cz Ref
Pz Ref
EKG

FIG. 4-44b

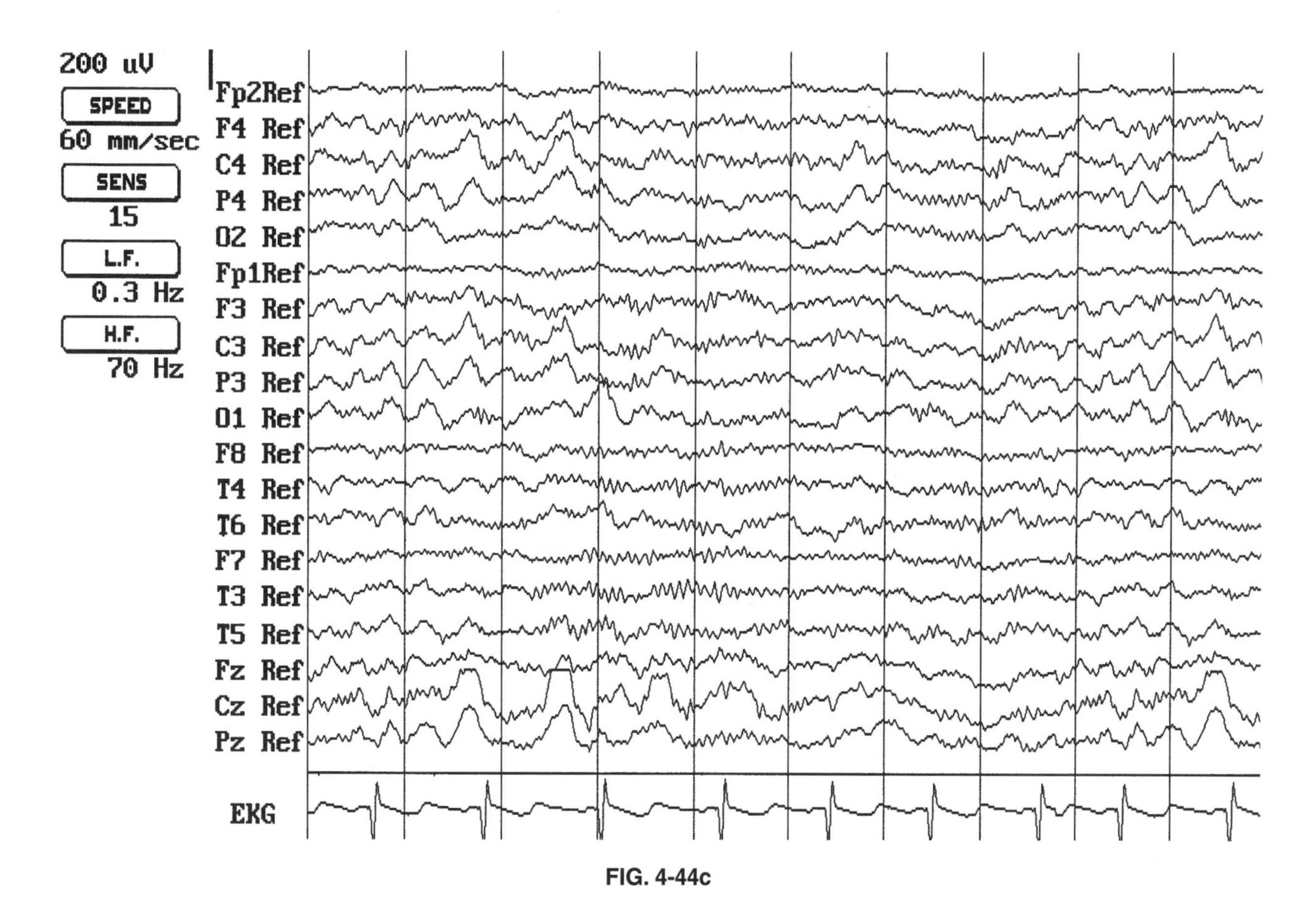
200 uV
SPEED
60 mm/sec
SENS
15
L.F.
0.3 Hz
H.F.
70 Hz
Fp2Ref
F4 Ref
C4 Ref
P4 Ref
O2 Ref
Fp1Ref
F3 Ref
C3 Ref
P3 Ref
O1 Ref
F8 Ref
T4 Ref
T6 Ref
F7 Ref
T3 Ref
T5 Ref
Fz Ref
Cz Ref
Pz Ref
EKG

FIG. 4-44c

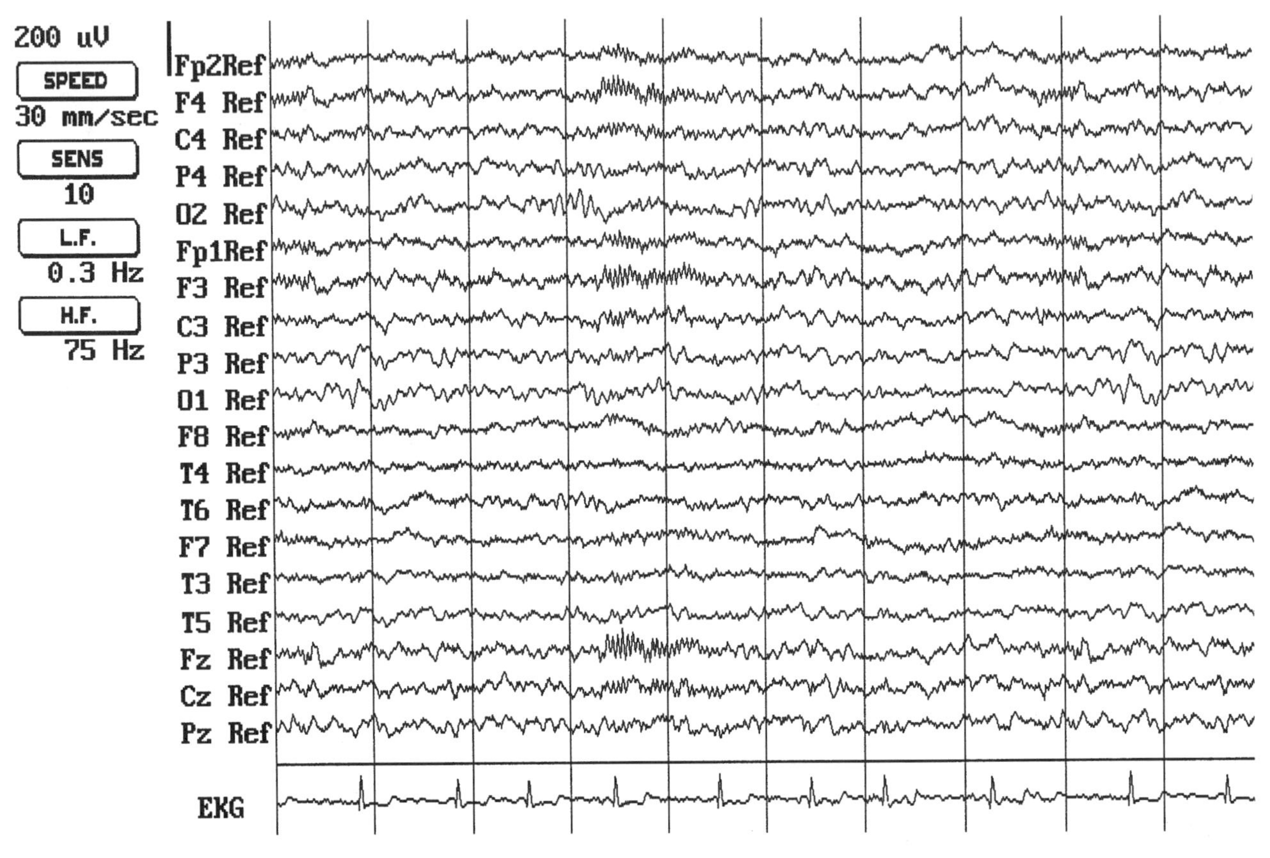

FIG. 4-45a,b,c,d Bianterior beta is seen on runs 1,2, and 3 and with a paper speed of 60 mm/s.

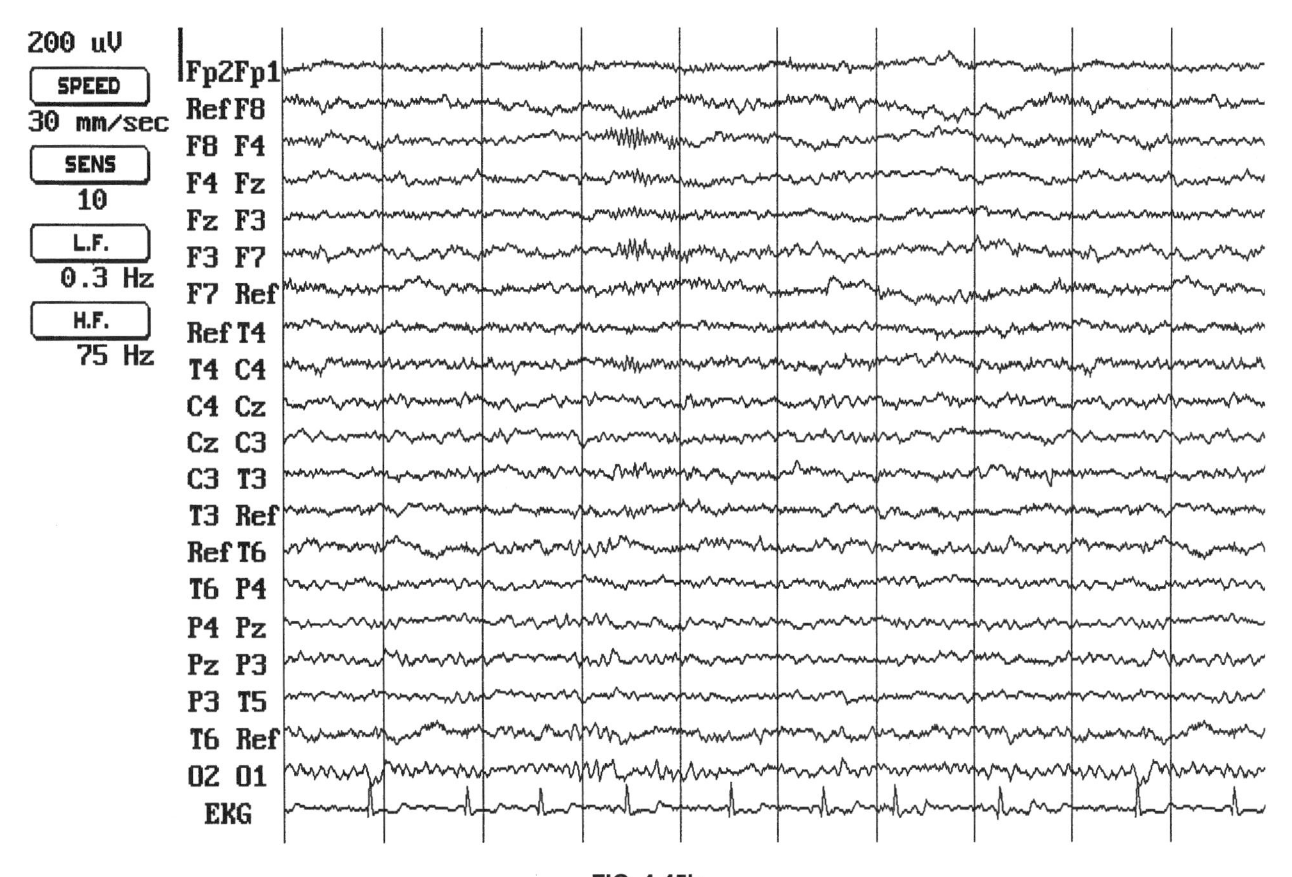
200 uV
SPEED
30 mm/sec
SENS
10
L.F.
0.3 Hz
H.F.
75 Hz
Fp2Fp1
Ref F8
F8 F4
F4 Fz
Fz F3
F3 F7
F7 Ref
Ref T4
T4 C4
C4 Cz
Cz C3
C3 T3
T3 Ref
Ref T6
T6 P4
P4 Pz
Pz P3
P3 T5
T6 Ref
O2 O1
EKG

FIG. 4-45b

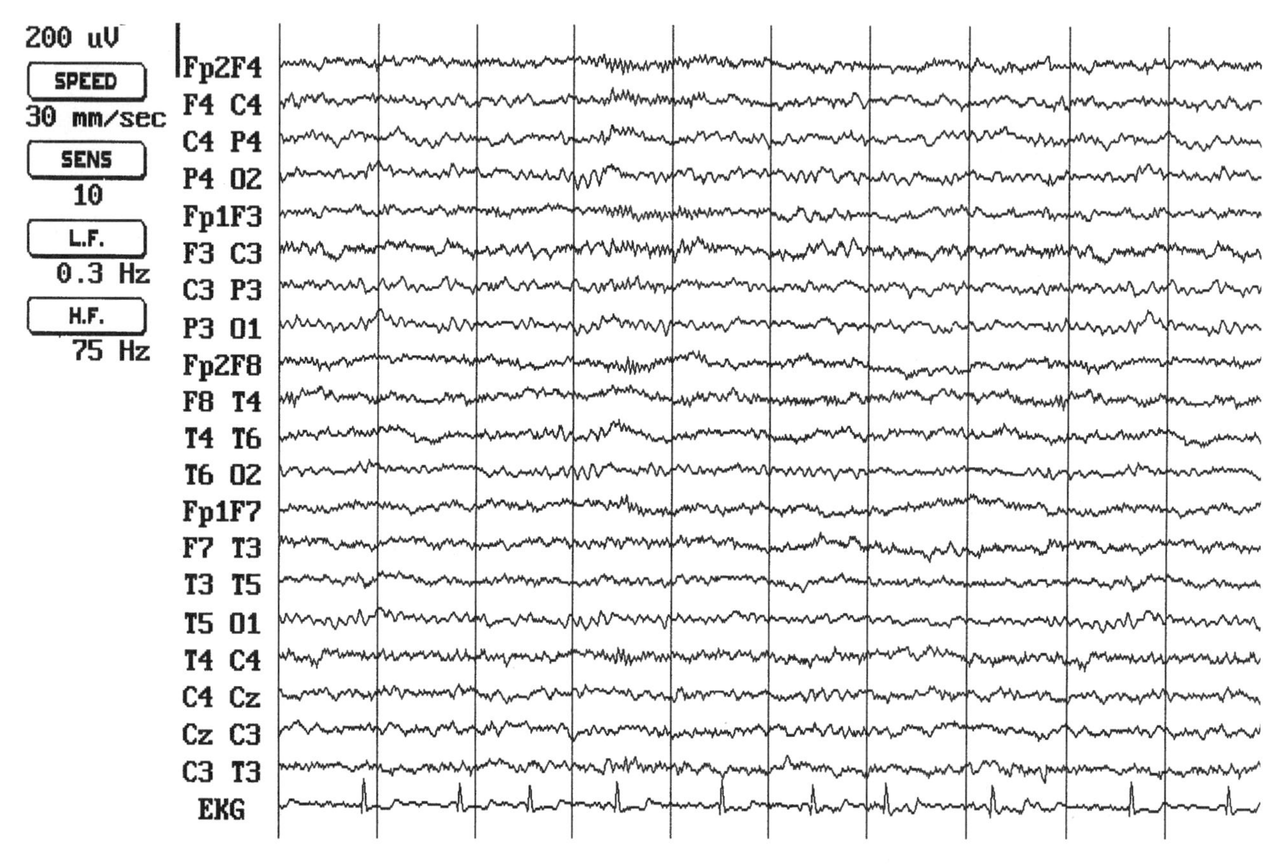
200 uV
SPEED
30 mm/sec
SENS
10
L.F.
0.3 Hz
H.F.
75 Hz
Fp2F4
F4 C4
C4 P4
P4 O2
Fp1F3
F3 C3
C3 P3
P3 O1
Fp2F8
F8 T4
T4 T6
T6 O2
Fp1F7
F7 T3
T3 T5
T5 O1
T4 C4
C4 Cz
Cz C3
C3 T3
EKG

FIG. 4-45c

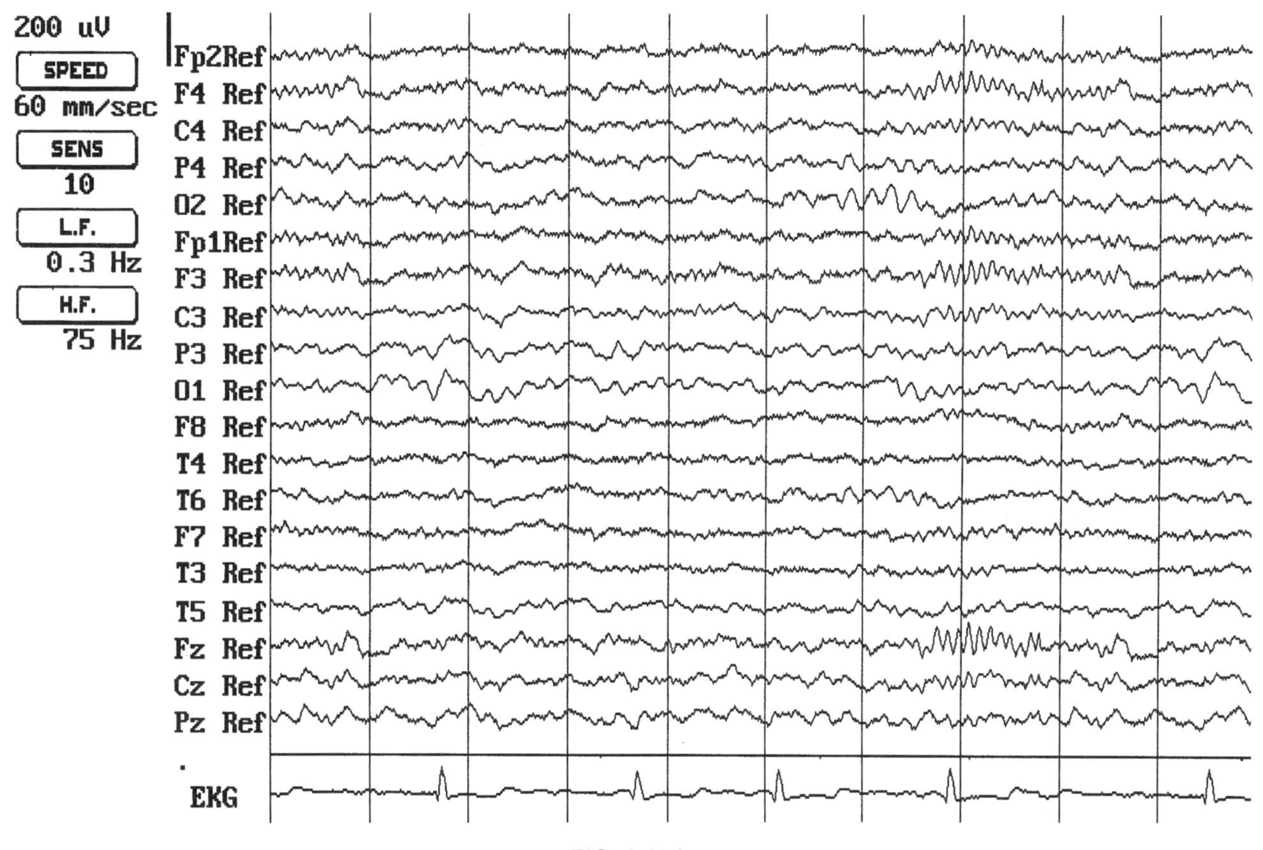
200 uV
SPEED
60 mm/sec
SENS
10
L.F.
0.3 Hz
H.F.
75 Hz
Fp2Ref
F4 Ref
C4 Ref
P4 Ref
O2 Ref
Fp1Ref
F3 Ref
C3 Ref
P3 Ref
O1 Ref
F8 Ref
T4 Ref
T6 Ref
F7 Ref
T3 Ref
T5 Ref
Fz Ref
Cz Ref
Pz Ref
EKG

FIG. 4-45d

Theta

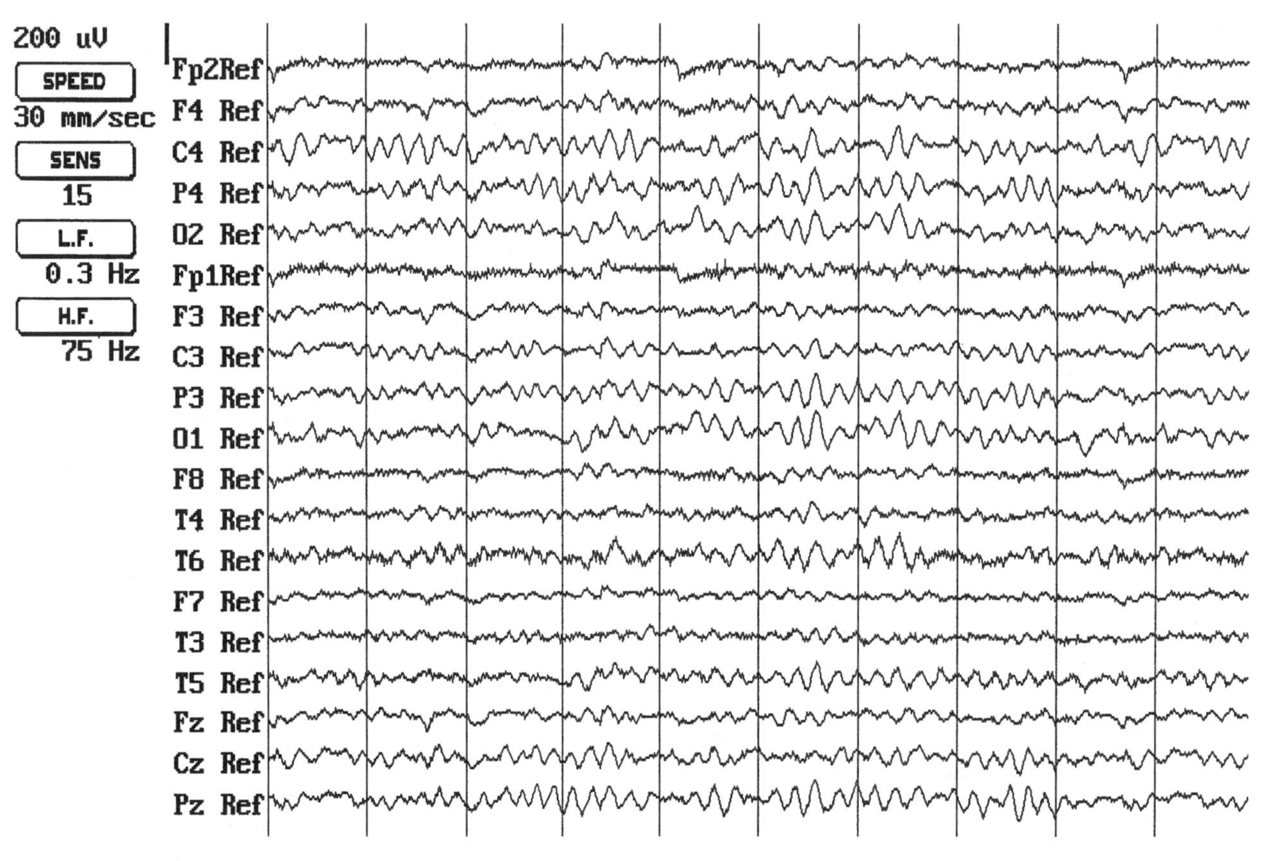

FIG. 4-46a,b,c Normal drowsiness showing diffuse theta maximum at right central parietal is seen on run 1. On run 2 there appears to be a right hemispheric dysrhythmia, while run 3 shows a right central temporal dysrhythmia. If the interpretation was limited to a particular montage, different localizations would result from the same data.

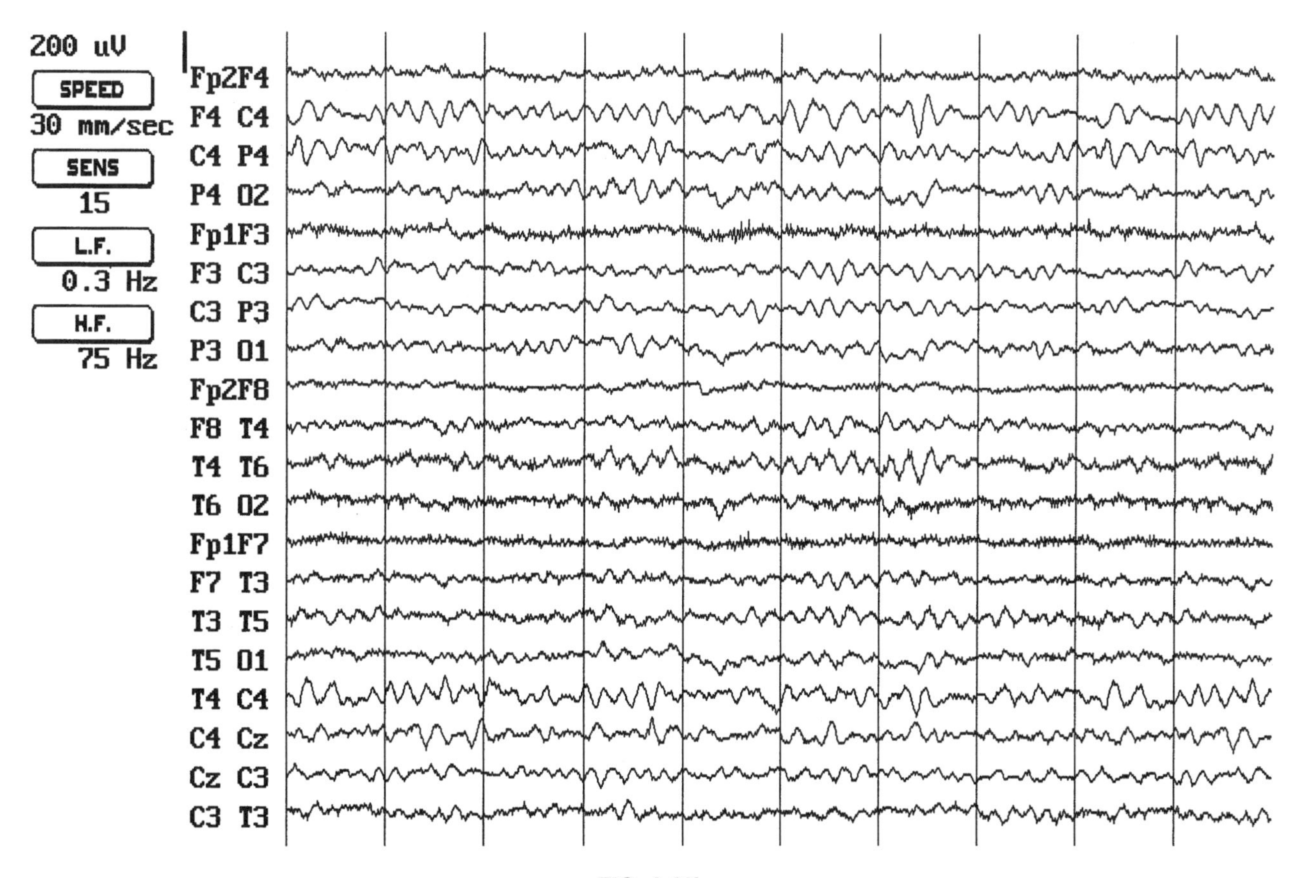
200 uV
SPEED
30 mm/sec
SENS
15
L.F.
0.3 Hz
H.F.
75 Hz
Fp2F4
F4 C4
C4 P4
P4 O2
Fp1F3
F3 C3
C3 P3
P3 O1
Fp2F8
F8 T4
T4 T6
T6 O2
Fp1F7
F7 T3
T3 T5
T5 O1
T4 C4
C4 Cz
Cz C3
C3 T3

FIG. 4-46b

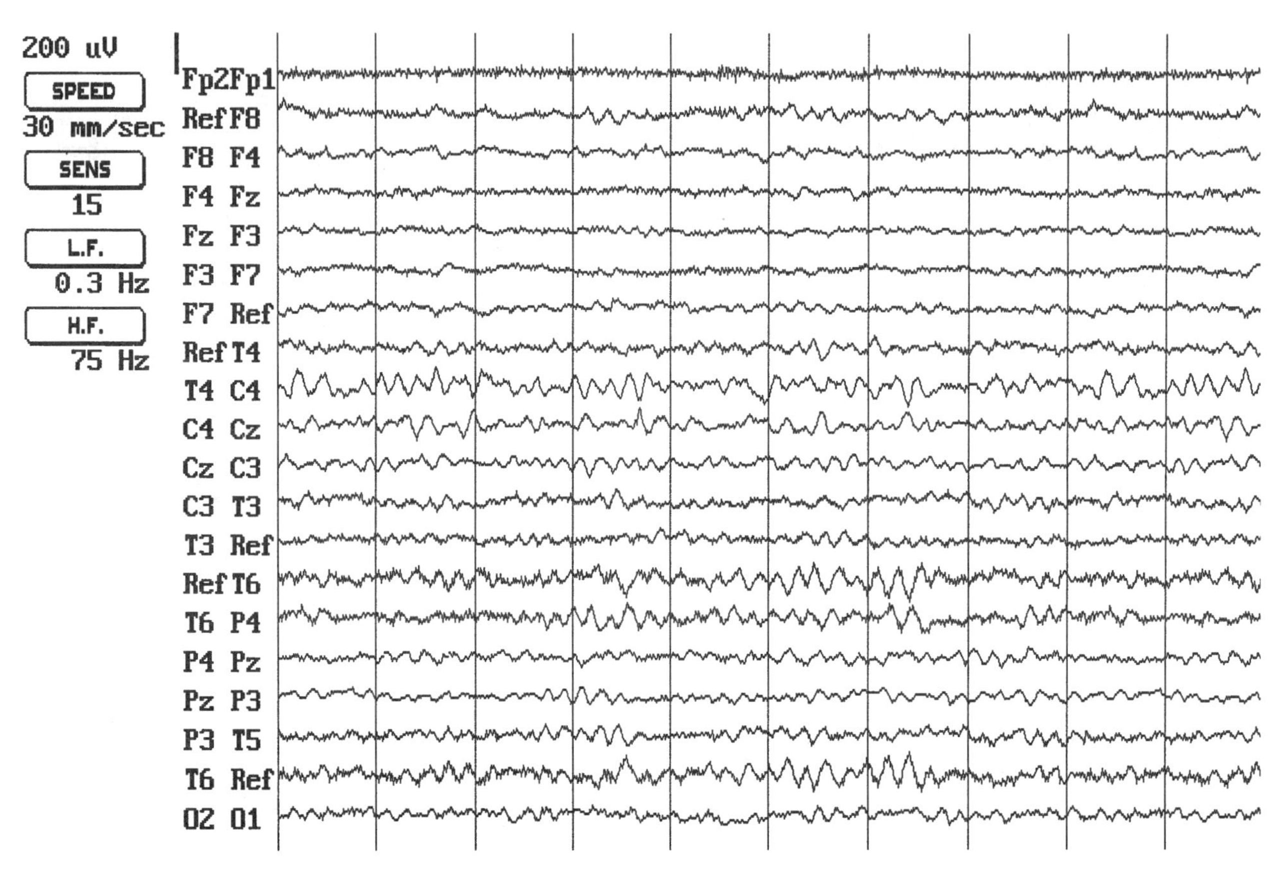
200 uV
SPEED
30 mm/sec
SENS
15
L.F.
0.3 Hz
H.F.
75 Hz
Fp2Fp1
Ref F8
F8 F4
F4 Fz
Fz F3
F3 F7
F7 Ref
Ref T4
T4 C4
C4 Cz
Cz C3
C3 T3
T3 Ref
Ref T6
T6 P4
P4 Pz
Pz P3
P3 T5
T6 Ref
O2 O1

FIG. 4-46c

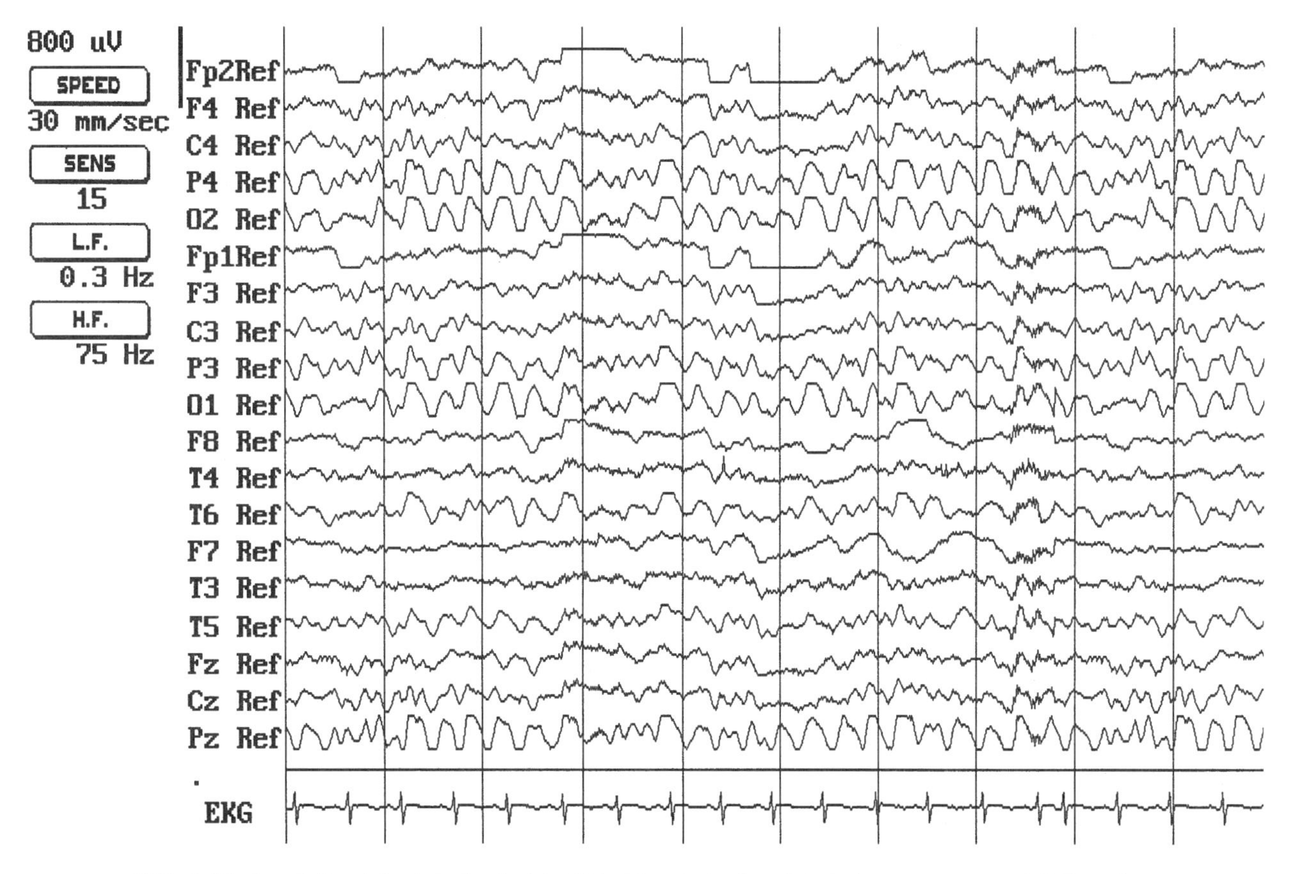

FIG. 4-47a,b,c,d Persistent rhythmic 4 to 5 Hz biposterior head theta is seen on runs 1,2,3, and 4. Run 1 with a slow paper speed enhances theta. Run 3 gives the worst localization.

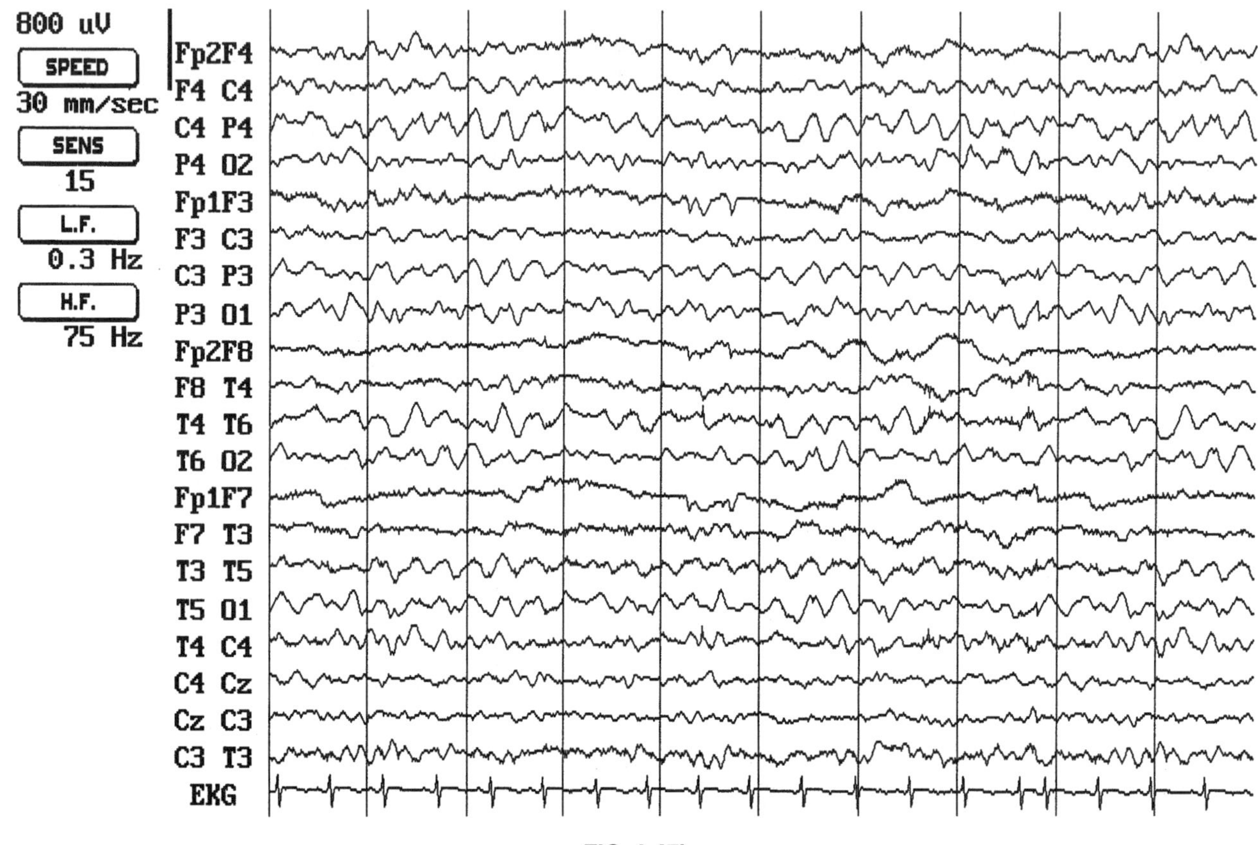
800 uV
SPEED
30 mm/sec
SENS
15
L.F.
0.3 Hz
H.F.
75 Hz
Fp2F4
F4 C4
C4 P4
P4 O2
Fp1F3
F3 C3
C3 P3
P3 O1
Fp2F8
F8 T4
T4 T6
T6 O2
Fp1F7
F7 T3
T3 T5
T5 O1
T4 C4
C4 Cz
Cz C3
C3 T3
EKG

FIG. 4-47b

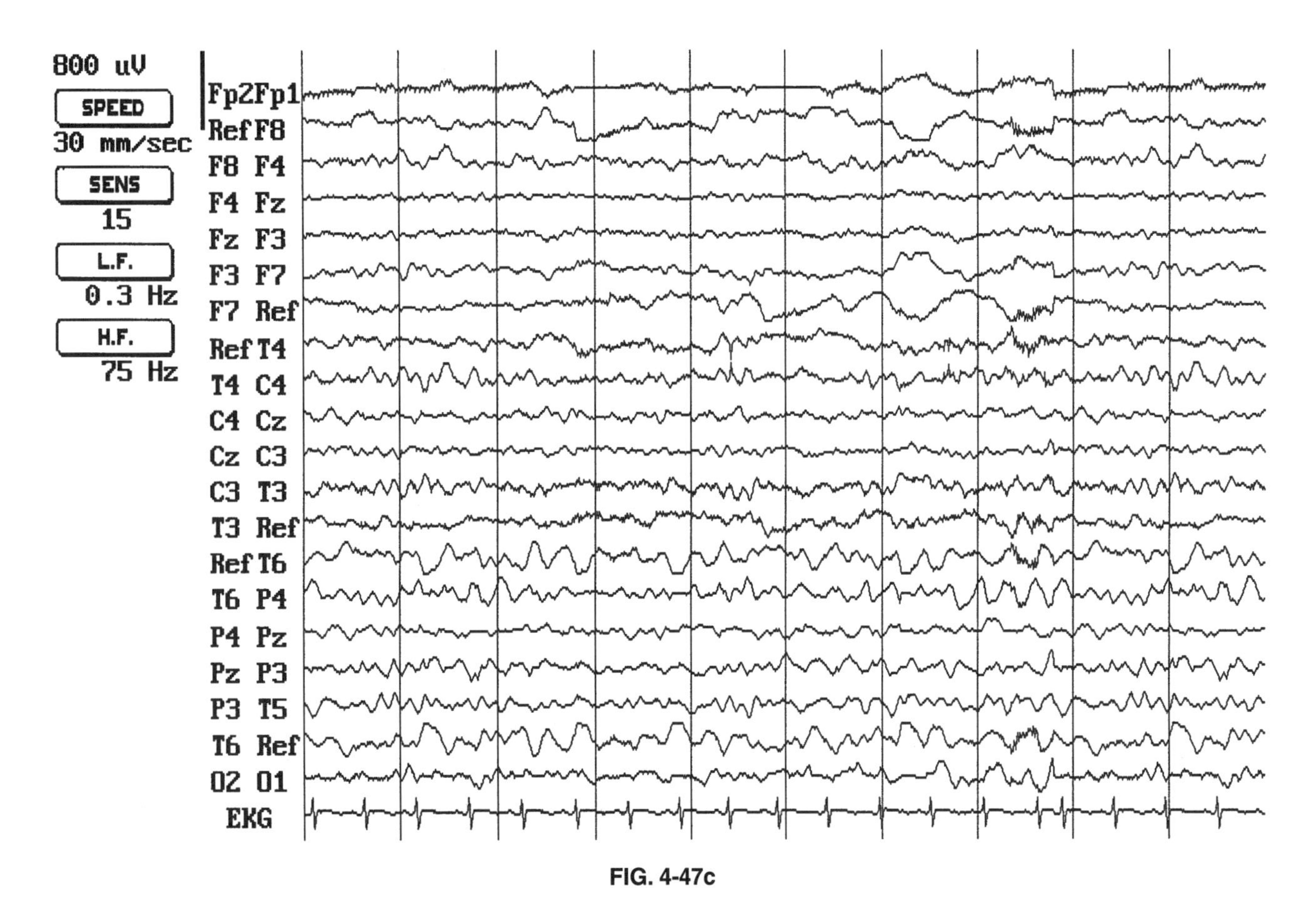
800 uV
SPEED
30 mm/sec
SENS
15
L.F.
0.3 Hz
H.F.
75 Hz
Fp2Fp1
Ref F8
F8 F4
F4 Fz
Fz F3
F3 F7
F7 Ref
Ref T4
T4 C4
C4 Cz
Cz C3
C3 T3
T3 Ref
Ref T6
T6 P4
P4 Pz
Pz P3
P3 T5
T6 Ref
O2 O1
EKG

FIG. 4-47c

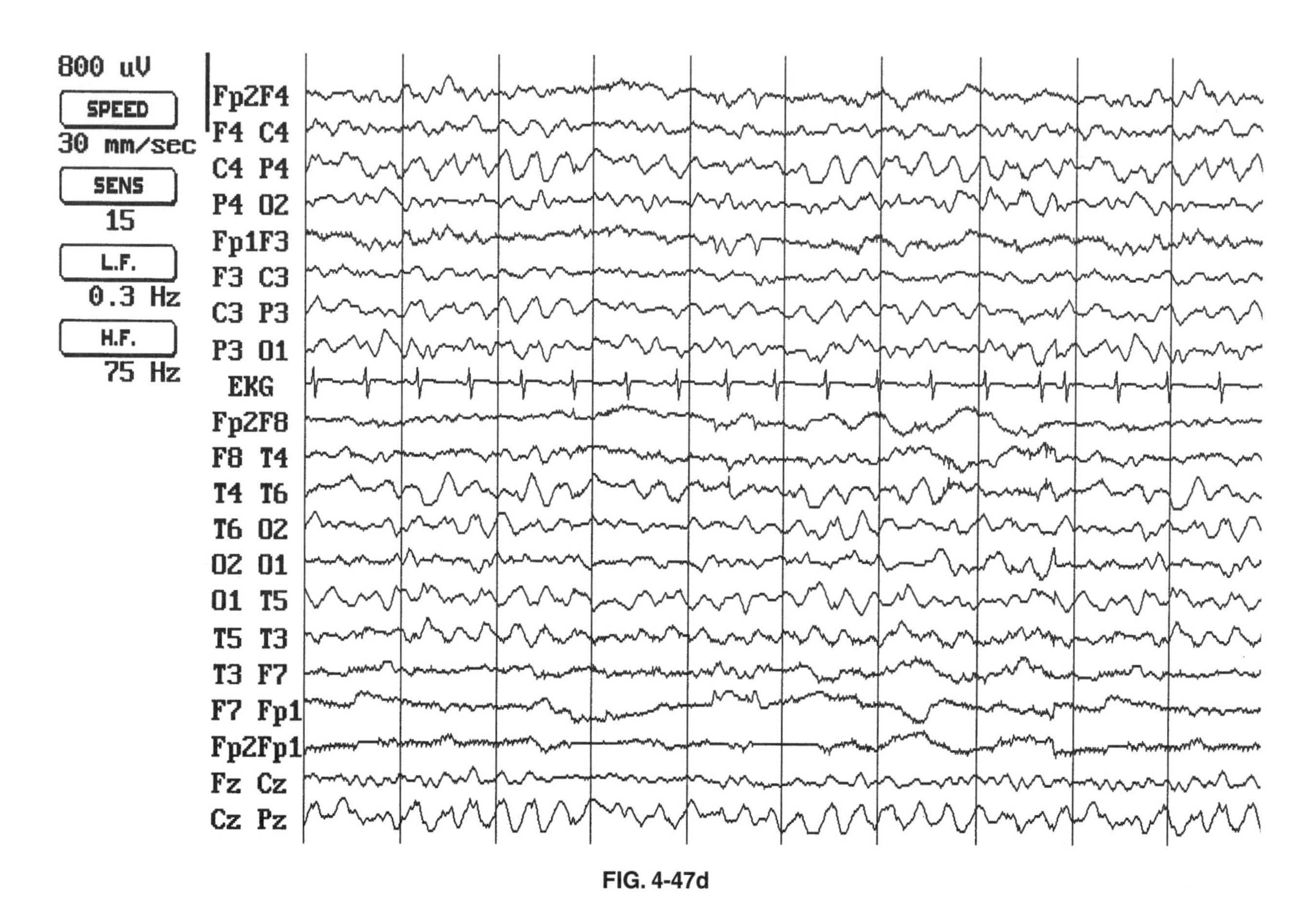
800 uV
SPEED
30 mm/sec
SENS
15
L.F.
0.3 Hz
H.F.
75 Hz
Fp2F4
F4 C4
C4 P4
P4 O2
Fp1F3
F3 C3
C3 P3
P3 O1
EKG
Fp2F8
F8 T4
T4 T6
T6 O2
O2 O1
O1 T5
T5 T3
T3 F7
F7 Fp1
Fp2Fp1
Fz Cz
Cz Pz

FIG. 4-47d

Delta

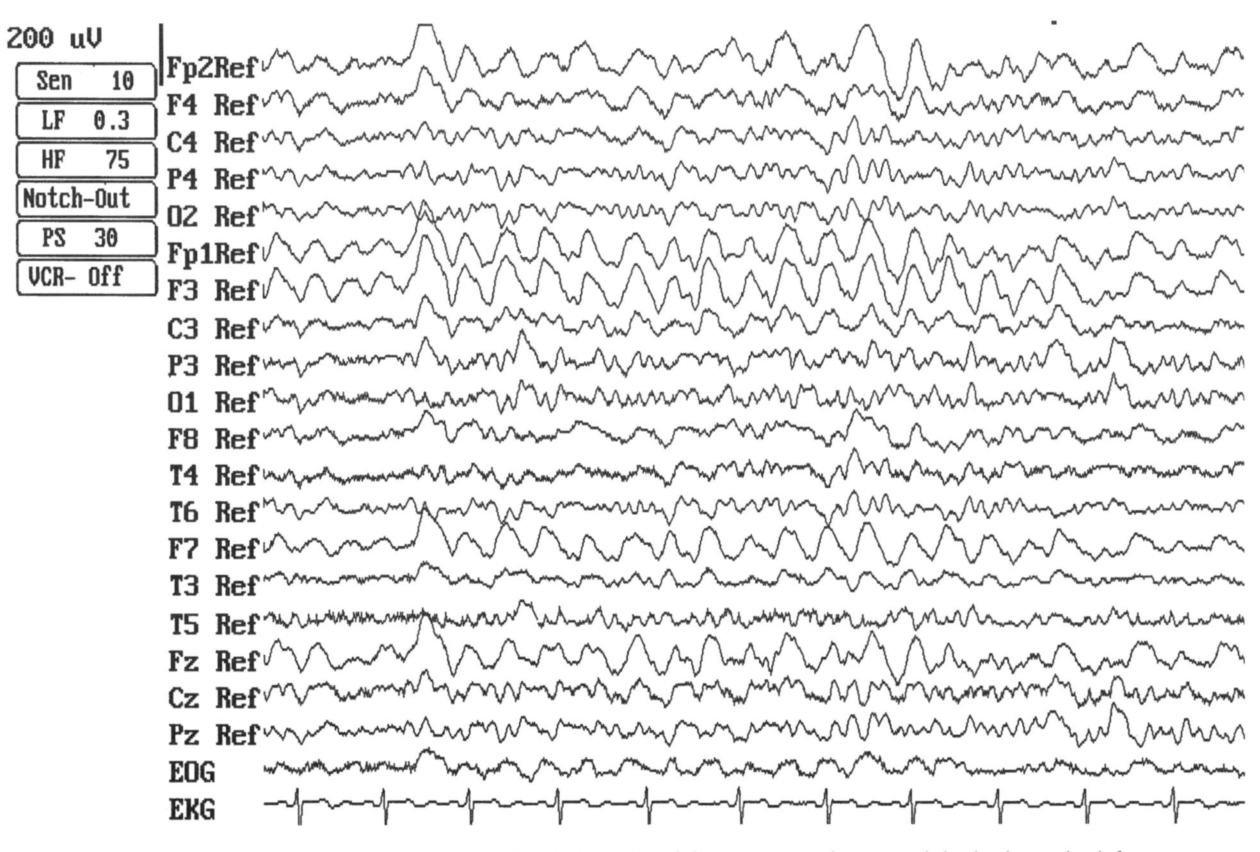

FIG. 4-48a,b,c This example shows a focal bianterior delta, more persistent and rhythmic on the left, more paroxysmal on the right, as seen on run 1 at 30 and 15 mm/s; run 4 is shown for comparison.

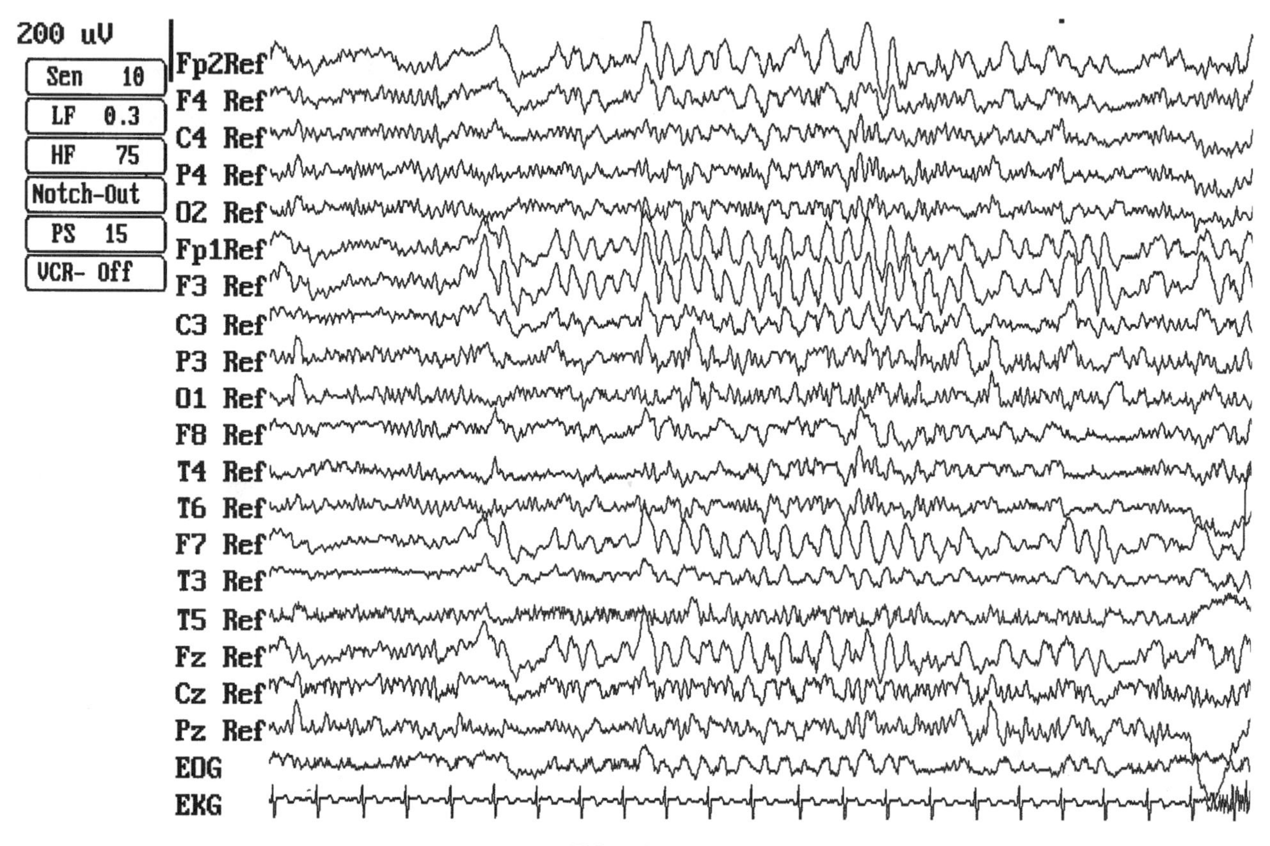
200 uV
Sen 10
LF 0.3
HF 75
Notch-Out
PS 15
VCR- Off
Fp2Ref
F4 Ref
C4 Ref
P4 Ref
O2 Ref
Fp1Ref
F3 Ref
C3 Ref
P3 Ref
O1 Ref
F8 Ref
T4 Ref
T6 Ref
F7 Ref
T3 Ref
T5 Ref
Fz Ref
Cz Ref
Pz Ref
EOG
EKG

FIG. 4-48b

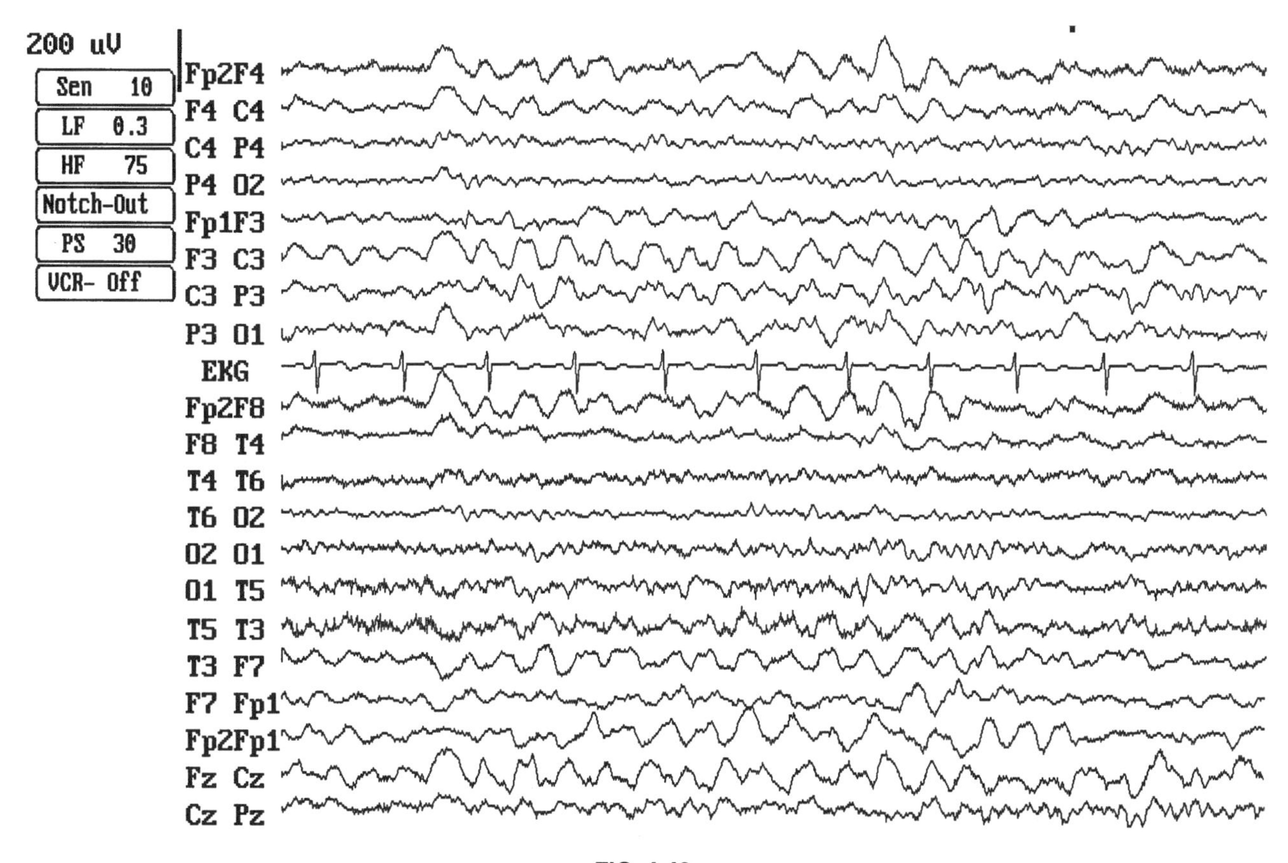
200 uV
Sen 10
LF 0.3
HF 75
Notch-Out
PS 30
VCR- Off
Fp2F4
F4 C4
C4 P4
P4 O2
Fp1F3
F3 C3
C3 P3
P3 O1
EKG
Fp2F8
F8 T4
T4 T6
T6 O2
O2 O1
O1 T5
T5 T3
T3 F7
F7 Fp1
Fp2Fp1
Fz Cz
Cz Pz

FIG. 4-48c

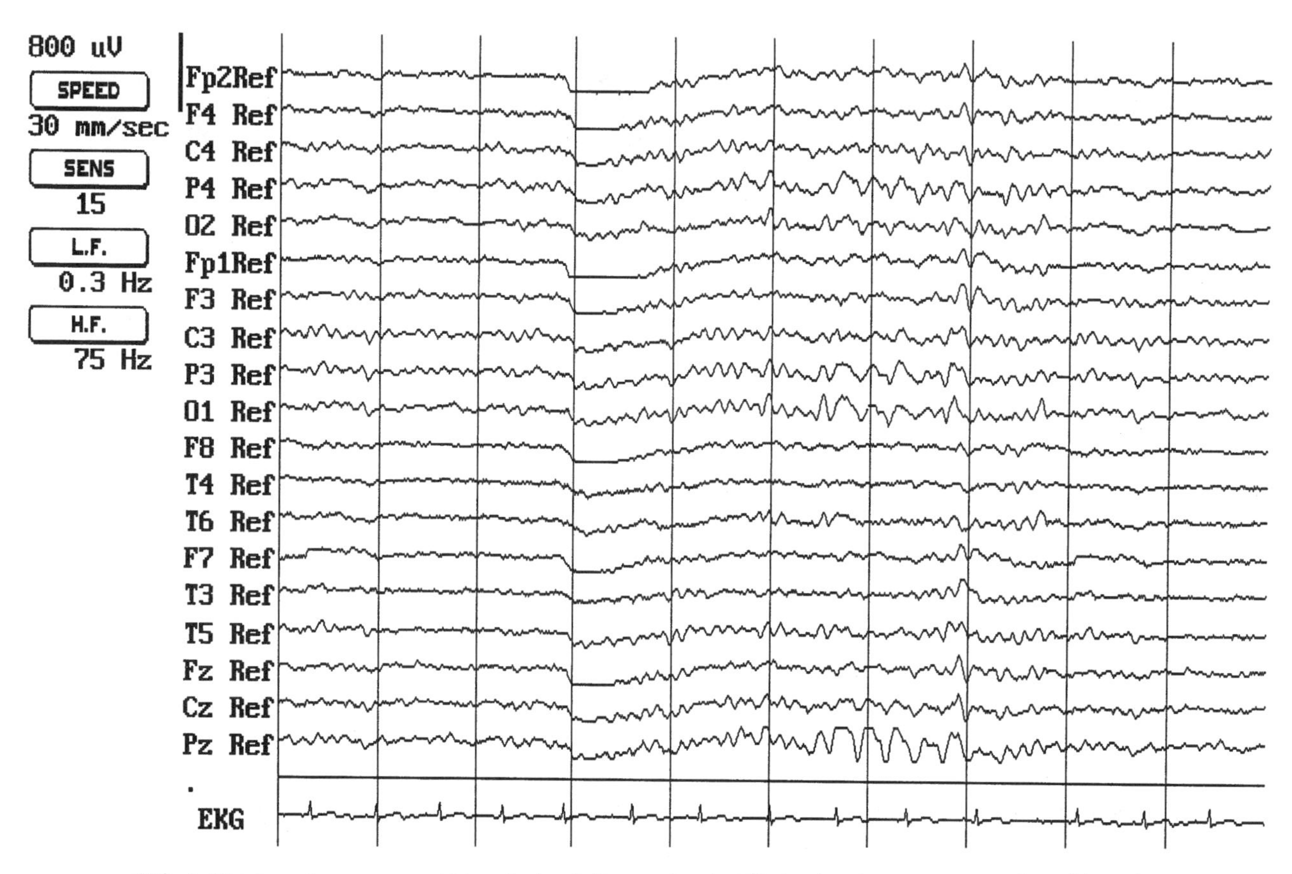

FIG. 4-49a,b,c A paroxysmal biposterior delta maximal at Pz is clearly seen on run 1 and is only seen on 1 channel (Cz-Pz) on run 4. There are misleading theta phase reversals at Pz on run 3.

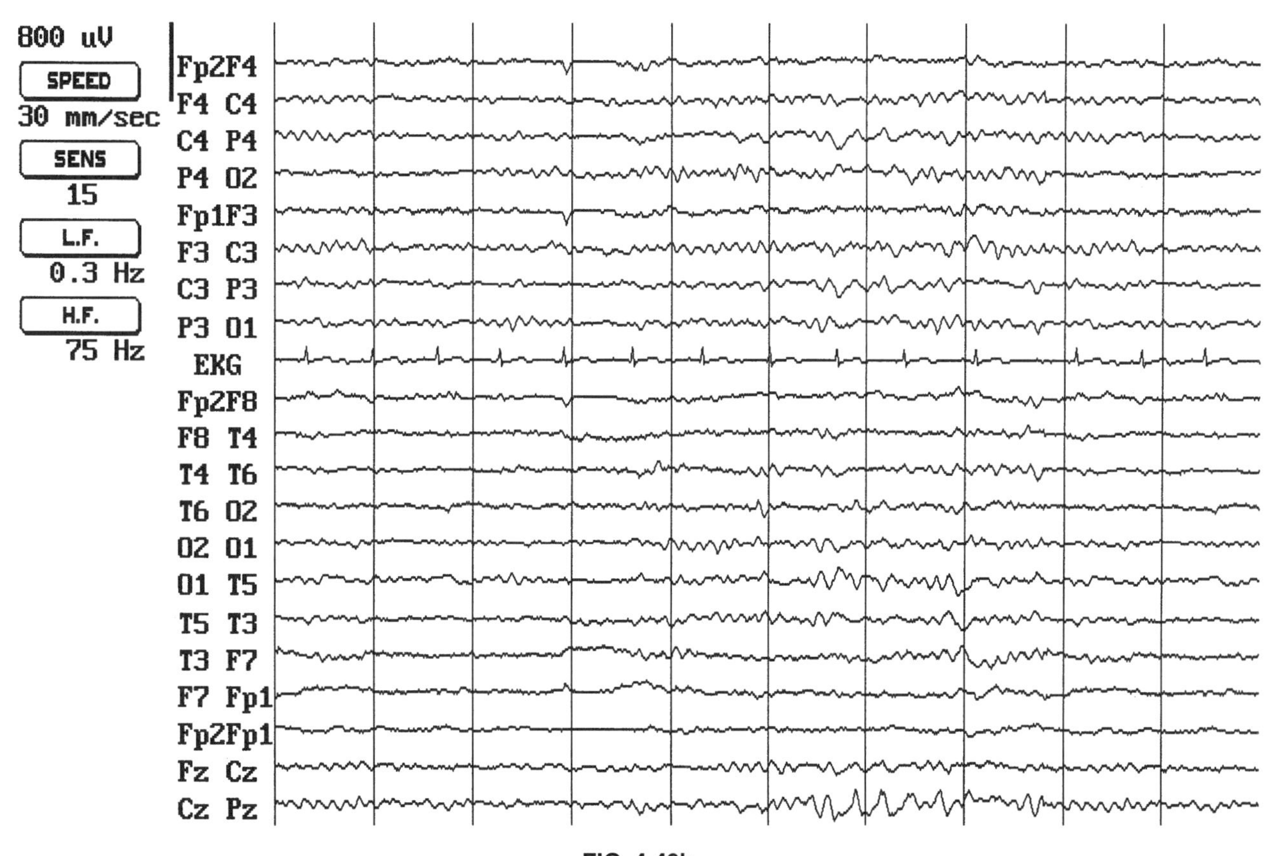
800 uV
SPEED
30 mm/sec
SENS
15
L.F.
0.3 Hz
H.F.
75 Hz
Fp2F4
F4 C4
C4 P4
P4 O2
Fp1F3
F3 C3
C3 P3
P3 O1
EKG
Fp2F8
F8 T4
T4 T6
T6 O2
O2 O1
O1 T5
T5 T3
T3 F7
F7 Fp1
Fp2Fp1
Fz Cz
Cz Pz

FIG. 4-49b

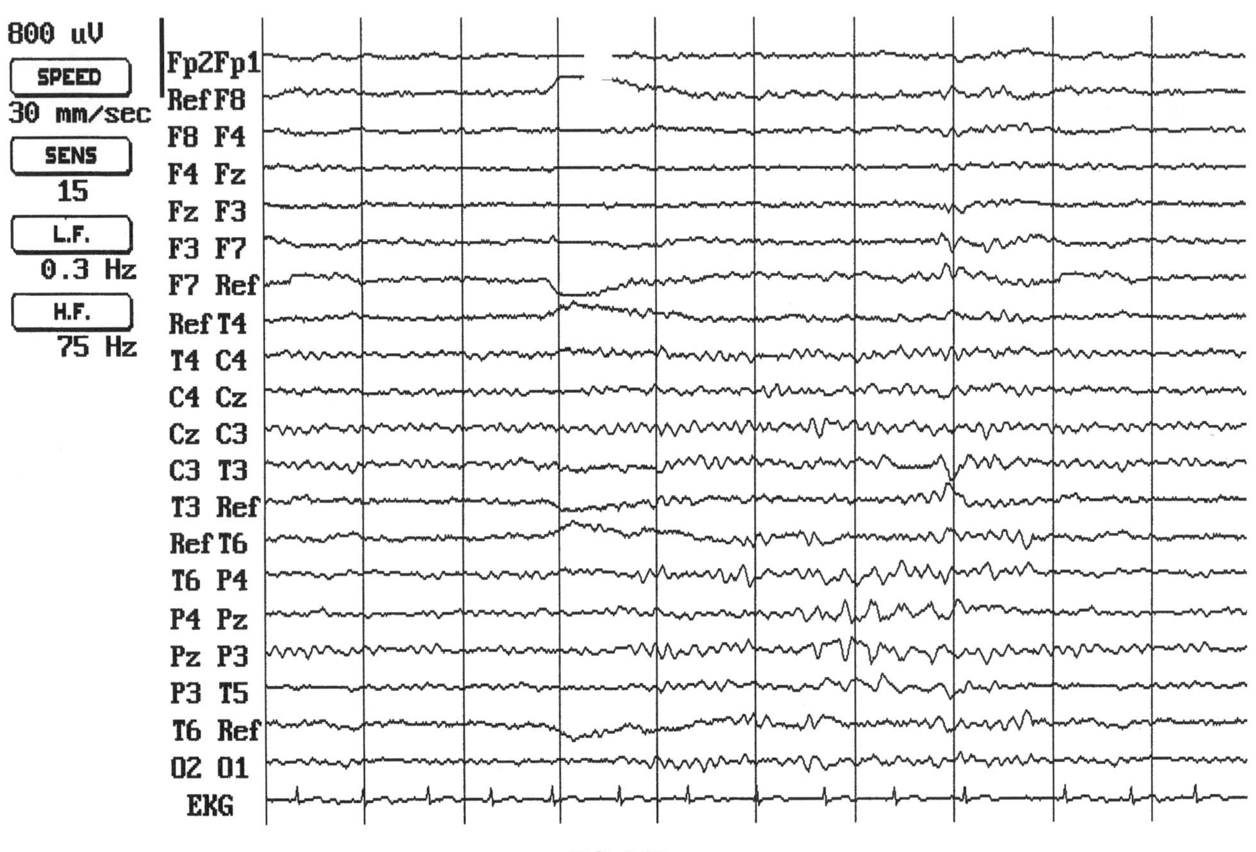
800 uV
SPEED
30 mm/sec
SENS
15
L.F.
0.3 Hz
H.F.
75 Hz
Fp2Fp1
Ref F8
F8 F4
F4 Fz
Fz F3
F3 F7
F7 Ref
Ref T4
T4 C4
C4 Cz
Cz C3
C3 T3
T3 Ref
Ref T6
T6 P4
P4 Pz
Pz P3
P3 T5
T6 Ref
O2 O1
EKG

FIG. 4-49c

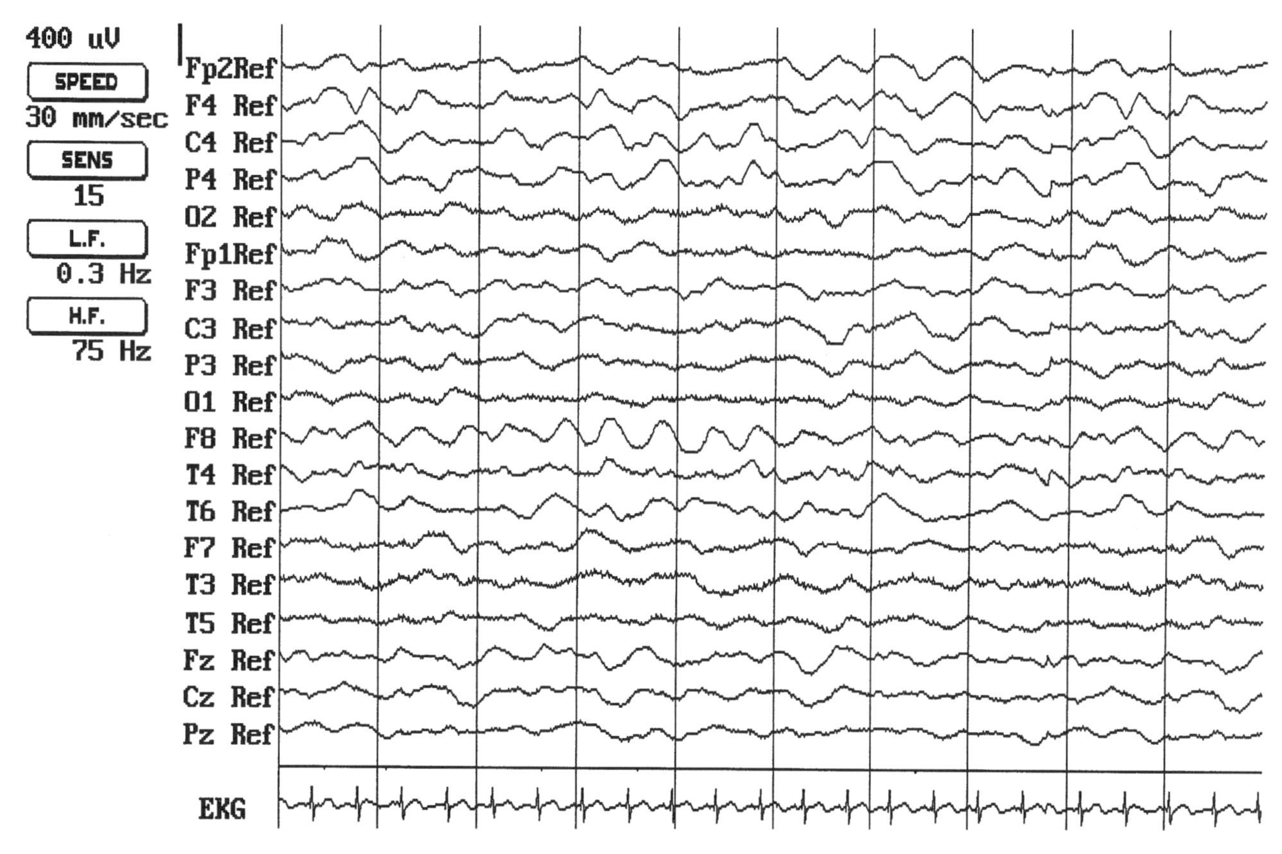

FIG. 4-50a,b,c,d This shows a poorly defined right sided delta on run 1 (better with slow PS). Run 3 shows a suggestion of two distinct delta frequencies, though run 2 shows them best: rhythmic fast delta at F8, and a slower delta maximal at C4.

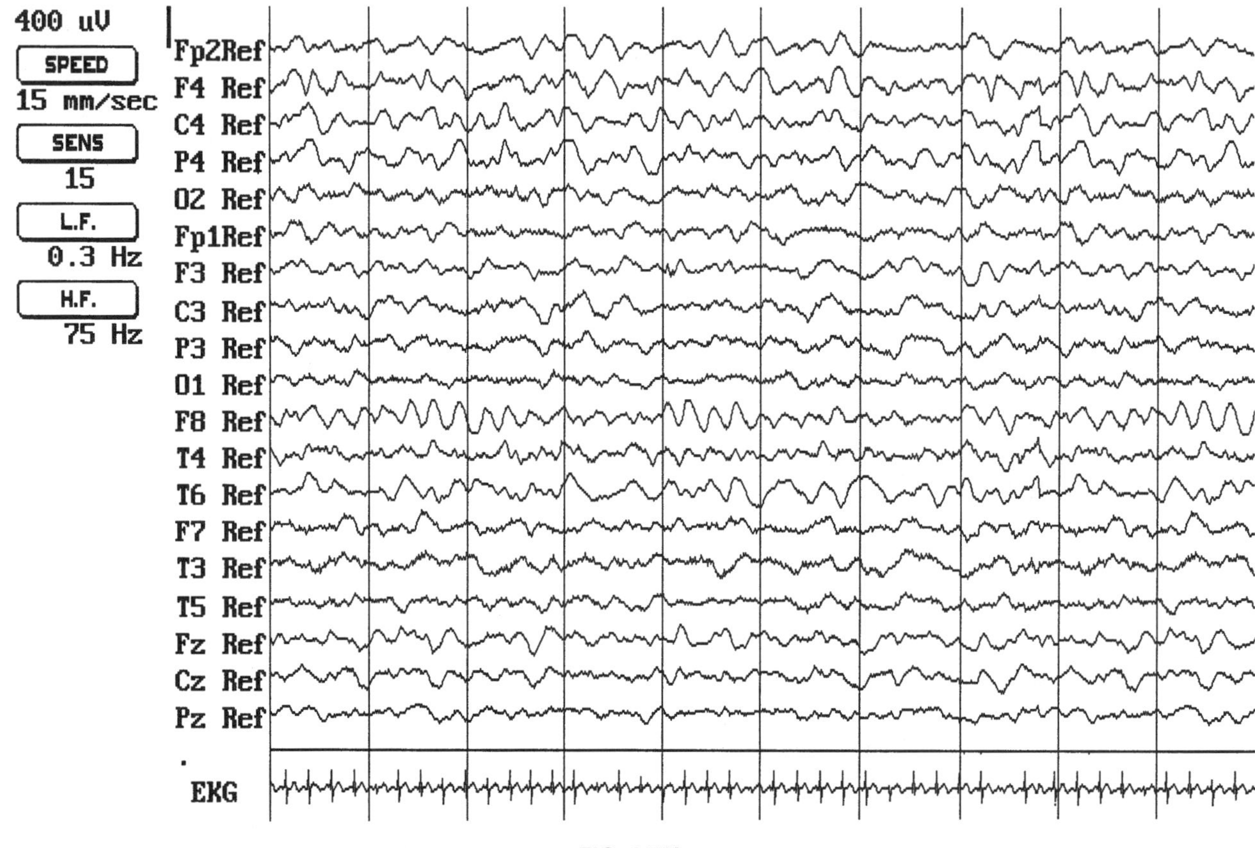
400 uV
SPEED
15 mm/sec
SENS
15
L.F.
0.3 Hz
H.F.
75 Hz
Fp2Ref
F4 Ref
C4 Ref
P4 Ref
O2 Ref
Fp1Ref
F3 Ref
C3 Ref
P3 Ref
O1 Ref
F8 Ref
T4 Ref
T6 Ref
F7 Ref
T3 Ref
T5 Ref
Fz Ref
Cz Ref
Pz Ref
EKG

FIG. 4-50b

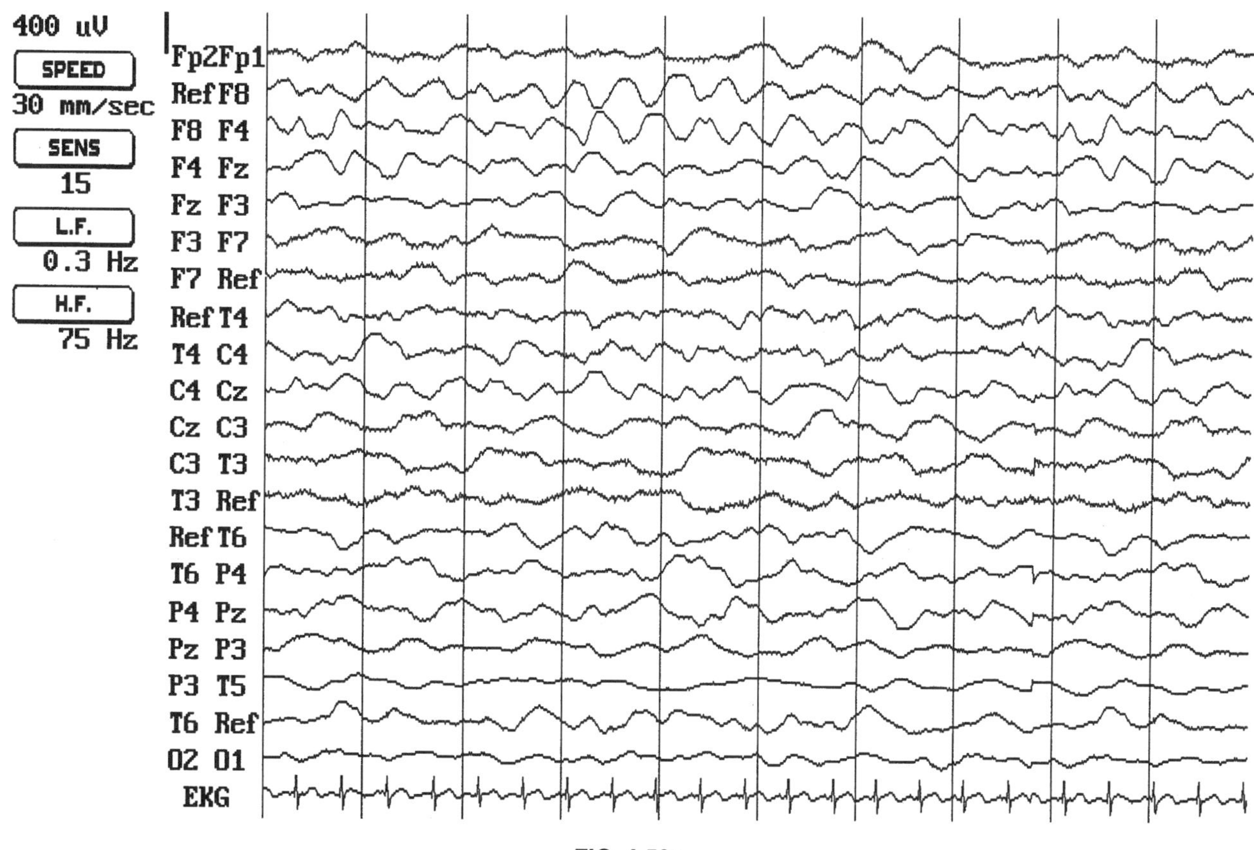
400 uV
SPEED
30 mm/sec
SENS
15
L.F.
0.3 Hz
H.F.
75 Hz
Fp2Fp1
Ref F8
F8 F4
F4 Fz
Fz F3
F3 F7
F7 Ref
Ref T4
T4 C4
C4 Cz
Cz C3
C3 T3
T3 Ref
Ref T6
T6 P4
P4 Pz
Pz P3
P3 T5
T6 Ref
O2 O1
EKG

FIG. 4-50c

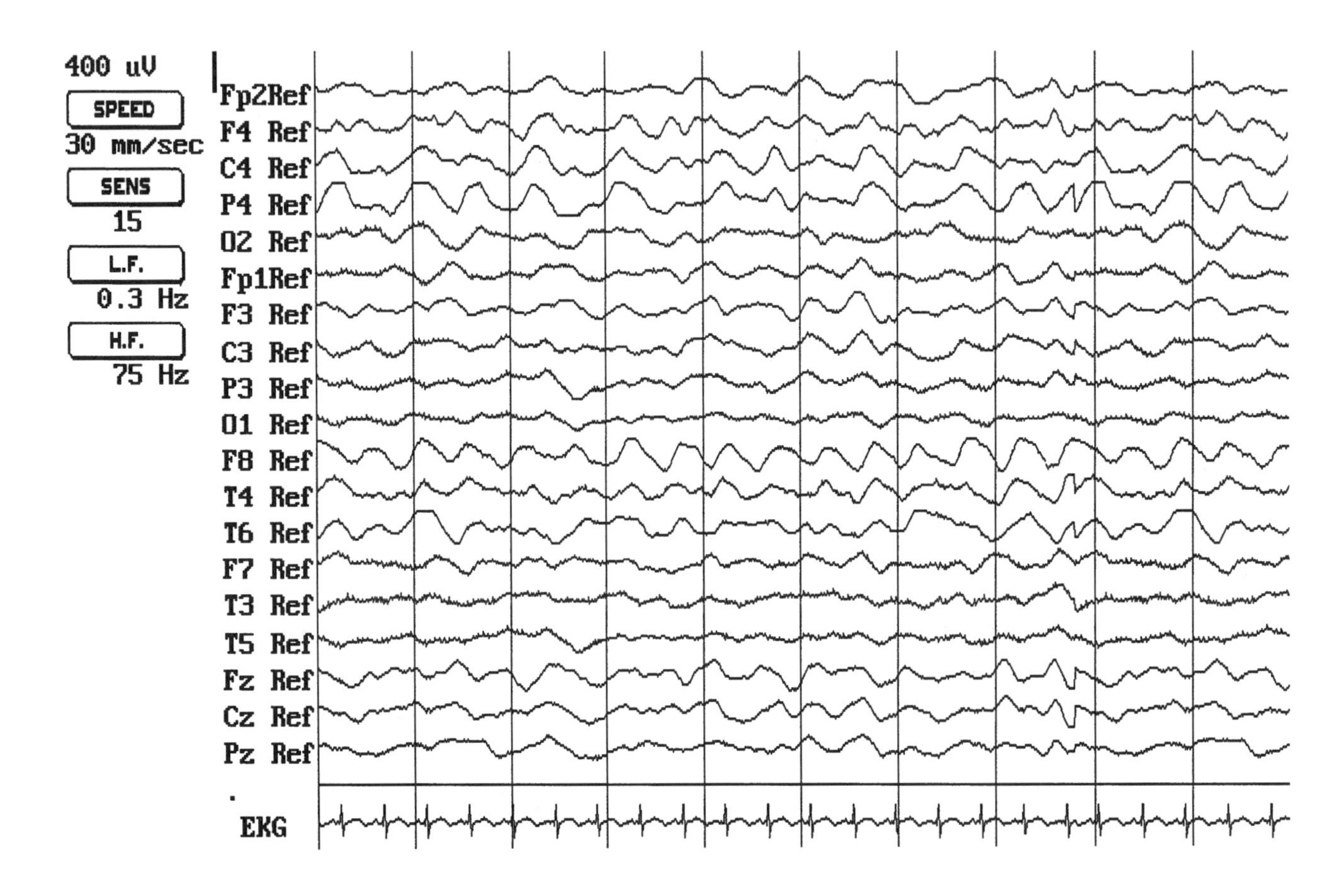
400 uV
SPEED
30 mm/sec
SENS
15
L.F.
0.3 Hz
H.F.
75 Hz
Fp2Ref
F4 Ref
C4 Ref
P4 Ref
O2 Ref
Fp1Ref
F3 Ref
C3 Ref
P3 Ref
O1 Ref
F8 Ref
T4 Ref
T6 Ref
F7 Ref
T3 Ref
T5 Ref
Fz Ref
Cz Ref
Pz Ref
EKG

FIG. 4-50d

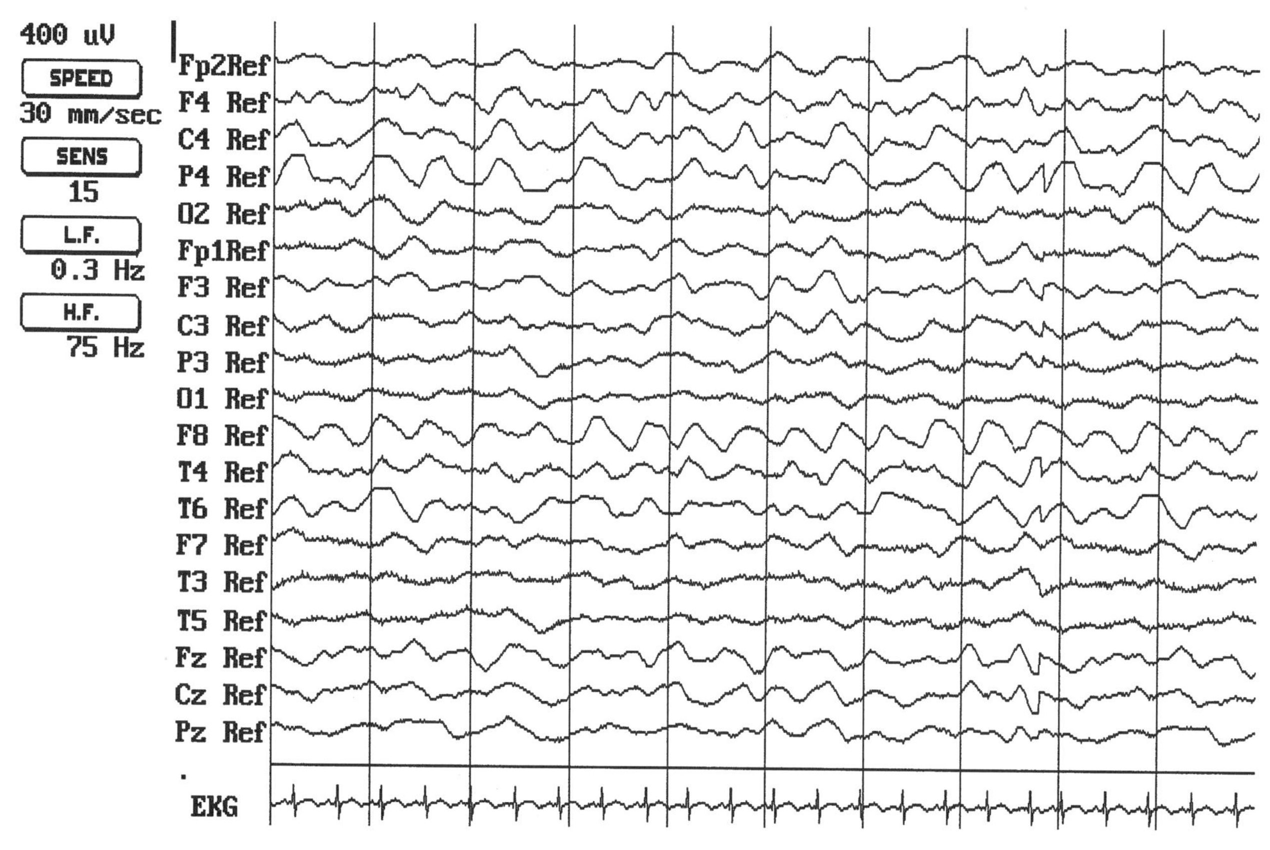

FIG. 4-51a,b,c Right frontal slowing is seen on run 1. Note the artifact at the 8th second. Faster delta phase reversals are seen at F8 and some slower delta at C4 are seen on run 2. These are most clear with PS for 15 mm/s.

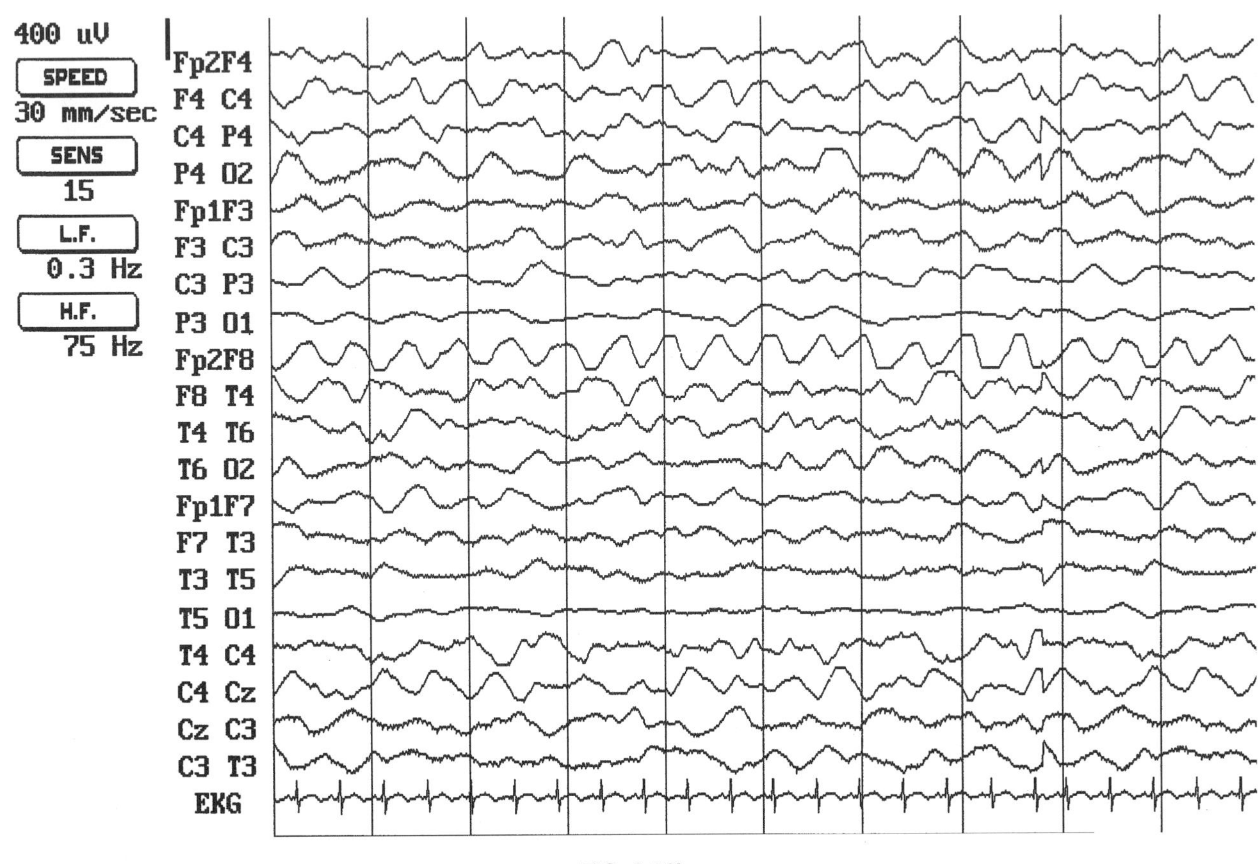
400 uV
SPEED
30 mm/sec
SENS
15
L.F.
0.3 Hz
H.F.
75 Hz
Fp2F4
F4 C4
C4 P4
P4 O2
Fp1F3
F3 C3
C3 P3
P3 O1
Fp2F8
F8 T4
T4 T6
T6 O2
Fp1F7
F7 T3
T3 T5
T5 O1
T4 C4
C4 Cz
Cz C3
C3 T3
EKG

FIG. 4-51b

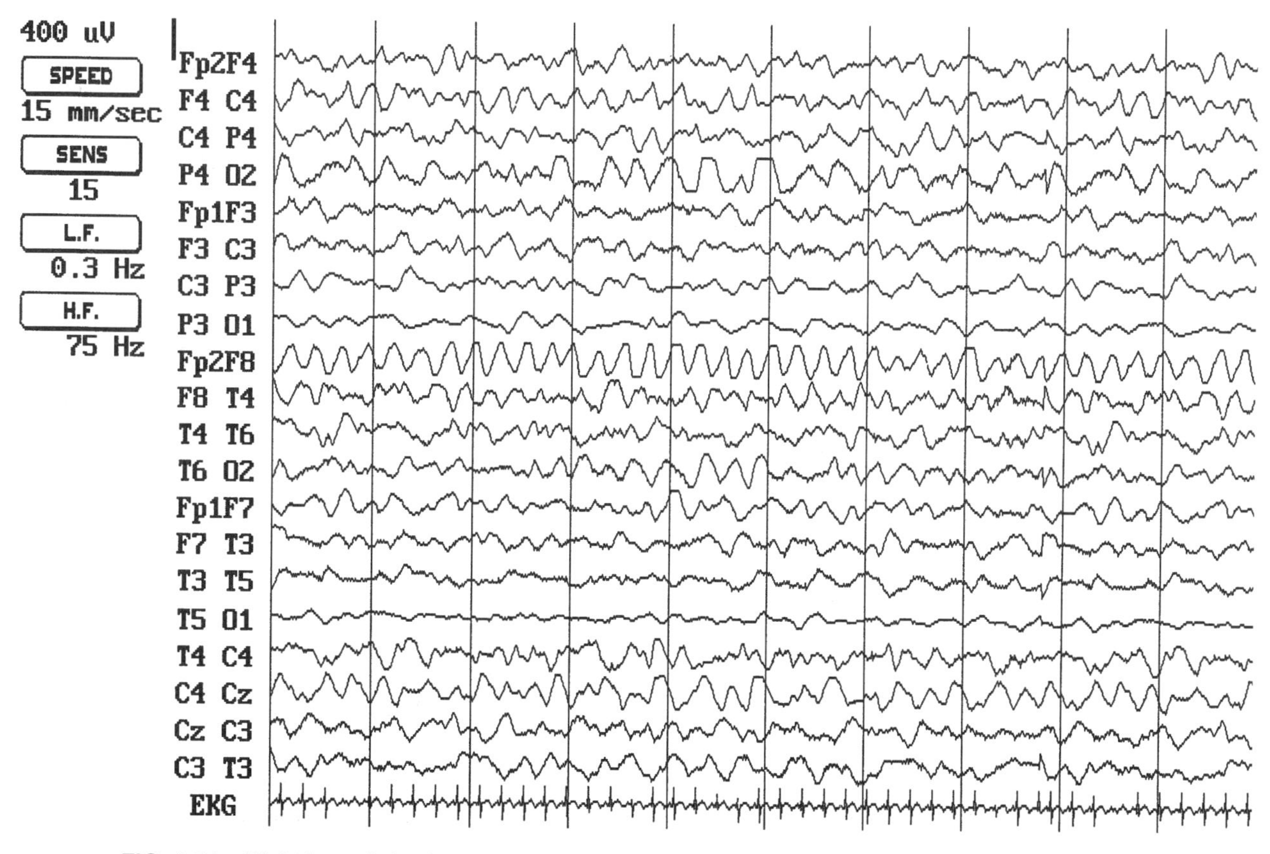

FIG. 4-51c Right frontal slowing is seen on run 1. Note the artifact at the 8th second. Faster delta phase reversals are seen at F8 and some slower delta at C4 are seen on run 2. These are most clear with PS for 15 mm/s.

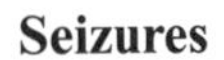

Seizures

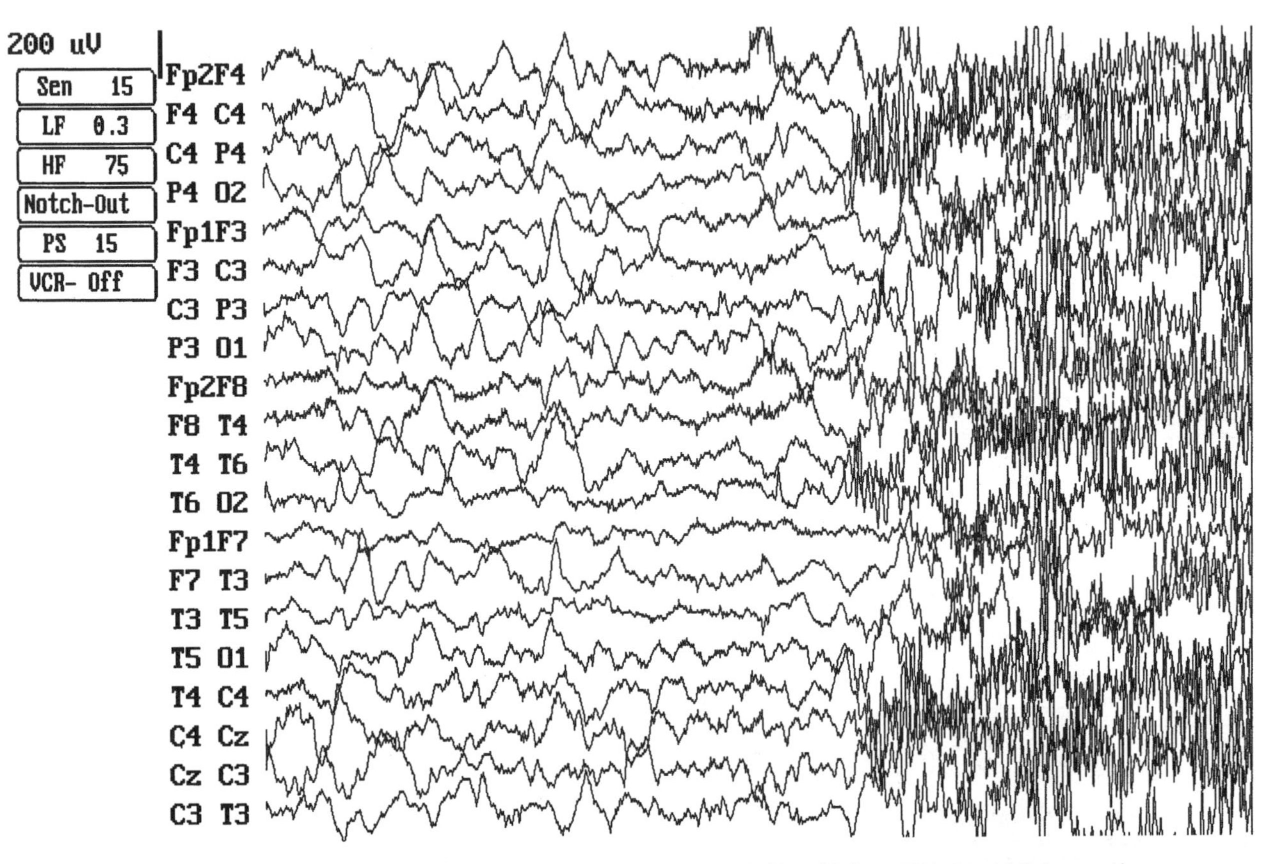

FIG. 4-52a,b,c,d A right hemispheric seizure is seen on run 2. Sensitivity = 15 is too high to see the seizure, but is good for seeing the preictal background. At sensitivity = 50, the ictal activity is seen better.

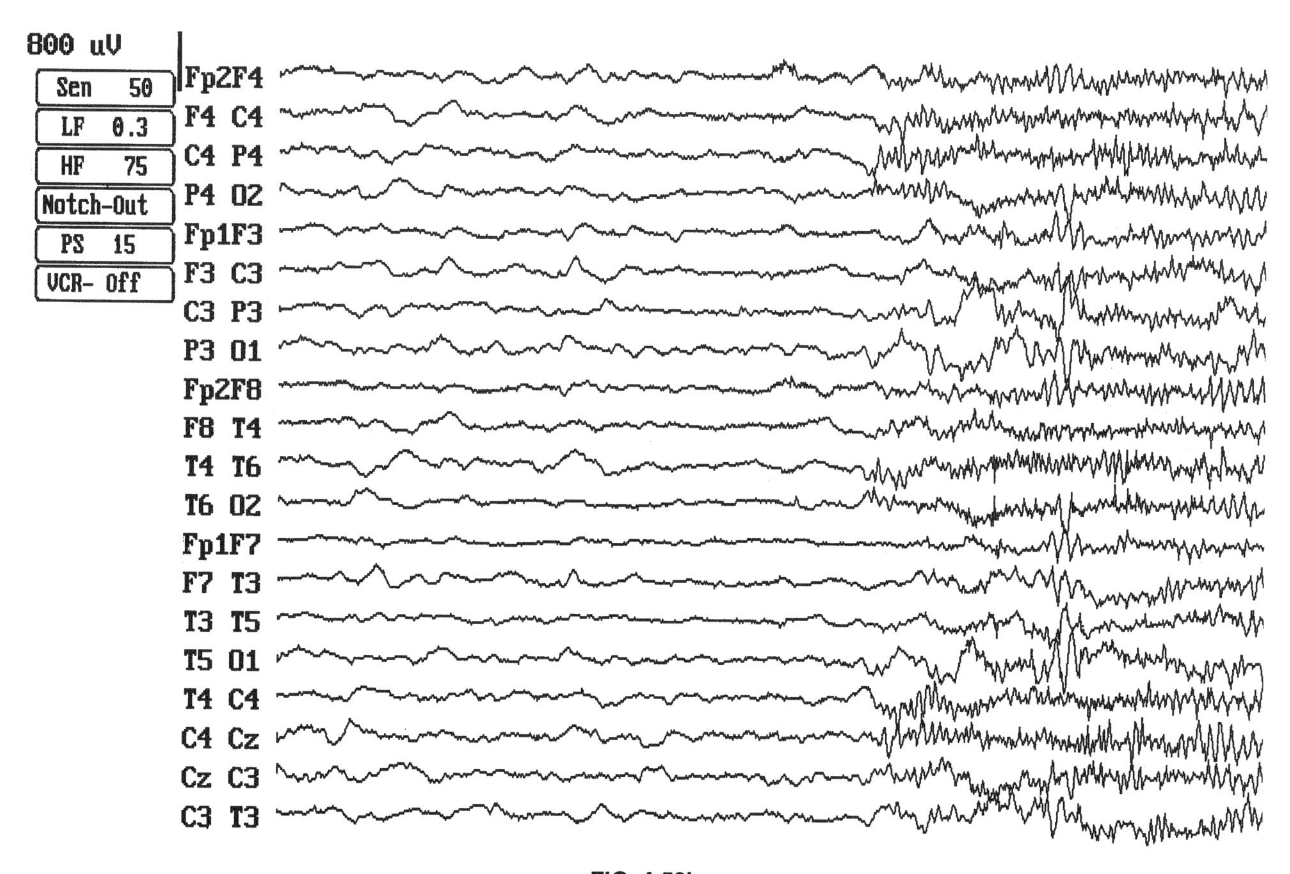
800 uV
Sen 50
LF 0.3
HF 75
Notch-Out
PS 15
VCR- Off
Fp2F4
F4 C4
C4 P4
P4 O2
Fp1F3
F3 C3
C3 P3
P3 O1
Fp2F8
F8 T4
T4 T6
T6 O2
Fp1F7
F7 T3
T3 T5
T5 O1
T4 C4
C4 Cz
Cz C3
C3 T3

FIG. 4-52b

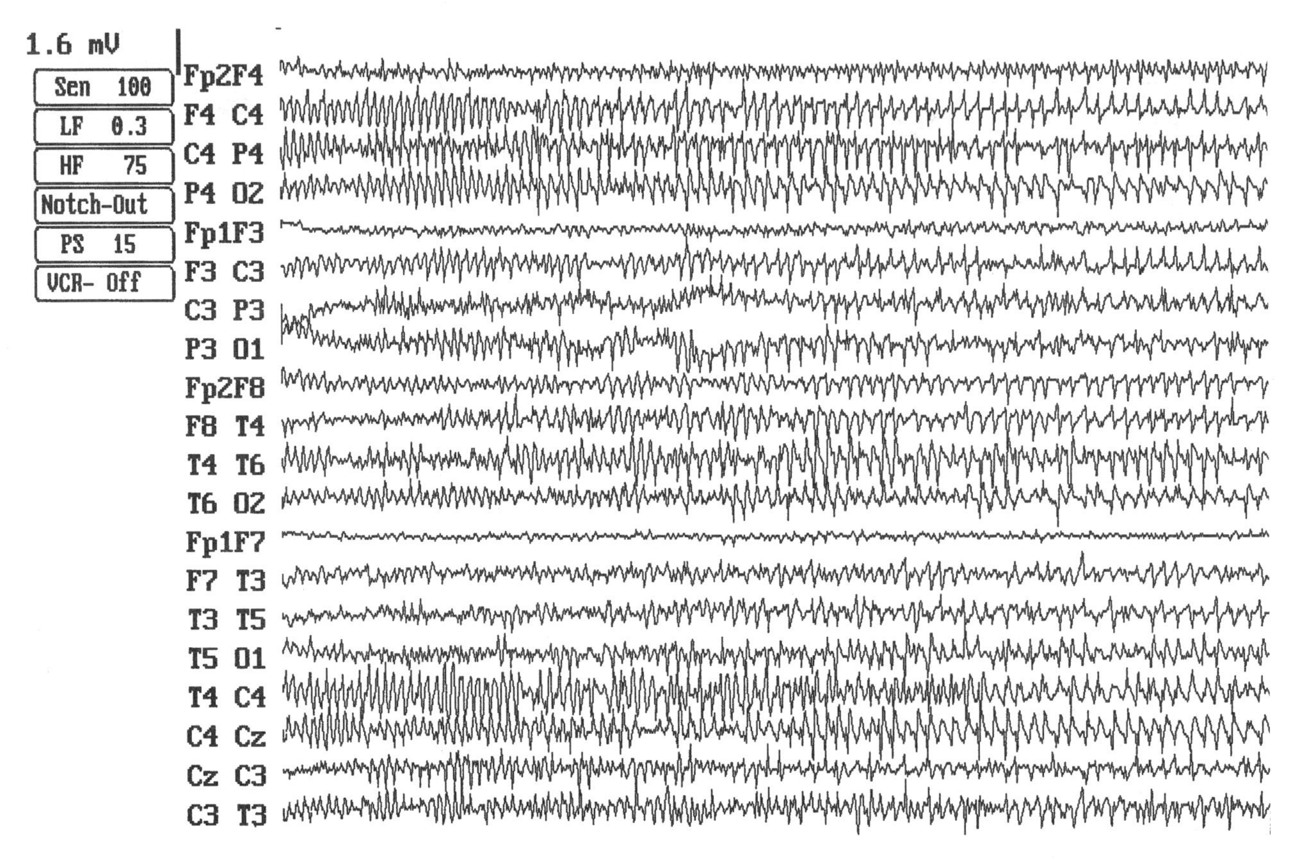
1.6 mV
Sen 100
LF 0.3
HF 75
Notch-Out
PS 15
VCR- Off
Fp2F4
F4 C4
C4 P4
P4 O2
Fp1F3
F3 C3
C3 P3
P3 O1
Fp2F8
F8 T4
T4 T6
T6 O2
Fp1F7
F7 T3
T3 T5
T5 O1
T4 C4
C4 Cz
Cz C3
C3 T3

FIG. 4-52c

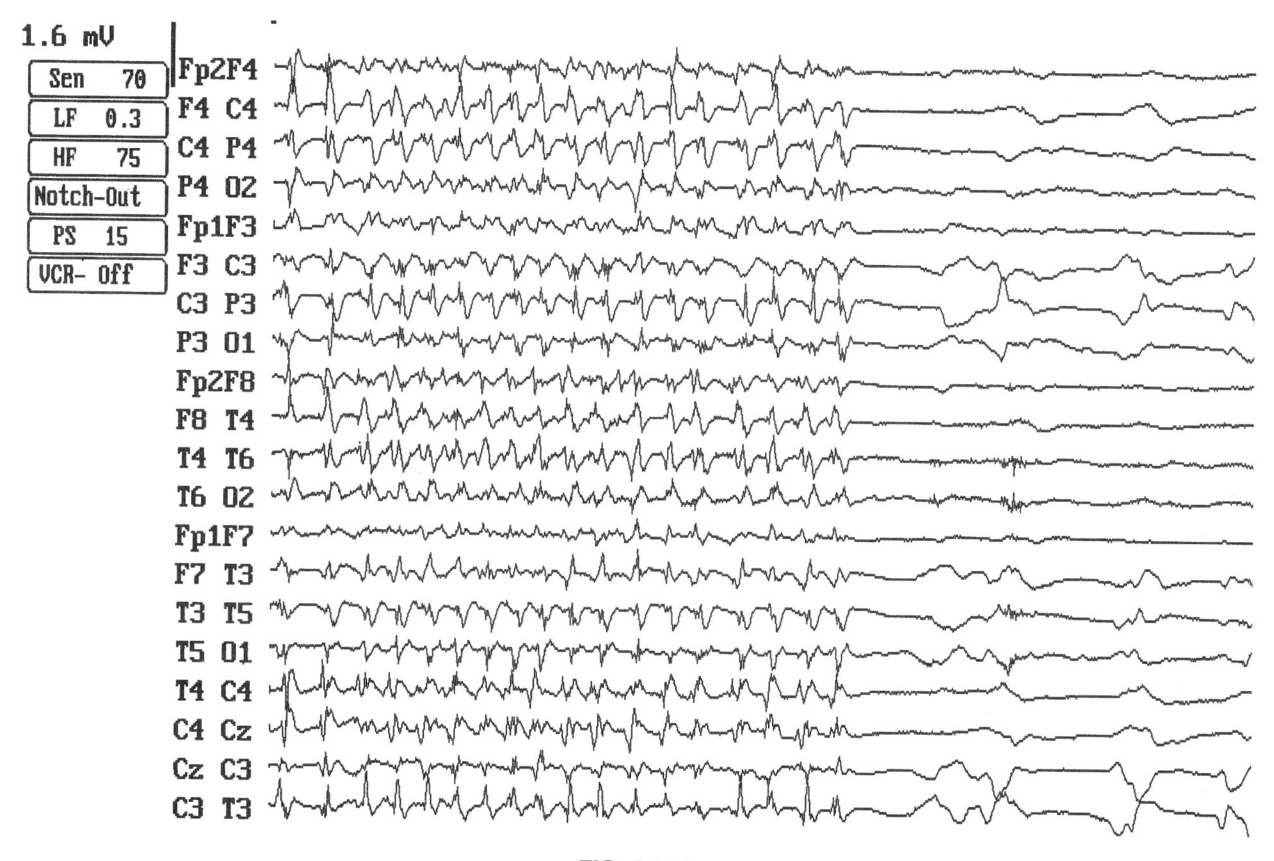
1.6 mV
Sen 70
LF 0.3
HF 75
Notch-Out
PS 15
VCR- Off
Fp2F4
F4 C4
C4 P4
P4 O2
Fp1F3
F3 C3
C3 P3
P3 O1
Fp2F8
F8 T4
T4 T6
T6 O2
Fp1F7
F7 T3
T3 T5
T5 O1
T4 C4
C4 Cz
Cz C3
C3 T3

FIG. 4-52d

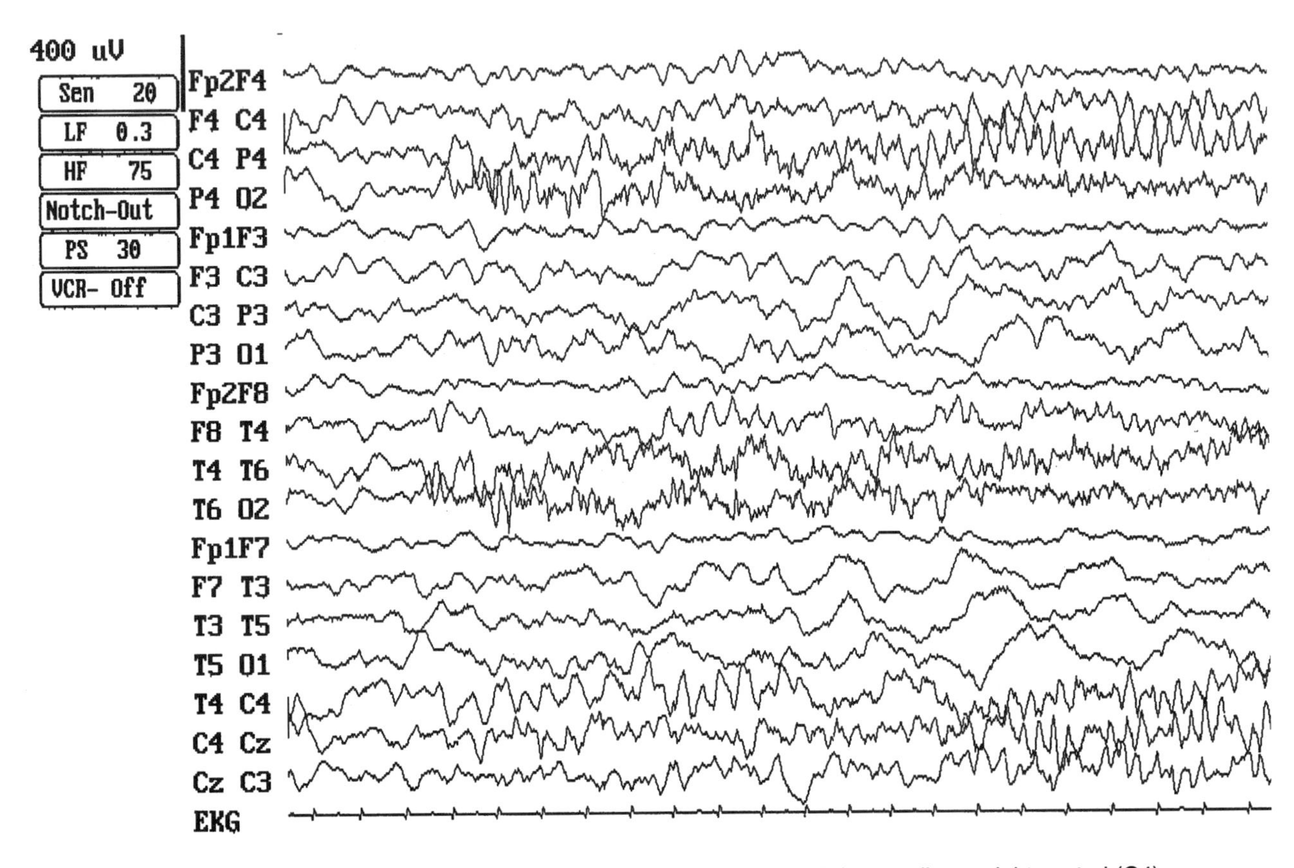

FIG. 4-53a,b,c,d This shows a right parietal temporal seizure (P4, T6) spreading to right central (C4) then to right temporal, later to the left hemisphere, ending with a strong ictal pattern at the left temporal area (run 2 throughout).

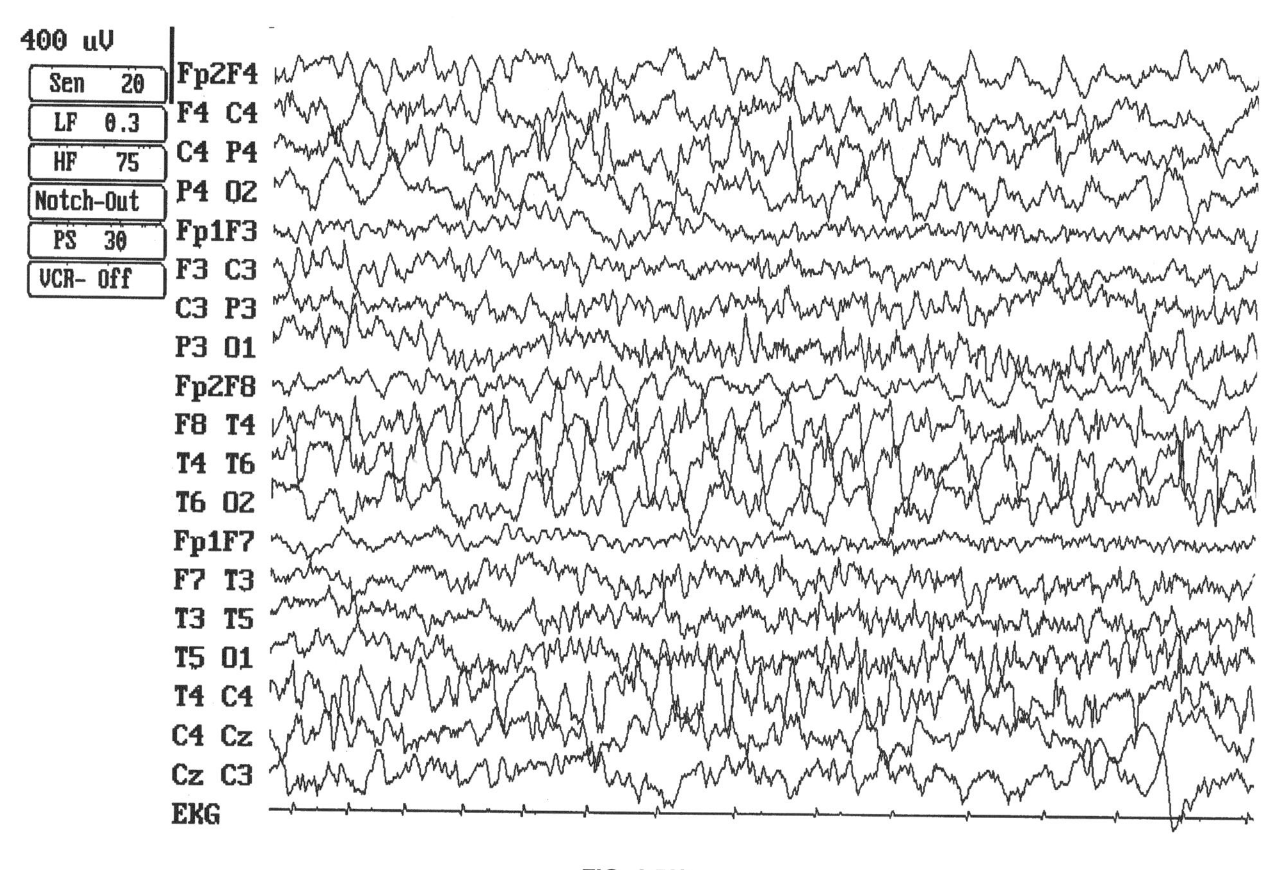
400 uV
Sen 20
LF 0.3
HF 75
Notch-Out
PS 30
VCR- Off
Fp2F4
F4 C4
C4 P4
P4 O2
Fp1F3
F3 C3
C3 P3
P3 O1
Fp2F8
F8 T4
T4 T6
T6 O2
Fp1F7
F7 T3
T3 T5
T5 O1
T4 C4
C4 Cz
Cz C3
EKG

FIG. 4-53b

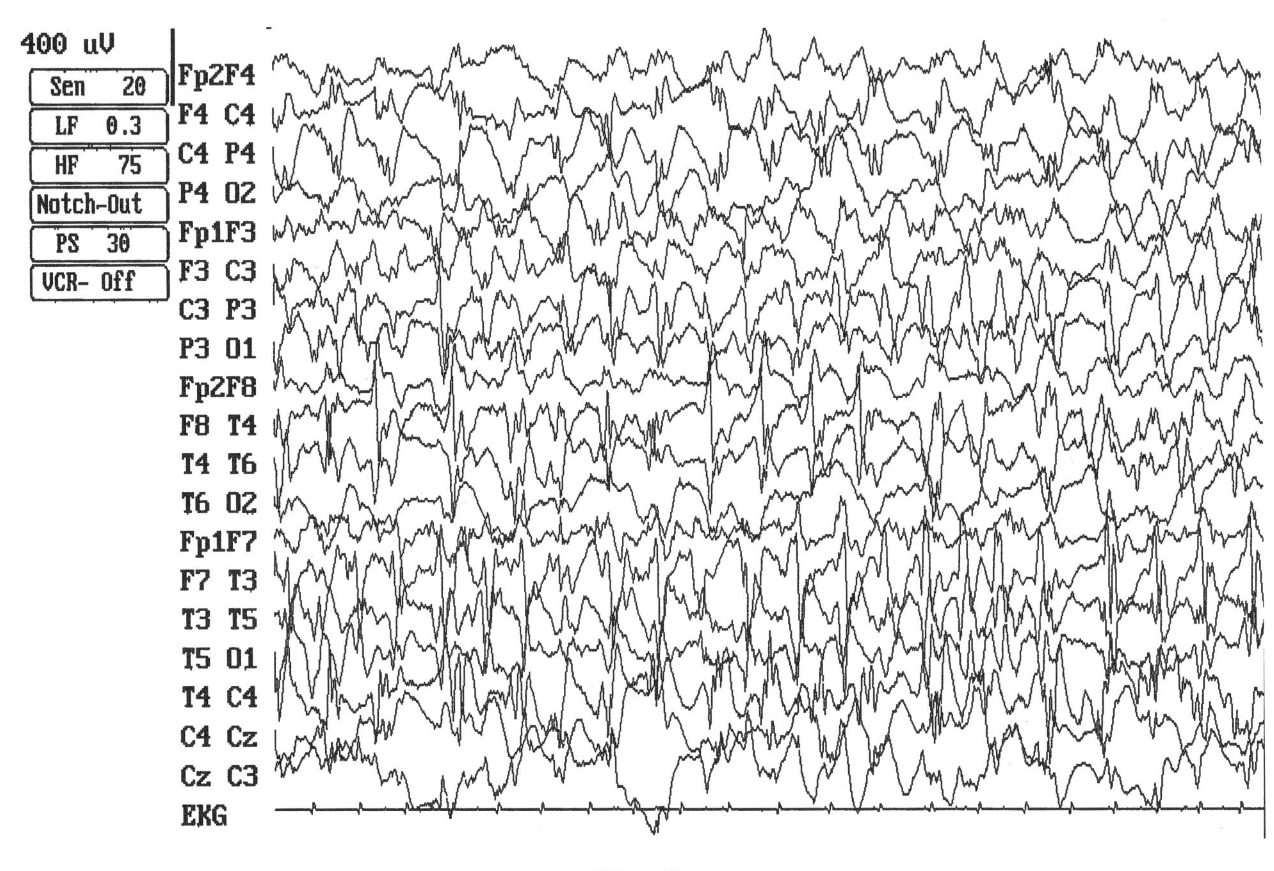
400 uV
Sen 20
LF 0.3
HF 75
Notch-Out
PS 30
VCR- Off
Fp2F4
F4 C4
C4 P4
P4 O2
Fp1F3
F3 C3
C3 P3
P3 O1
Fp2F8
F8 T4
T4 T6
T6 O2
Fp1F7
F7 T3
T3 T5
T5 O1
T4 C4
C4 Cz
Cz C3
EKG

FIG. 4-53c

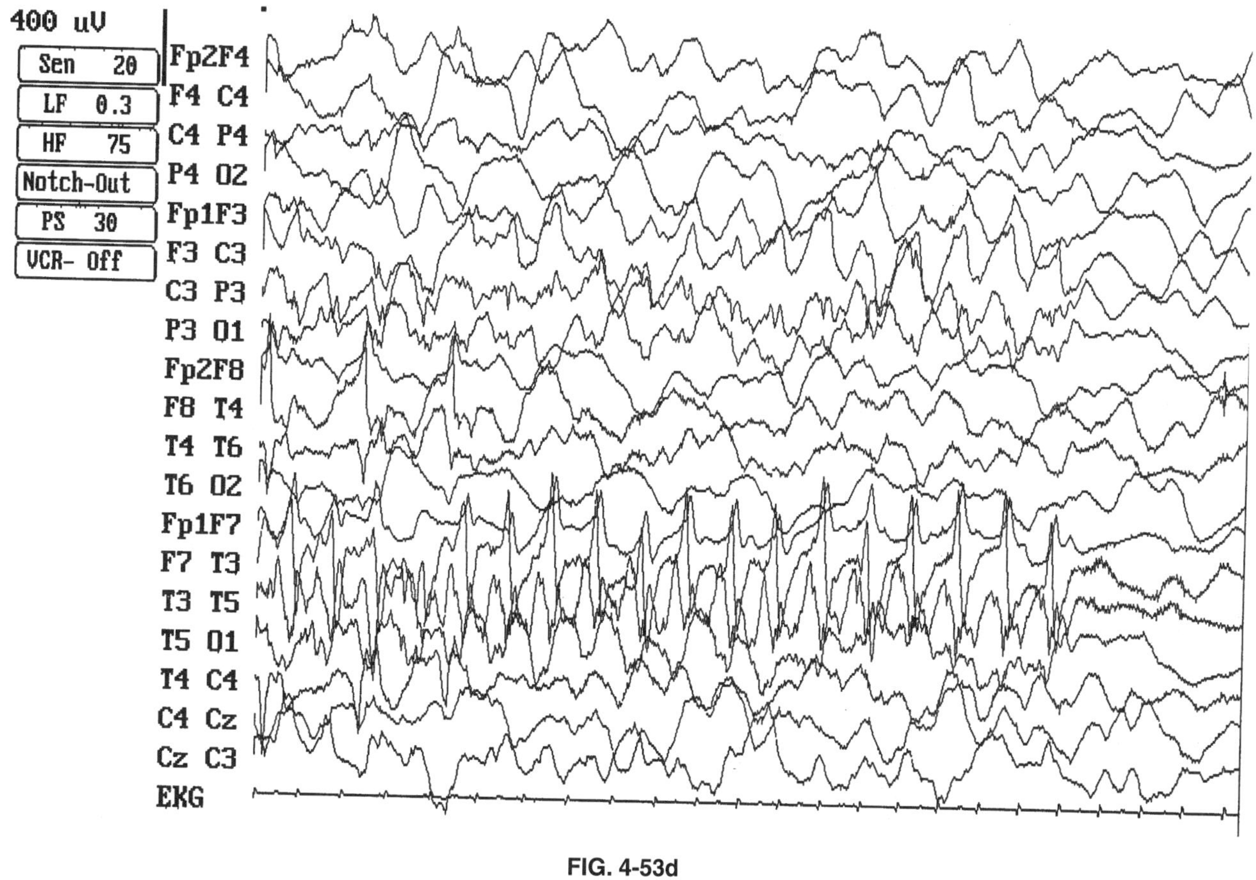
400 uV
Sen 20
LF 0.3
HF 75
Notch-Out
PS 30
VCR- Off
Fp2F4
F4 C4
C4 P4
P4 O2
Fp1F3
F3 C3
C3 P3
P3 O1
Fp2F8
F8 T4
T4 T6
T6 O2
Fp1F7
F7 T3
T3 T5
T5 O1
T4 C4
C4 Cz
Cz C3
EKG

FIG. 4-53d

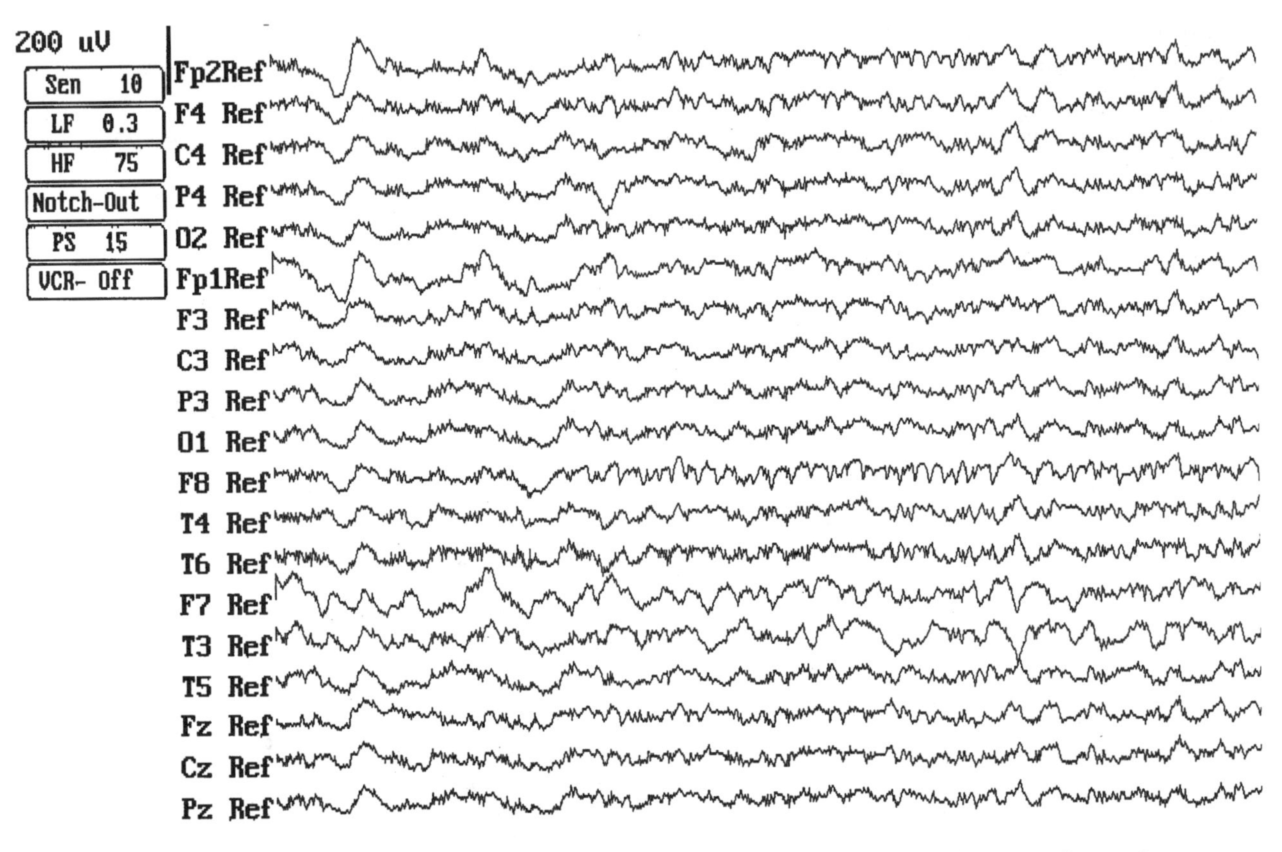

FIG. 4-54a,b,c This shows a right anterior temporal seizure vaguely seen at F8 on run 1. On run 2 the ictal onset is seen much better. The development of the ictal pattern is shown 10 s later.

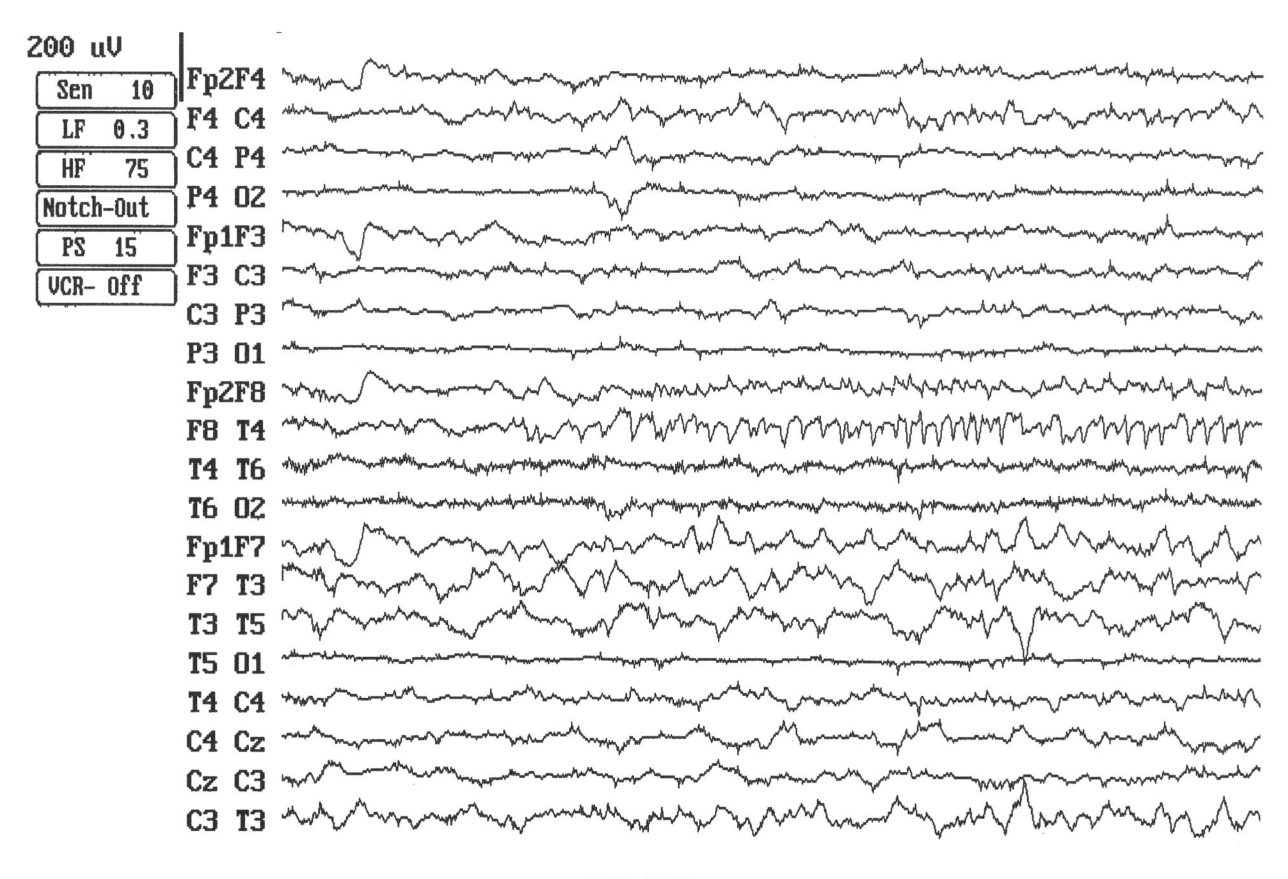
200 uV
Sen 10
LF 0.3
HF 75
Notch-Out
PS 15
VCR- Off
Fp2F4
F4 C4
C4 P4
P4 O2
Fp1F3
F3 C3
C3 P3
P3 O1
Fp2F8
F8 T4
T4 T6
T6 O2
Fp1F7
F7 T3
T3 T5
T5 O1
T4 C4
C4 Cz
Cz C3
C3 T3

FIG. 4-54b

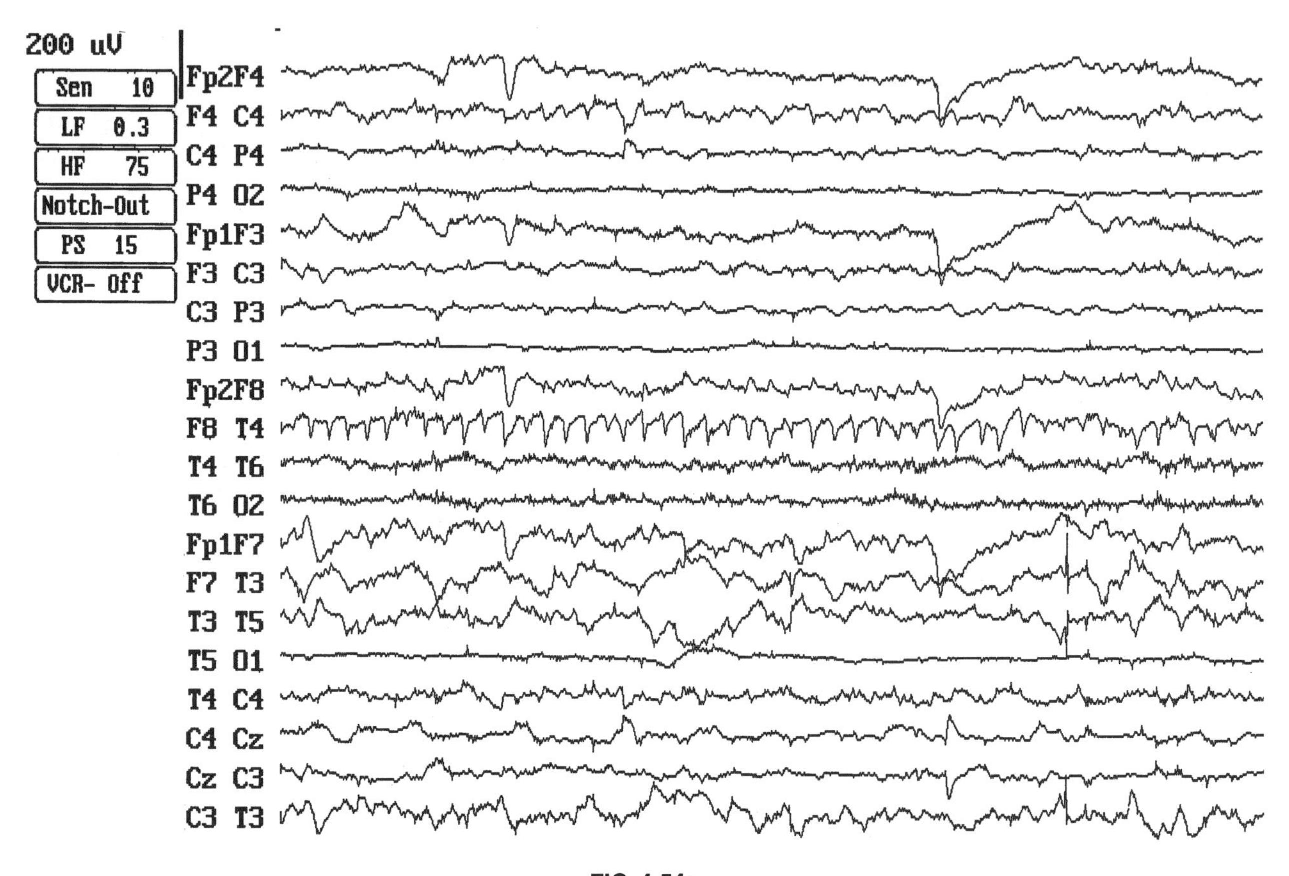
200 uV
Sen 10
LF 0.3
HF 75
Notch-Out
PS 15
VCR- Off
Fp2F4
F4 C4
C4 P4
P4 O2
Fp1F3
F3 C3
C3 P3
P3 O1
Fp2F8
F8 T4
T4 T6
T6 O2
Fp1F7
F7 T3
T3 T5
T5 O1
T4 C4
C4 Cz
Cz C3
C3 T3

FIG. 4-54c

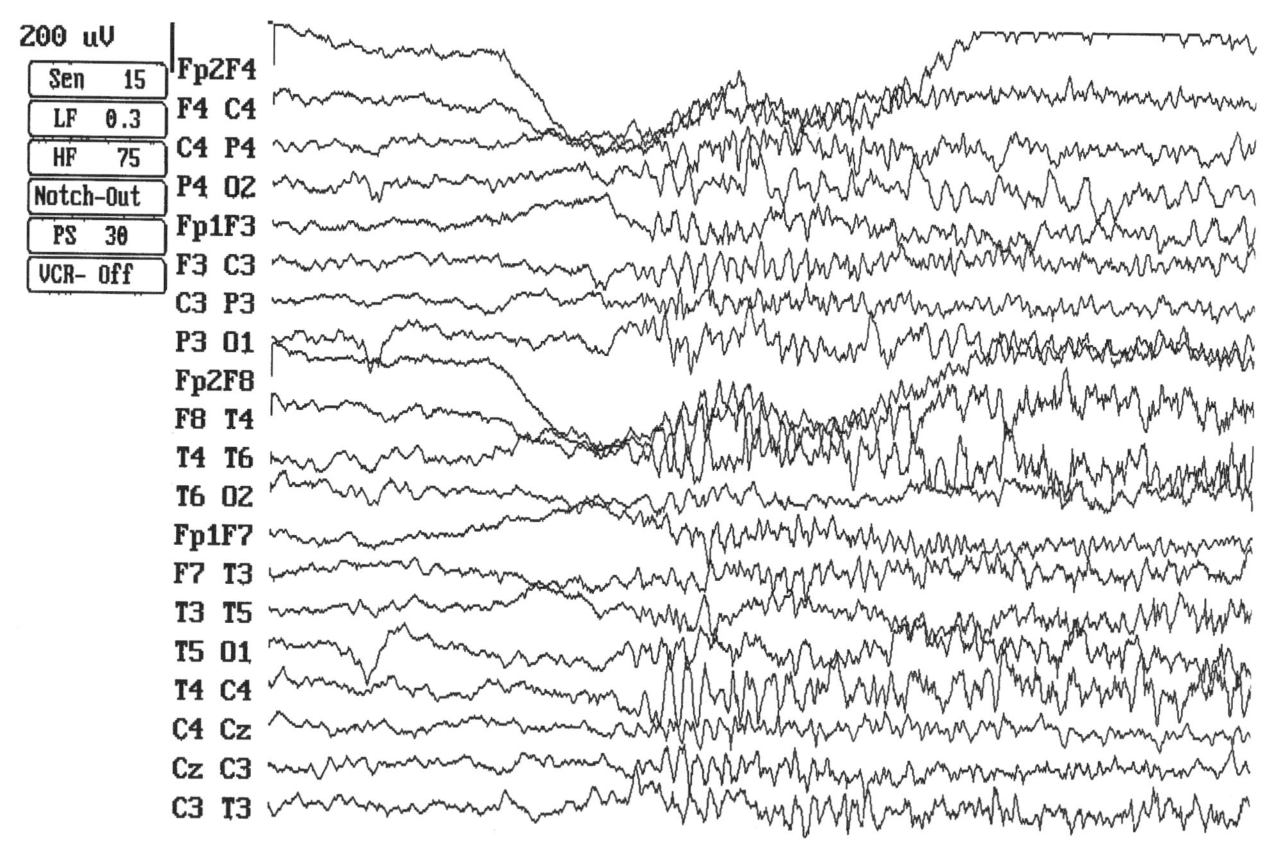

FIG. 4-55a,b,c,d,e This example shows a generalized seizure consisting of diffuse theta then delta. Run 2 shows the eye movements obscuring the ictal onset, whereas run 1 shows the onset better. Subsequent ictal development continues on run 2 without problems with the ictus ending at P3.

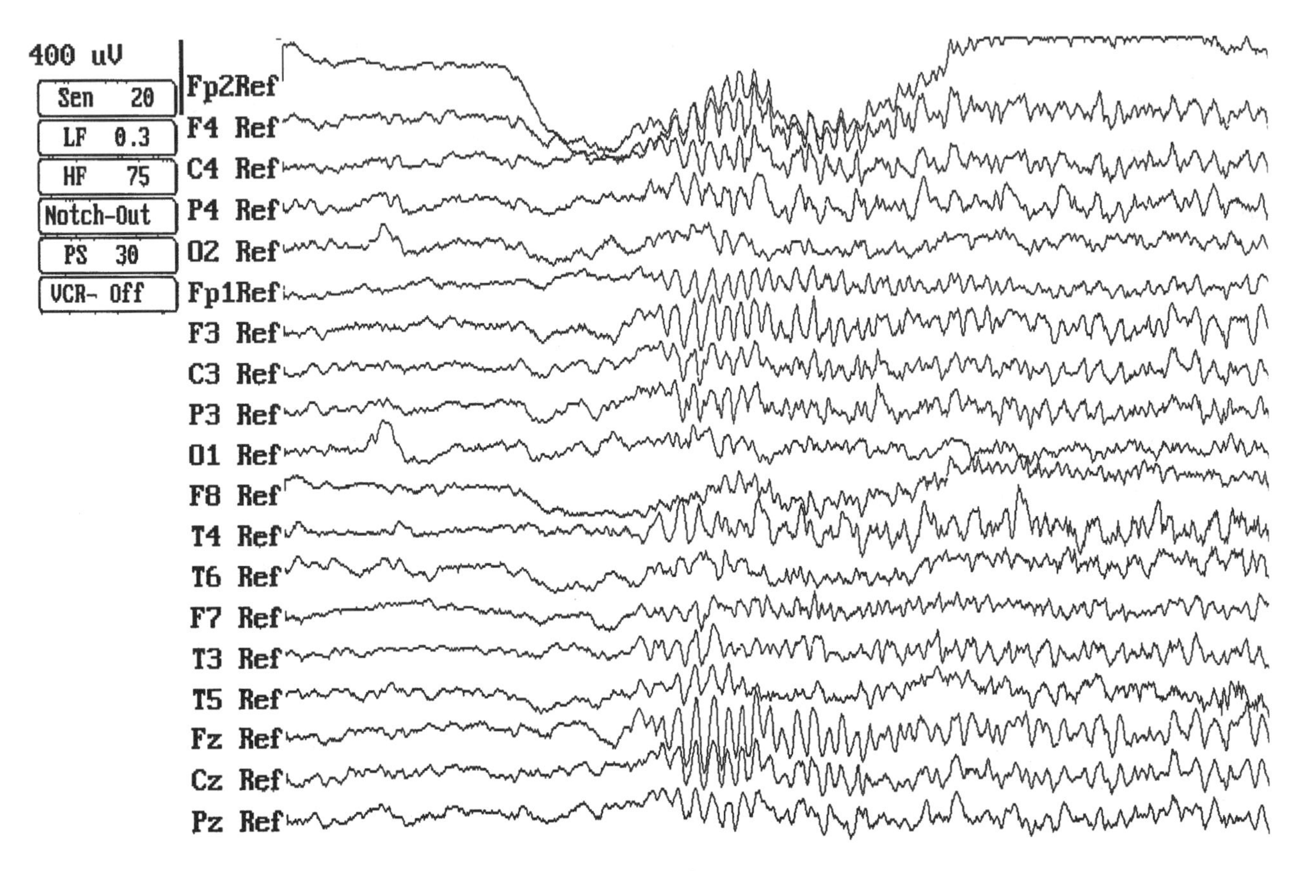
400 uV
Sen 20
LF 0.3
HF 75
Notch-Out
PS 30
VCR- Off
Fp2Ref
F4 Ref
C4 Ref
P4 Ref
O2 Ref
Fp1Ref
F3 Ref
C3 Ref
P3 Ref
O1 Ref
F8 Ref
T4 Ref
T6 Ref
F7 Ref
T3 Ref
T5 Ref
Fz Ref
Cz Ref
Pz Ref

FIG. 4-55b

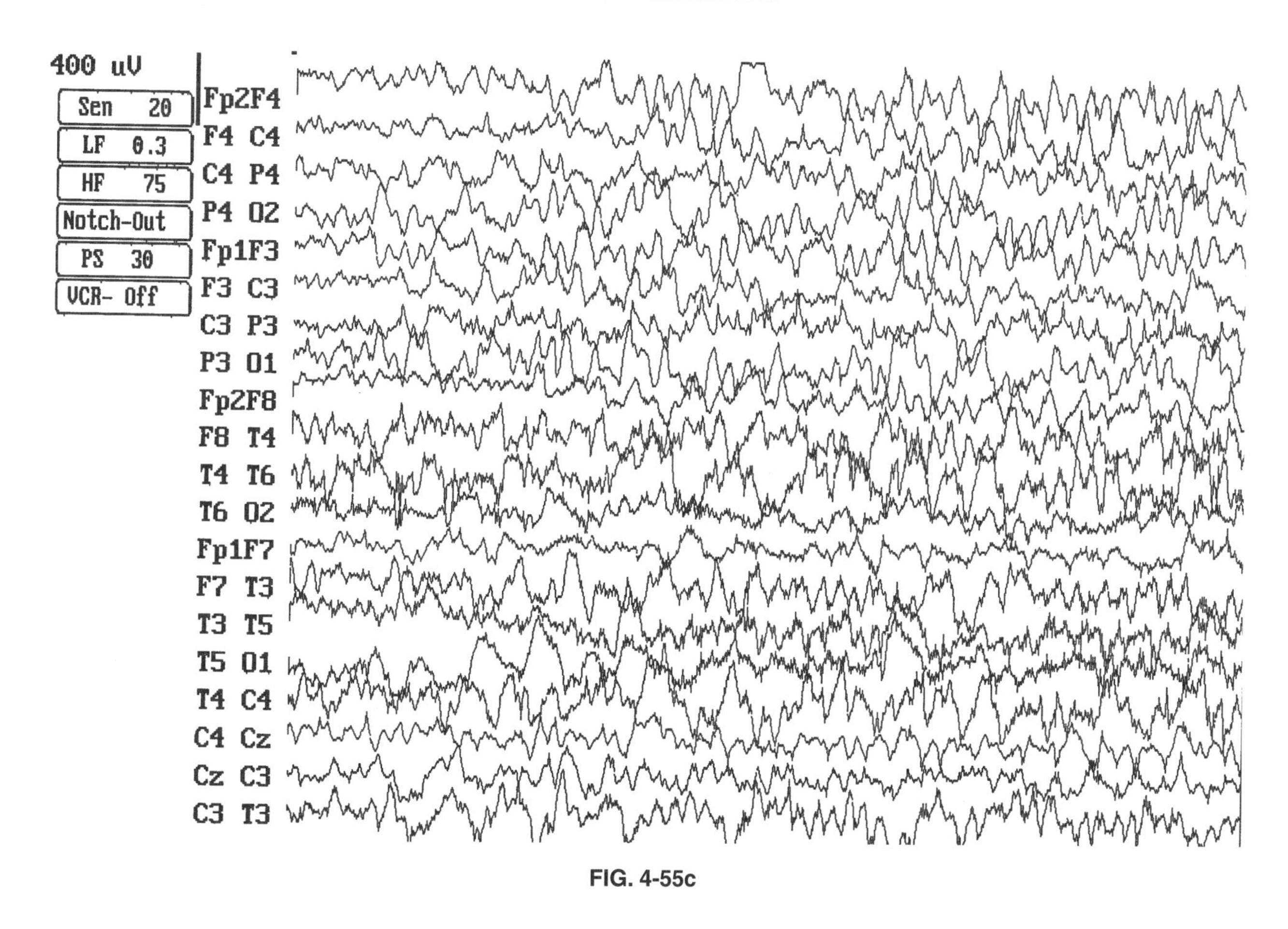
400 uV
Sen 20
LF 0.3
HF 75
Notch-Out
PS 30
VCR- Off
Fp2F4
F4 C4
C4 P4
P4 O2
Fp1F3
F3 C3
C3 P3
P3 O1
Fp2F8
F8 T4
T4 T6
T6 O2
Fp1F7
F7 T3
T3 T5
T5 O1
T4 C4
C4 Cz
Cz C3
C3 T3

FIG. 4-55c

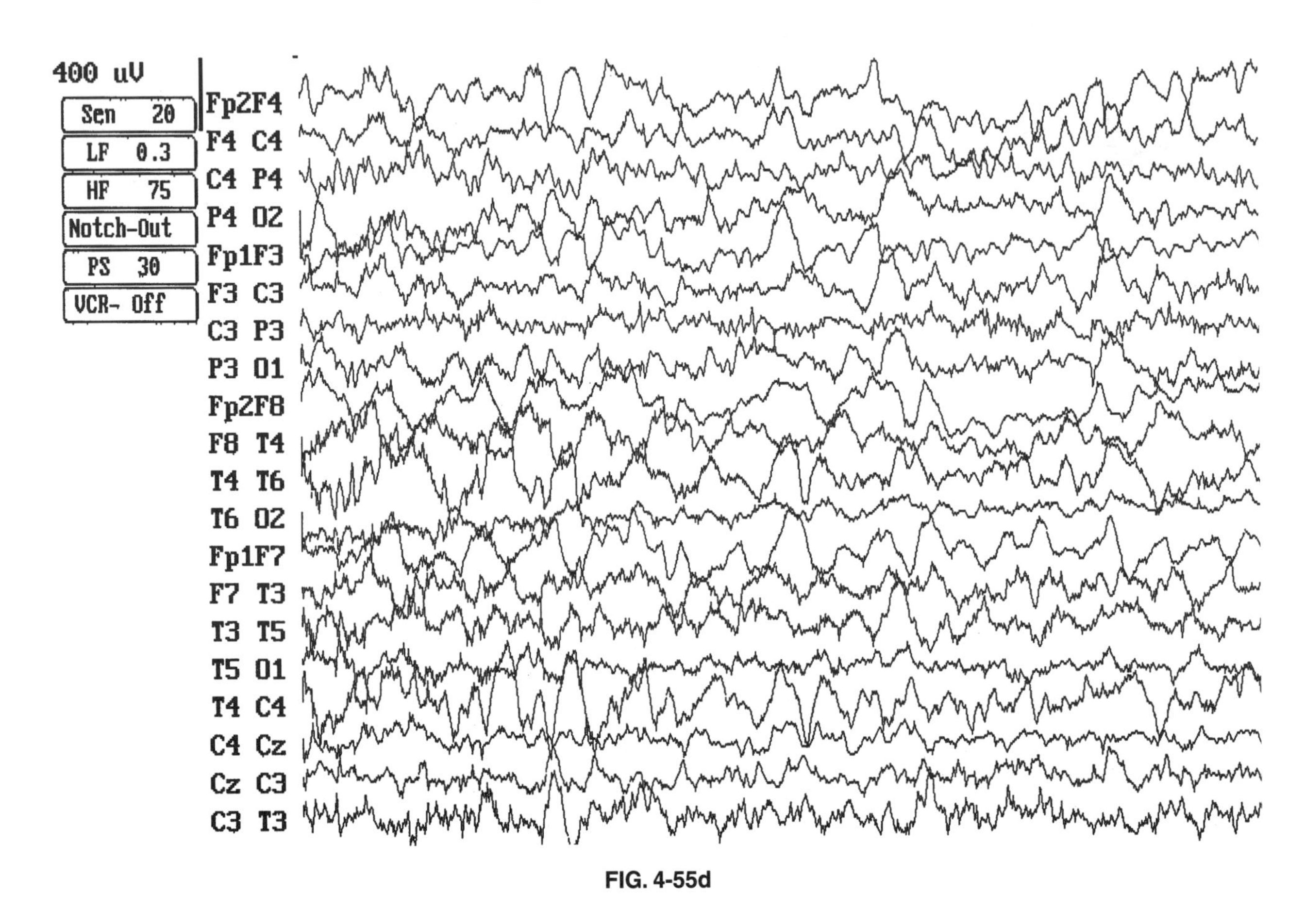
400 uV
Sen 20
LF 0.3
HF 75
Notch-Out
PS 30
VCR- Off
Fp2F4
F4 C4
C4 P4
P4 O2
Fp1F3
F3 C3
C3 P3
P3 O1
Fp2F8
F8 T4
T4 T6
T6 O2
Fp1F7
F7 T3
T3 T5
T5 O1
T4 C4
C4 Cz
Cz C3
C3 T3

FIG. 4-55d

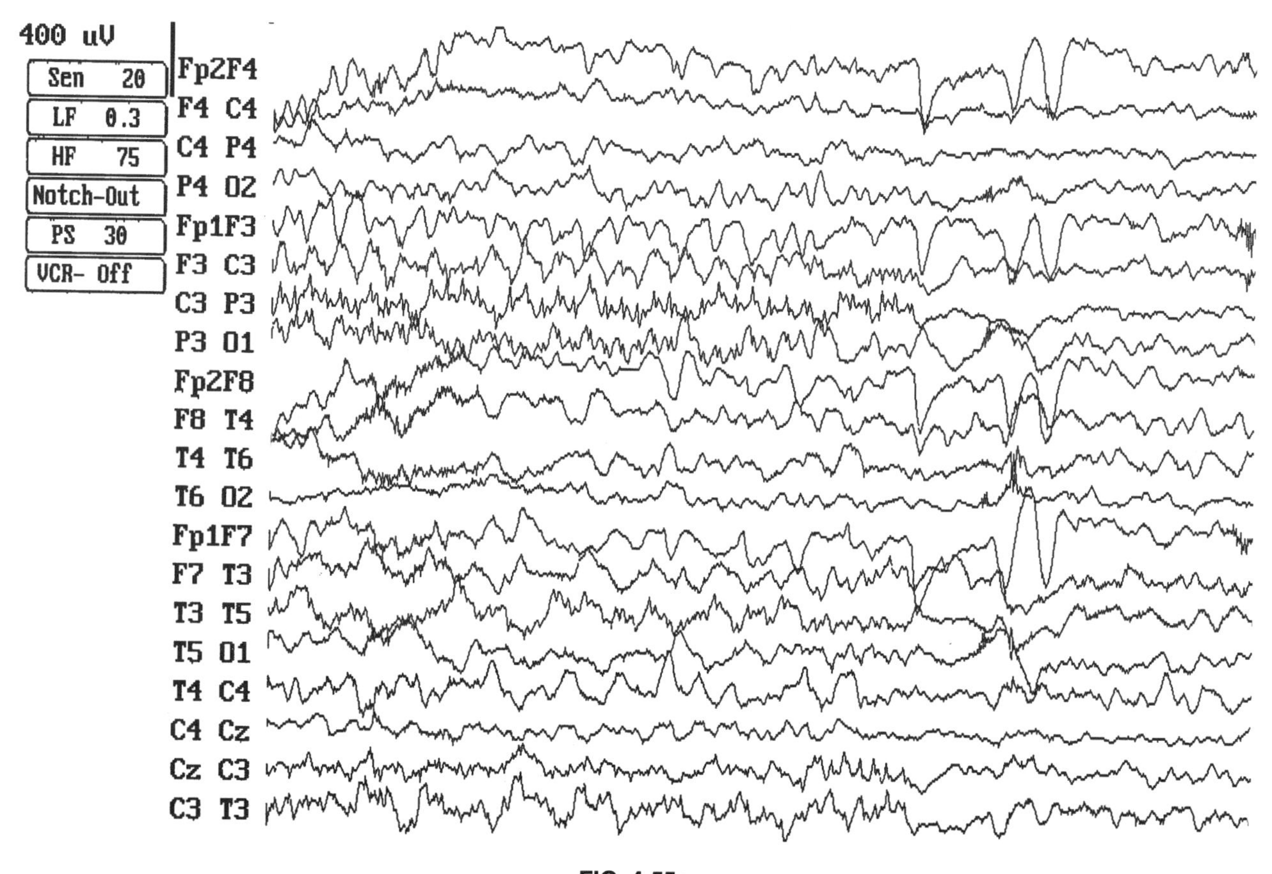
400 uV
Sen 20
LF 0.3
HF 75
Notch-Out
PS 30
VCR- Off
Fp2F4
F4 C4
C4 P4
P4 O2
Fp1F3
F3 C3
C3 P3
P3 O1
Fp2F8
F8 T4
T4 T6
T6 O2
Fp1F7
F7 T3
T3 T5
T5 O1
T4 C4
C4 Cz
Cz C3
C3 T3

FIG. 4-55e

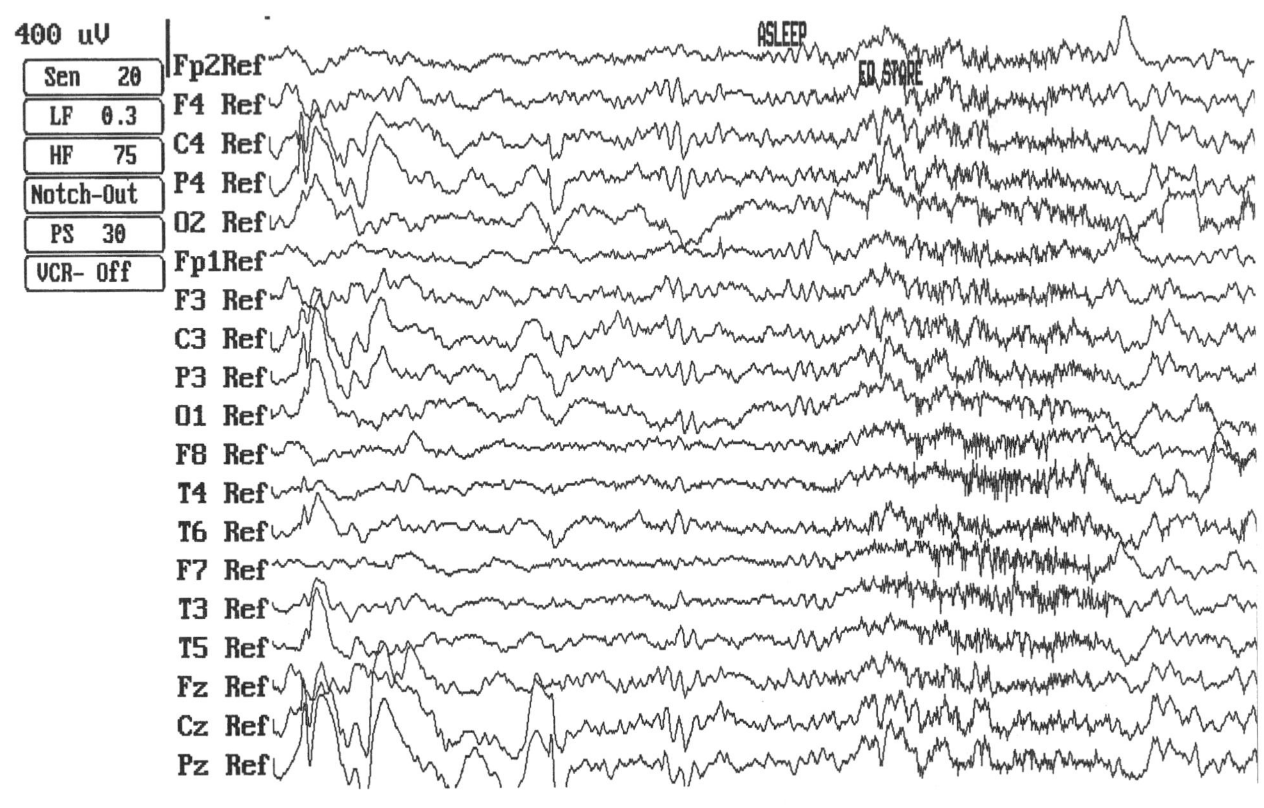

FIG. 4-56a,b,c,d,e This is a generalized tonic clonic seizure showing the use of different sensitivities during the entire seizure (all run 1). First, the ictal onset was recorded at sensitivity = 20, and then increasing the sensitivity to 30 and 50 to accommodate the higher amplitude activity. At ictal offset, sensitivity = 30 is used to see the offset background clearly.

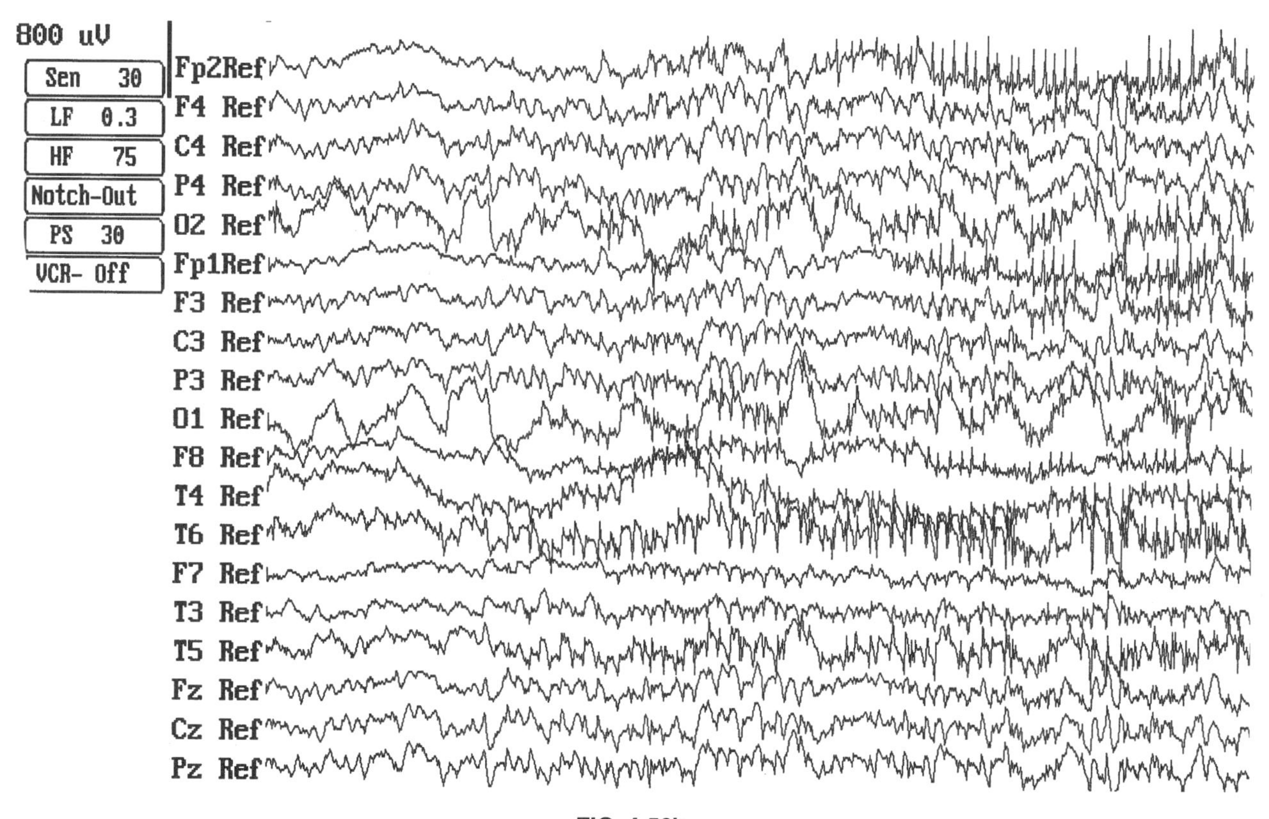
800 uV
Sen 30
LF 0.3
HF 75
Notch-Out
PS 30
VCR- Off
Fp2Ref
F4 Ref
C4 Ref
P4 Ref
O2 Ref
Fp1Ref
F3 Ref
C3 Ref
P3 Ref
O1 Ref
F8 Ref
T4 Ref
T6 Ref
F7 Ref
T3 Ref
T5 Ref
Fz Ref
Cz Ref
Pz Ref

FIG. 4-56b

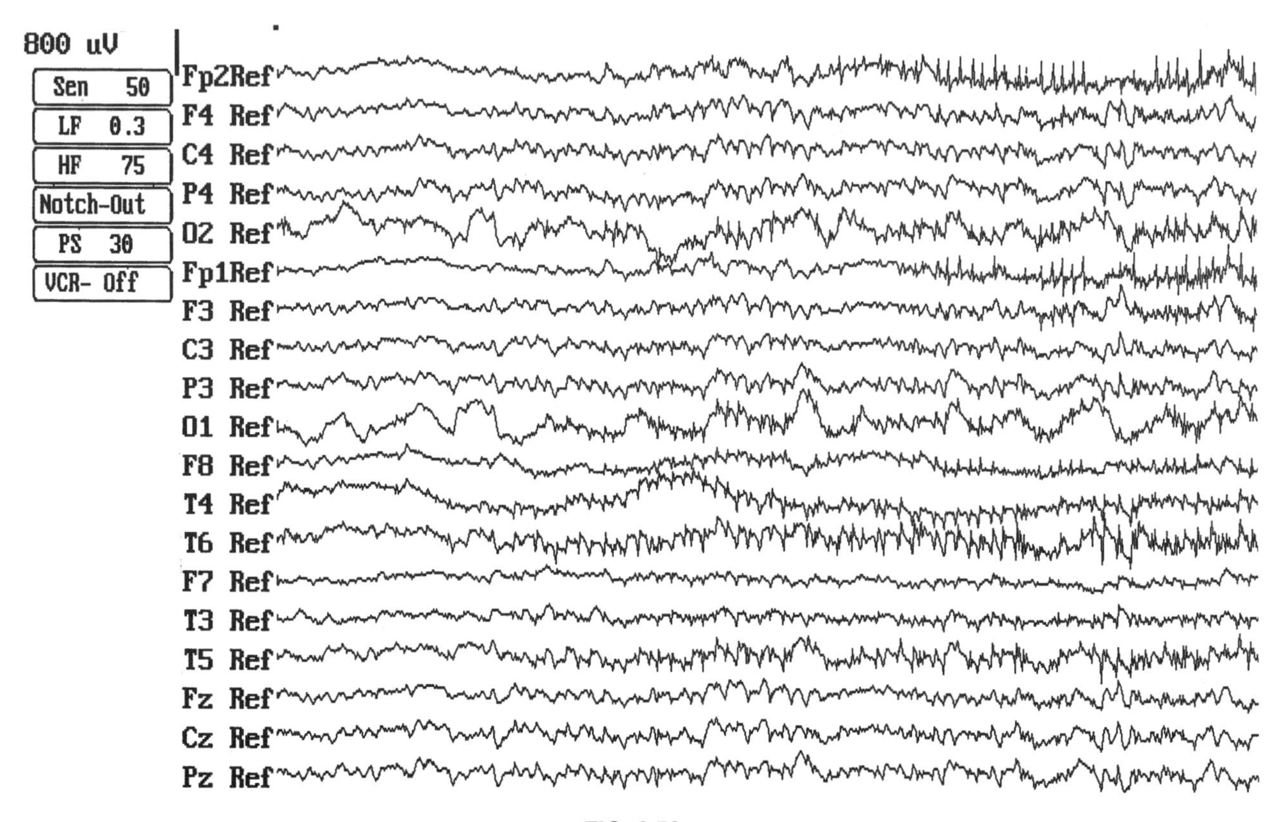
800 uV
Sen 50
LF 0.3
HF 75
Notch-Out
PS 30
VCR- Off
Fp2Ref
F4 Ref
C4 Ref
P4 Ref
O2 Ref
Fp1Ref
F3 Ref
C3 Ref
P3 Ref
O1 Ref
F8 Ref
T4 Ref
T6 Ref
F7 Ref
T3 Ref
T5 Ref
Fz Ref
Cz Ref
Pz Ref

FIG. 4-56c

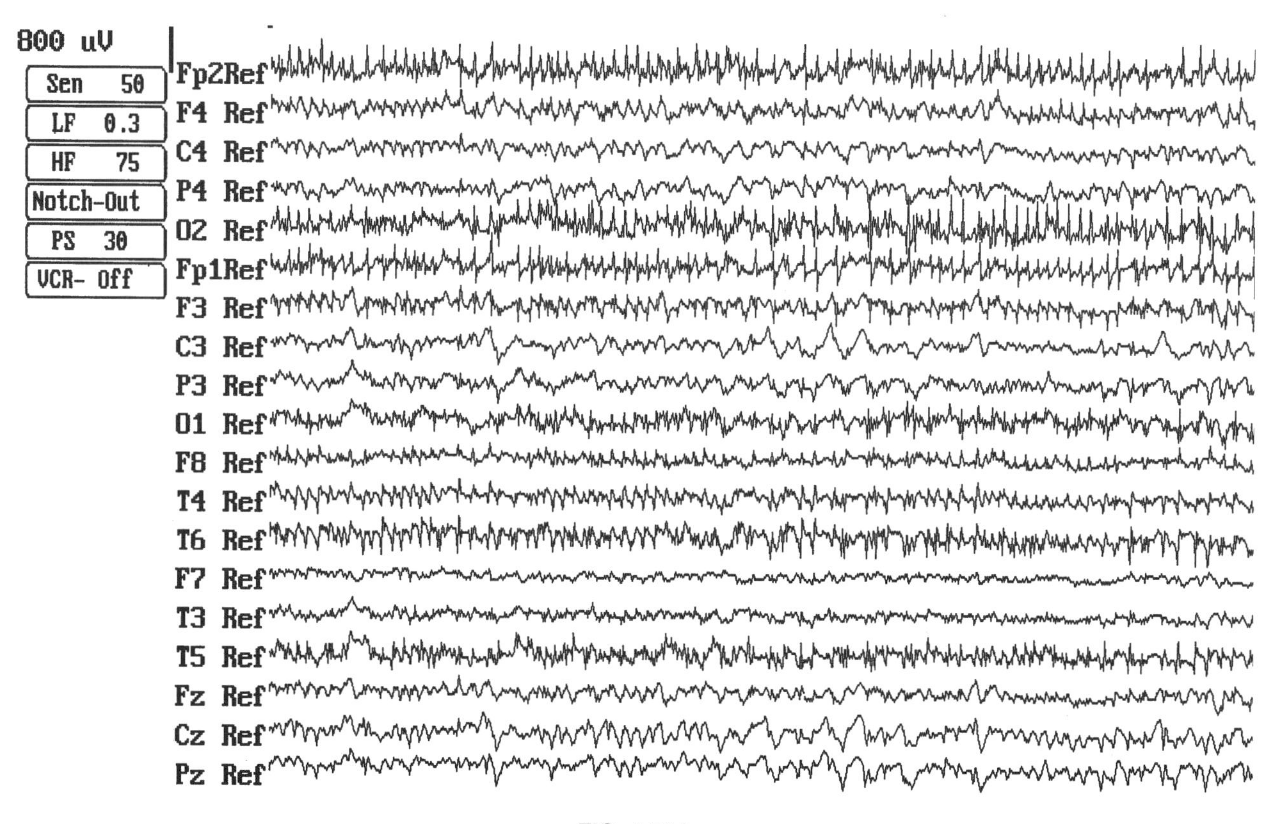
800 uV
Sen 50
LF 0.3
HF 75
Notch-Out
PS 30
VCR- Off
Fp2Ref
F4 Ref
C4 Ref
P4 Ref
O2 Ref
Fp1Ref
F3 Ref
C3 Ref
P3 Ref
O1 Ref
F8 Ref
T4 Ref
T6 Ref
F7 Ref
T3 Ref
T5 Ref
Fz Ref
Cz Ref
Pz Ref

FIG. 4-56d

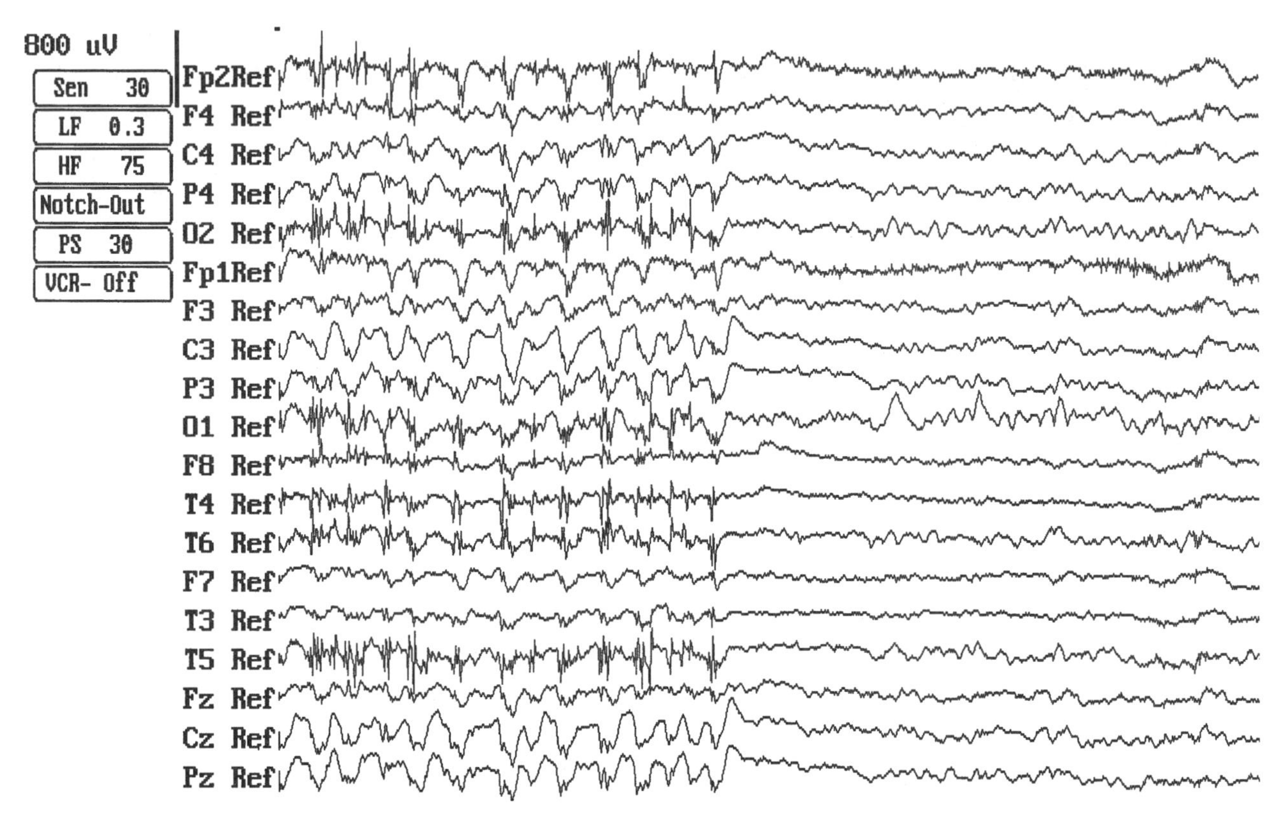
800 uV
Sen 30
LF 0.3
HF 75
Notch-Out
PS 30
VCR- Off
Fp2Ref
F4 Ref
C4 Ref
P4 Ref
O2 Ref
Fp1Ref
F3 Ref
C3 Ref
P3 Ref
O1 Ref
F8 Ref
T4 Ref
T6 Ref
F7 Ref
T3 Ref
T5 Ref
Fz Ref
Cz Ref
Pz Ref

FIG. 4-56e

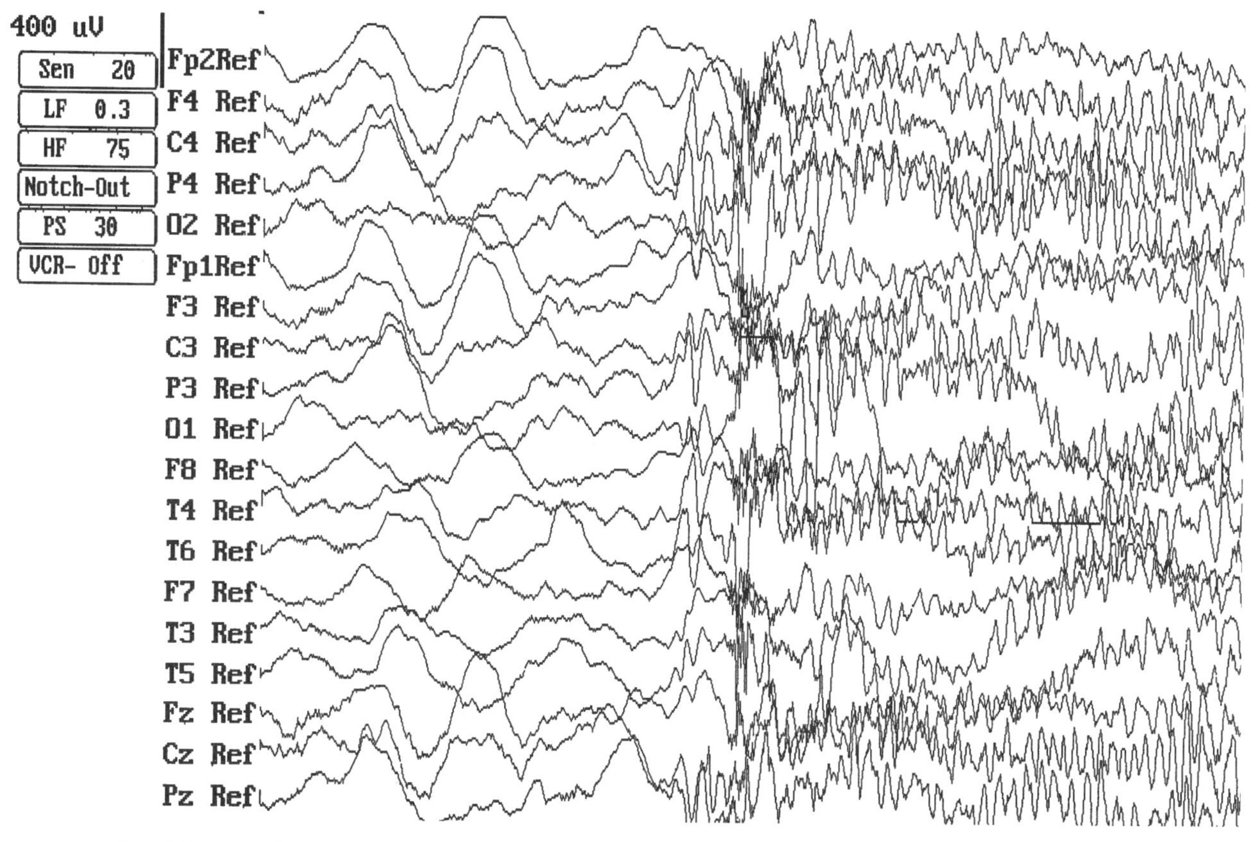

FIG. 4-57a,b,c,d,e,f,g,h In this generalized tonic clonic seizure the ictal onset is seen at sensitivity = 20 and 50. Note the slightly earlier right sided onset. The development of ictus required sensitivity = 100 to avoid clipping. Despite sensitivity = 100 (e) there was some amplifier saturation seen at C4 (flat top and bottom of large waveforms). To appreciate the markedly suppressed offset background, sensitivity = 20 is required.

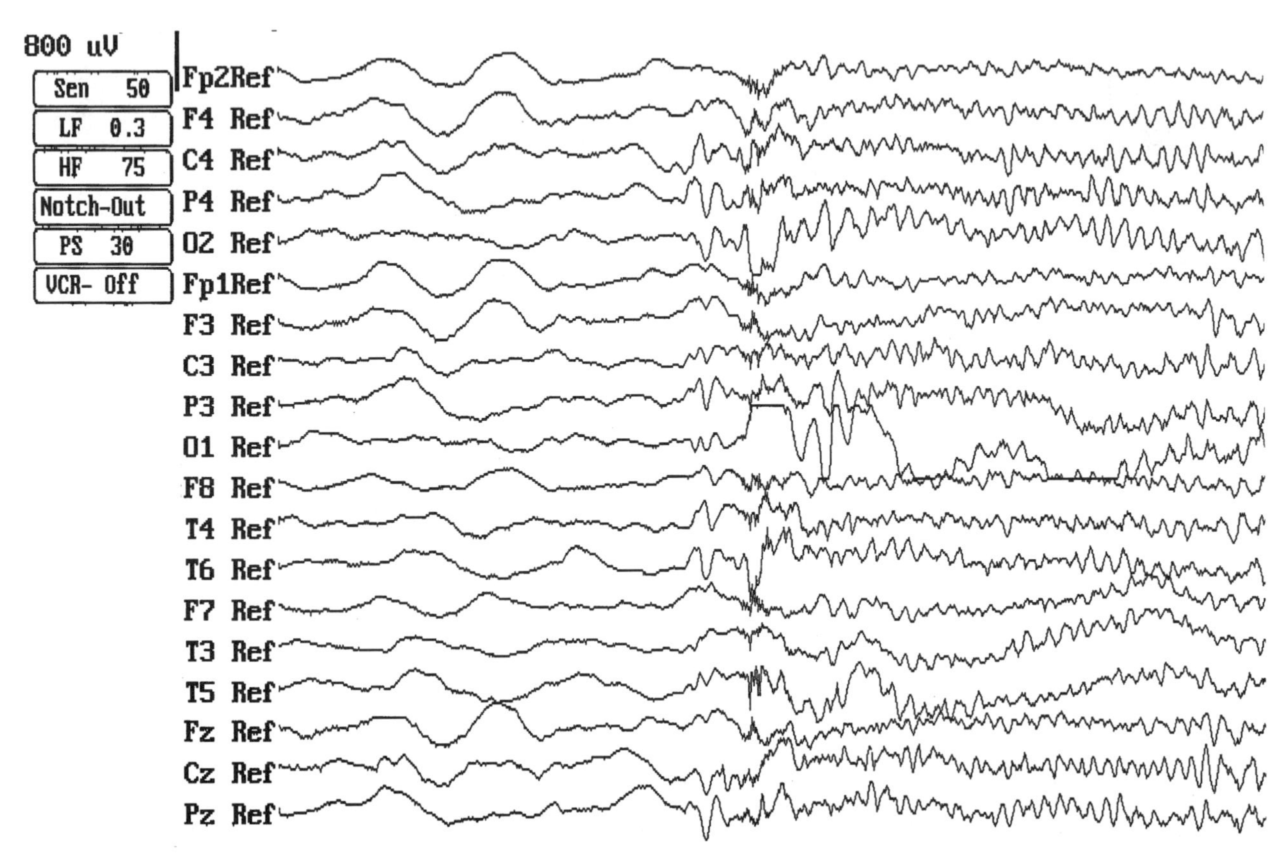
800 uV
Sen 50
LF 0.3
HF 75
Notch-Out
PS 30
VCR- Off
Fp2Ref
F4 Ref
C4 Ref
P4 Ref
O2 Ref
Fp1Ref
F3 Ref
C3 Ref
P3 Ref
O1 Ref
F8 Ref
T4 Ref
T6 Ref
F7 Ref
T3 Ref
T5 Ref
Fz Ref
Cz Ref
Pz Ref

FIG. 4-57b

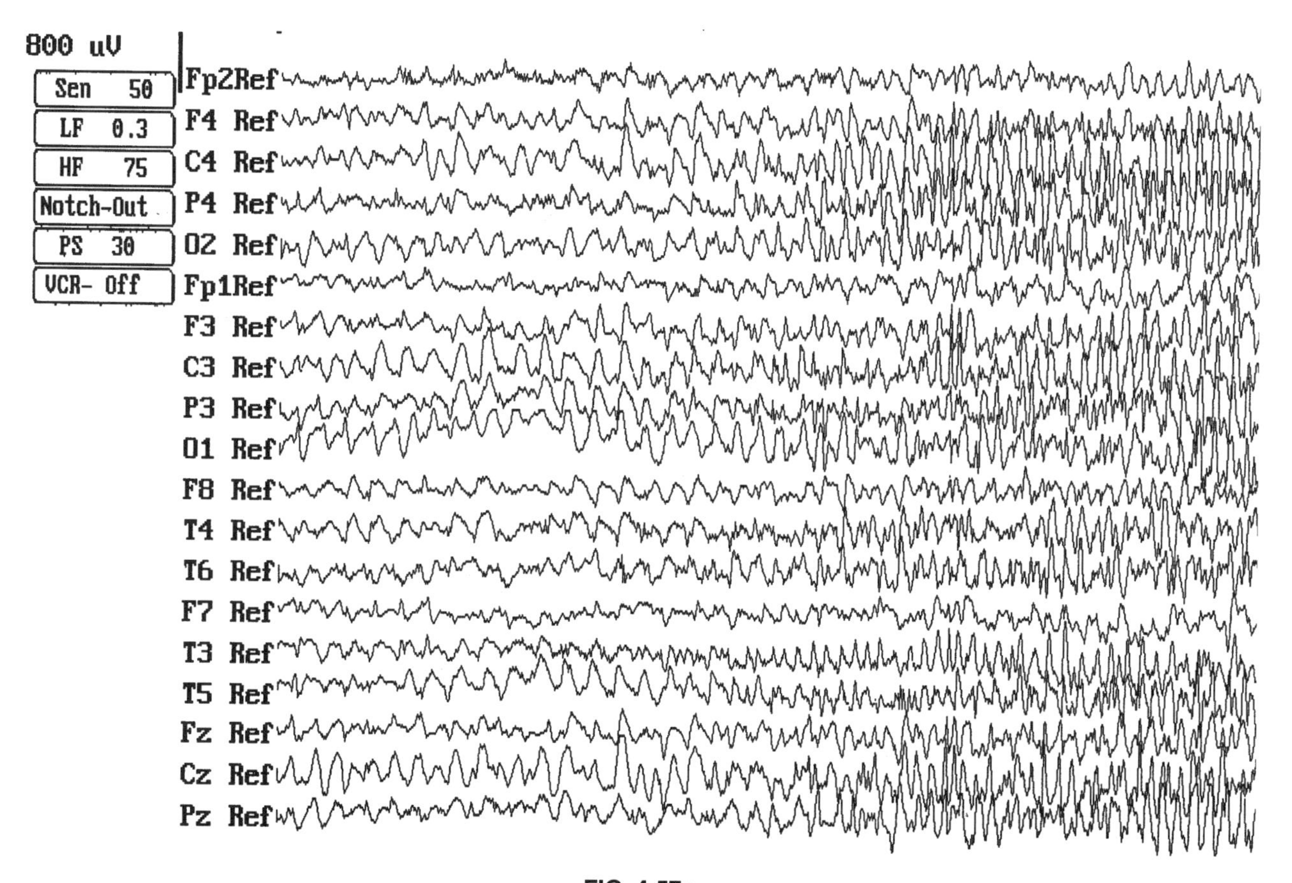
800 uV
Sen 50
LF 0.3
HF 75
Notch-Out
PS 30
VCR- Off
Fp2Ref
F4 Ref
C4 Ref
P4 Ref
O2 Ref
Fp1Ref
F3 Ref
C3 Ref
P3 Ref
O1 Ref
F8 Ref
T4 Ref
T6 Ref
F7 Ref
T3 Ref
T5 Ref
Fz Ref
Cz Ref
Pz Ref

FIG. 4-57c

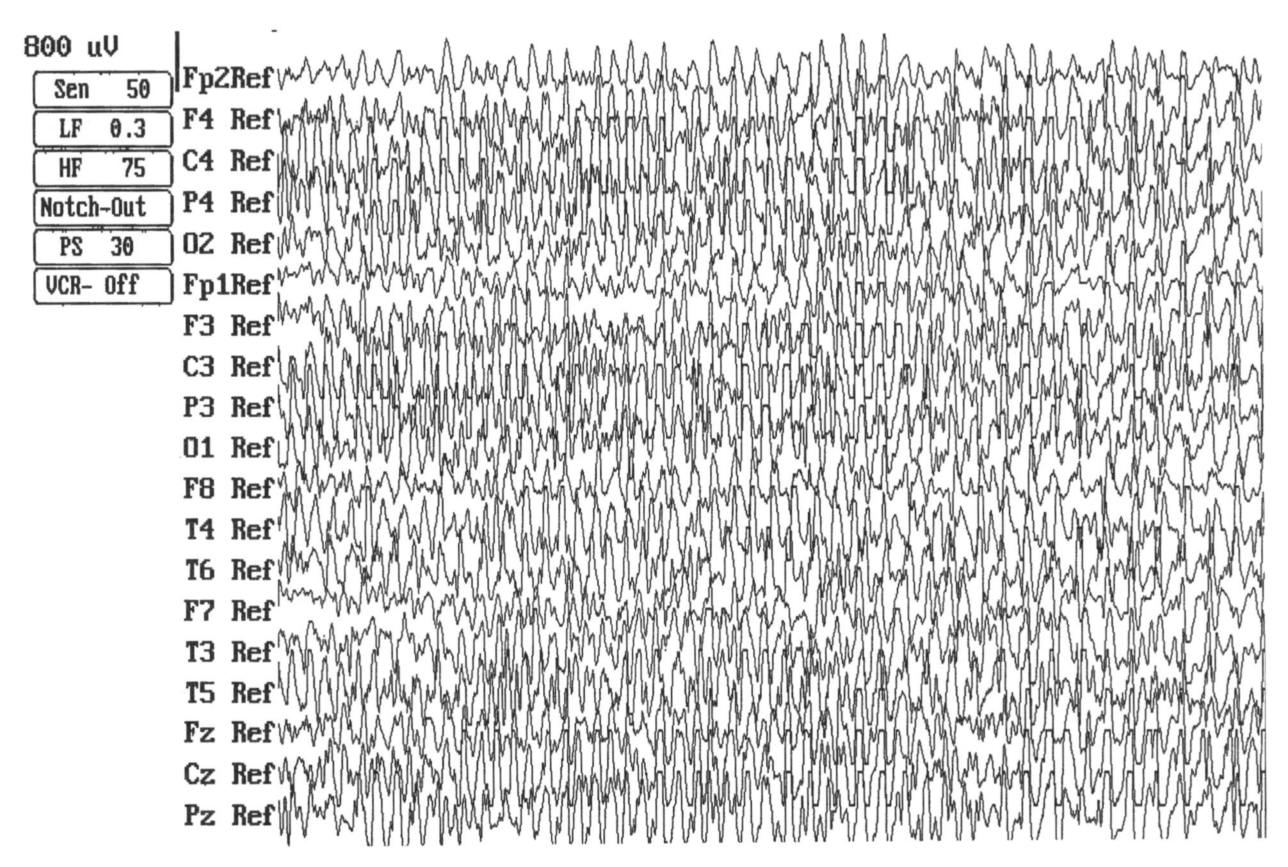
800 uV
Sen 50
LF 0.3
HF 75
Notch-Out
PS 30
VCR- Off
Fp2Ref
F4 Ref
C4 Ref
P4 Ref
O2 Ref
Fp1Ref
F3 Ref
C3 Ref
P3 Ref
O1 Ref
F8 Ref
T4 Ref
T6 Ref
F7 Ref
T3 Ref
T5 Ref
Fz Ref
Cz Ref
Pz Ref

FIG. 4-57d

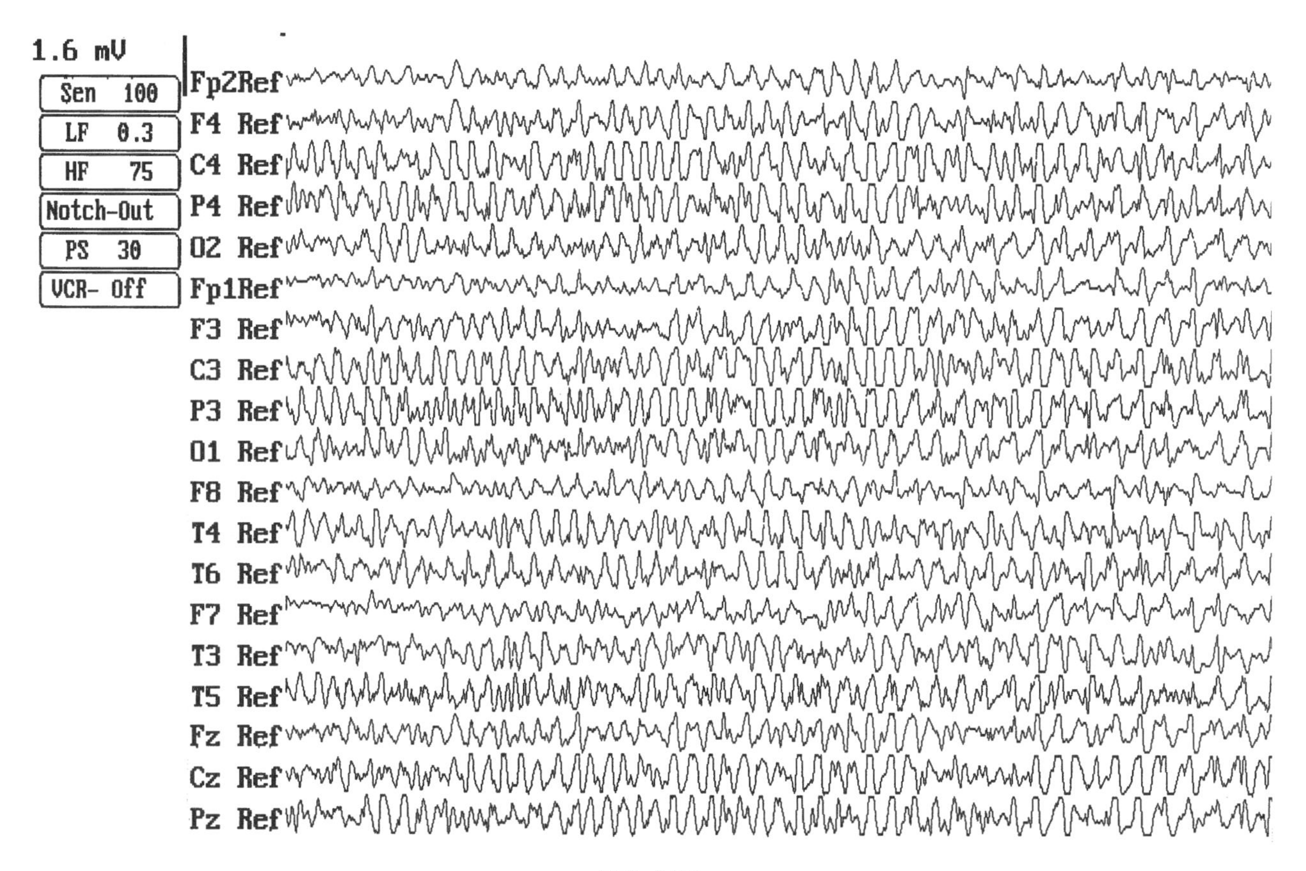
1.6 mV
Sen 100
LF 0.3
HF 75
Notch-Out
PS 30
VCR- Off
Fp2Ref
F4 Ref
C4 Ref
P4 Ref
O2 Ref
Fp1Ref
F3 Ref
C3 Ref
P3 Ref
O1 Ref
F8 Ref
T4 Ref
T6 Ref
F7 Ref
T3 Ref
T5 Ref
Fz Ref
Cz Ref
Pz Ref

FIG. 4-57e

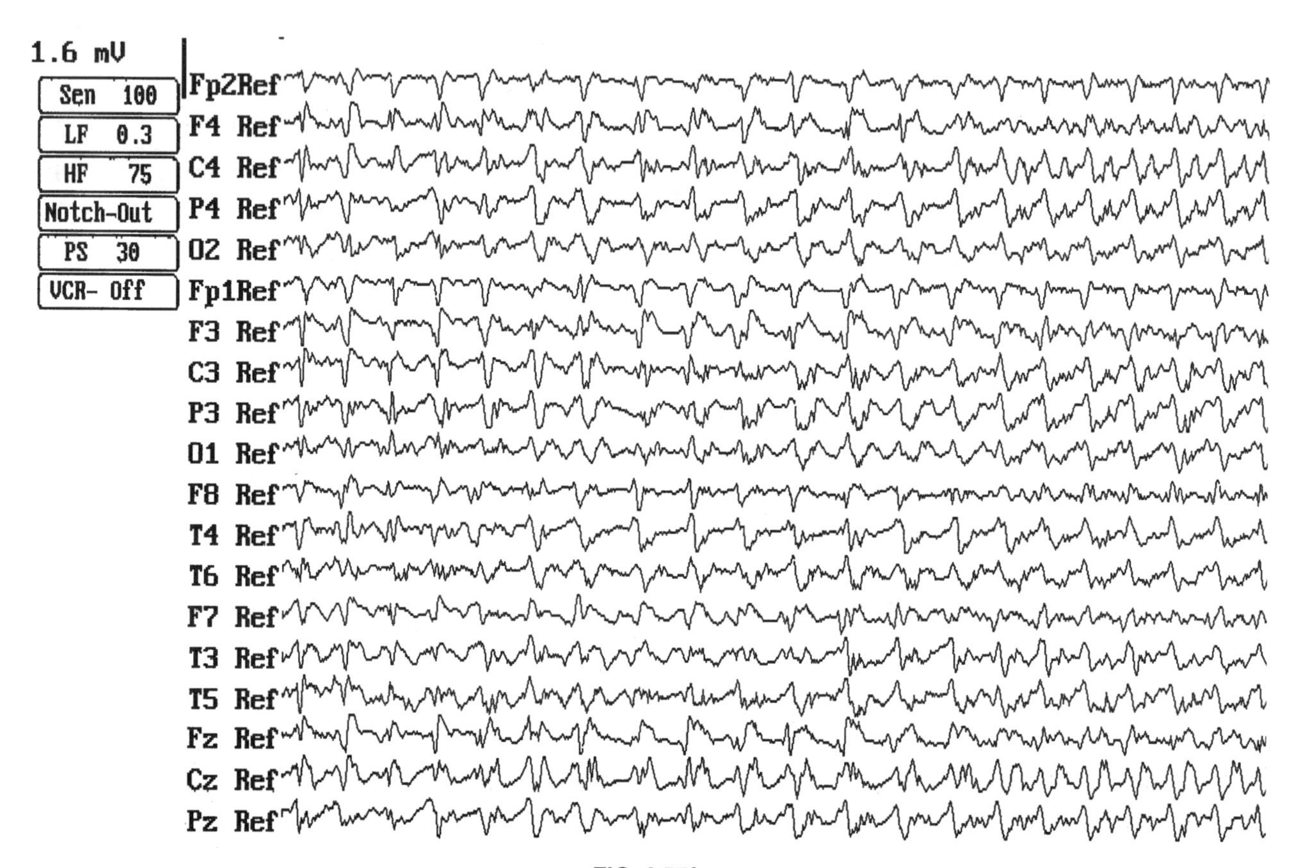
1.6 mV
Sen 100
LF 0.3
HF 75
Notch-Out
PS 30
VCR- Off
Fp2Ref
F4 Ref
C4 Ref
P4 Ref
O2 Ref
Fp1Ref
F3 Ref
C3 Ref
P3 Ref
O1 Ref
F8 Ref
T4 Ref
T6 Ref
F7 Ref
T3 Ref
T5 Ref
Fz Ref
Cz Ref
Pz Ref

FIG. 4-57f

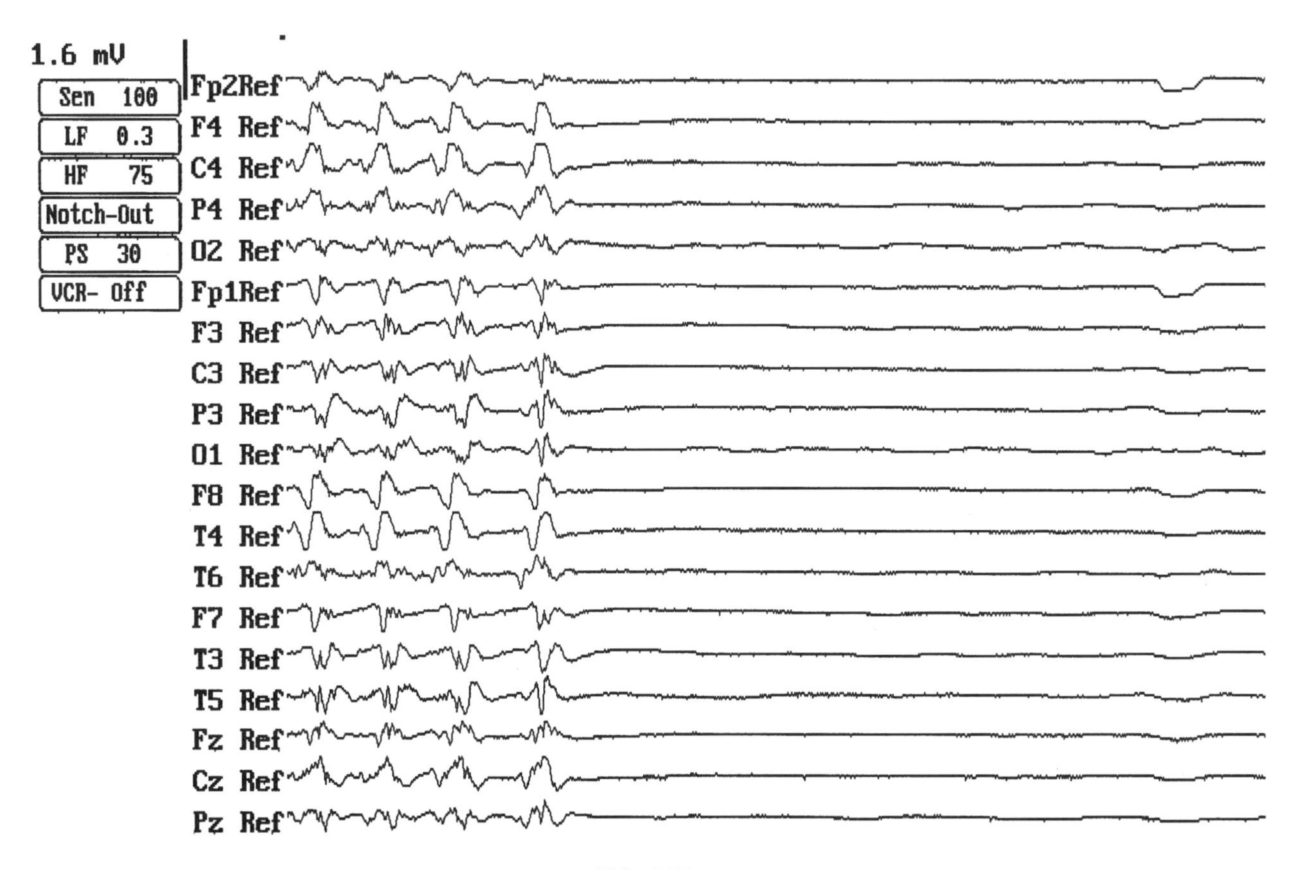
1.6 mV
Sen 100
LF 0.3
HF 75
Notch-Out
PS 30
VCR- Off
Fp2Ref
F4 Ref
C4 Ref
P4 Ref
O2 Ref
Fp1Ref
F3 Ref
C3 Ref
P3 Ref
O1 Ref
F8 Ref
T4 Ref
T6 Ref
F7 Ref
T3 Ref
T5 Ref
Fz Ref
Cz Ref
Pz Ref

FIG. 4-57g

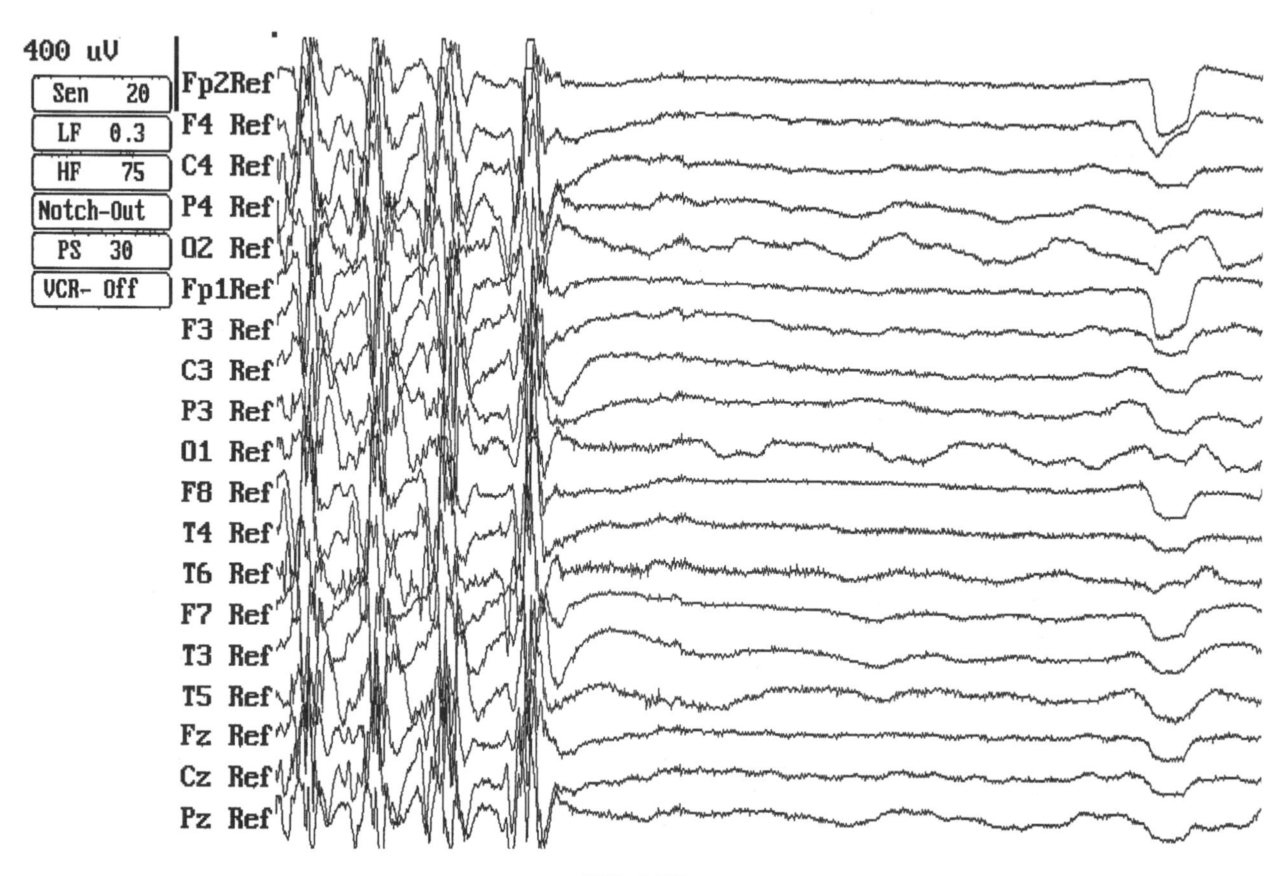
400 uV
Sen 20
LF 0.3
HF 75
Notch-Out
PS 30
VCR- Off
Fp2Ref
F4 Ref
C4 Ref
P4 Ref
O2 Ref
Fp1Ref
F3 Ref
C3 Ref
P3 Ref
O1 Ref
F8 Ref
T4 Ref
T6 Ref
F7 Ref
T3 Ref
T5 Ref
Fz Ref
Cz Ref
Pz Ref

FIG. 4-57h

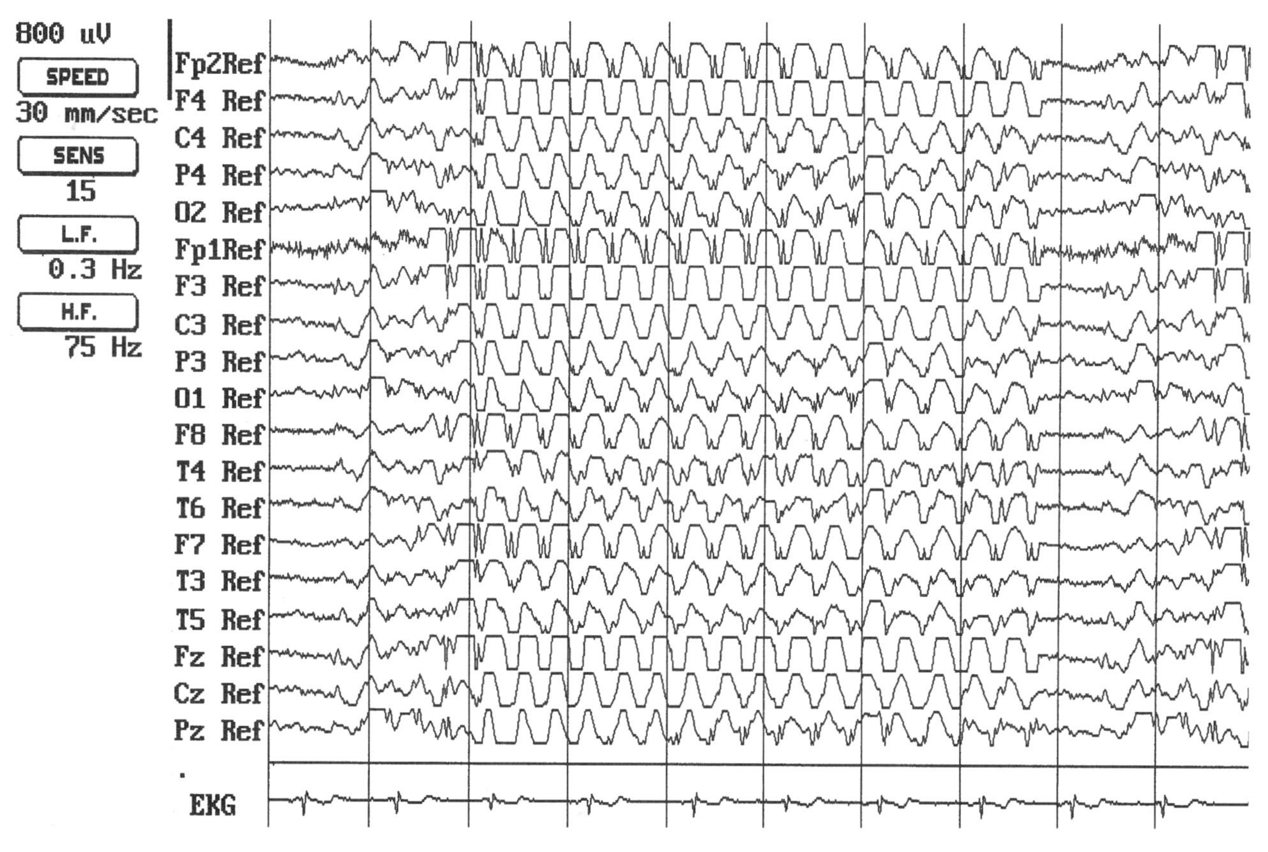

FIG. 4-58 A generalized 3/s spike and wave was recorded at 8 bits with too high sensitivity. Note the amplifier clipped waves that cannot be corrected by changing the display sensitivity.

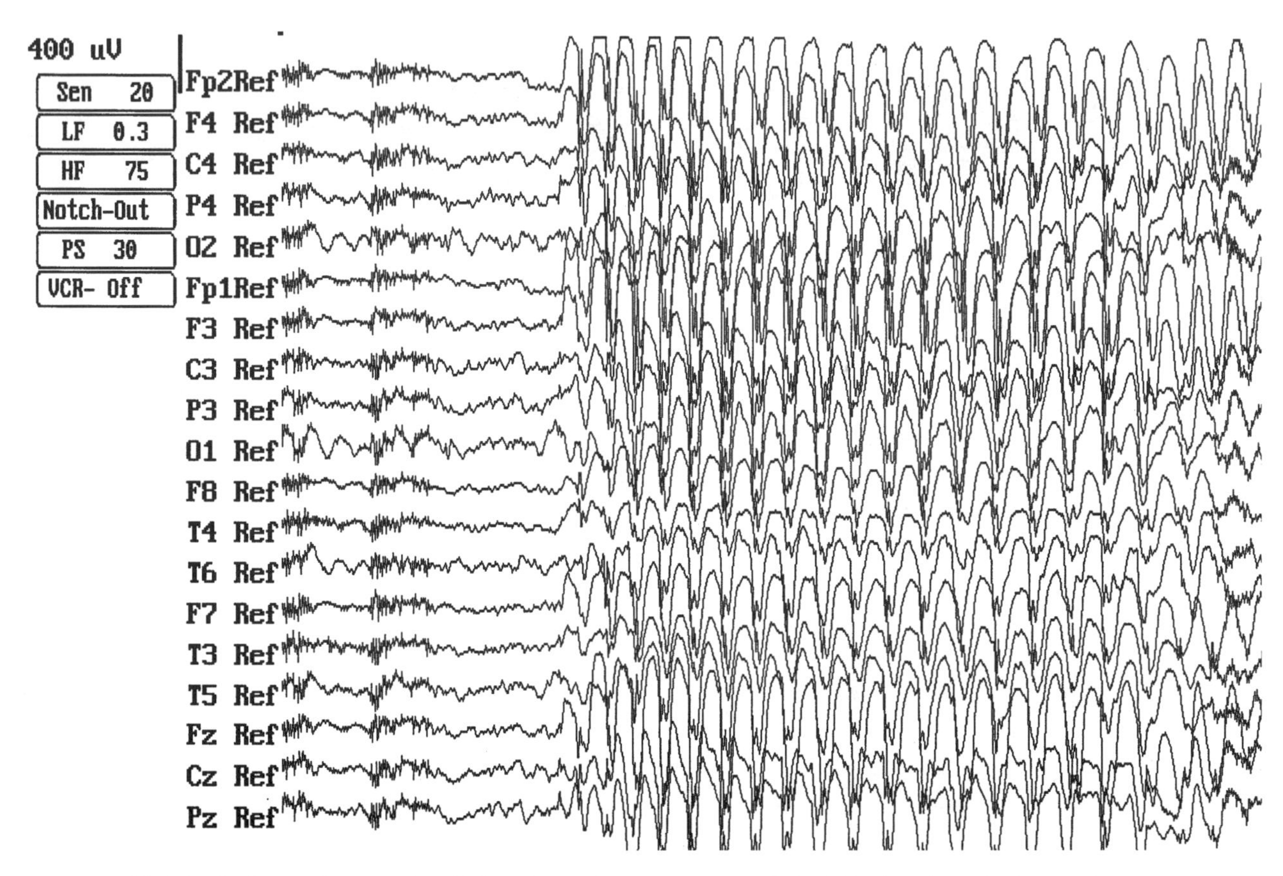

FIG. 4-59a,b,c,d A generalized 3/s spike and wave was recorded at 11 bits, then displayed at sensitivities of 20 and 50 to show the absence of clipping. The same data is shown on run 2 for comparison.

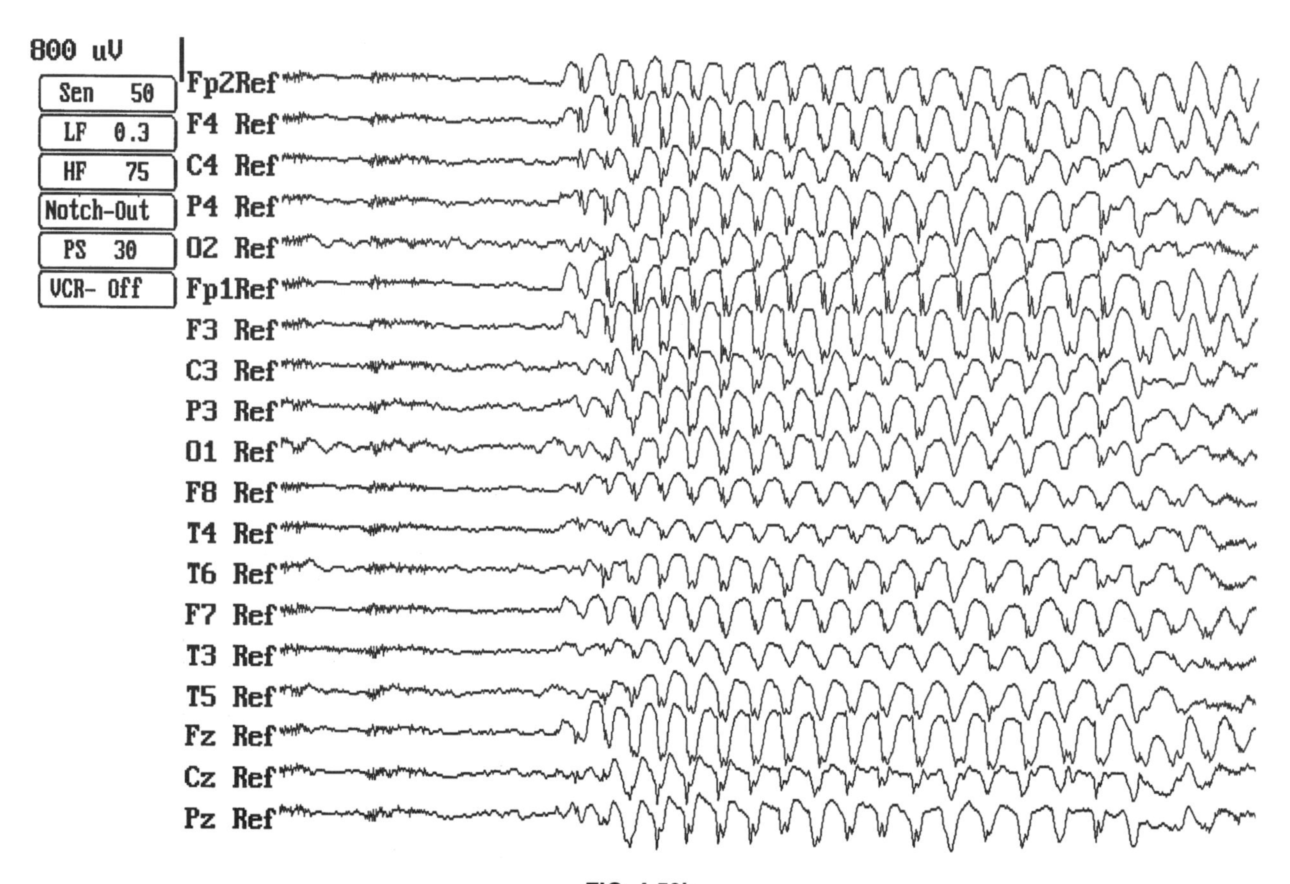
800 uV
Sen 50
LF 0.3
HF 75
Notch-Out
PS 30
VCR- Off
Fp2Ref
F4 Ref
C4 Ref
P4 Ref
O2 Ref
Fp1Ref
F3 Ref
C3 Ref
P3 Ref
O1 Ref
F8 Ref
T4 Ref
T6 Ref
F7 Ref
T3 Ref
T5 Ref
Fz Ref
Cz Ref
Pz Ref

FIG. 4-59b

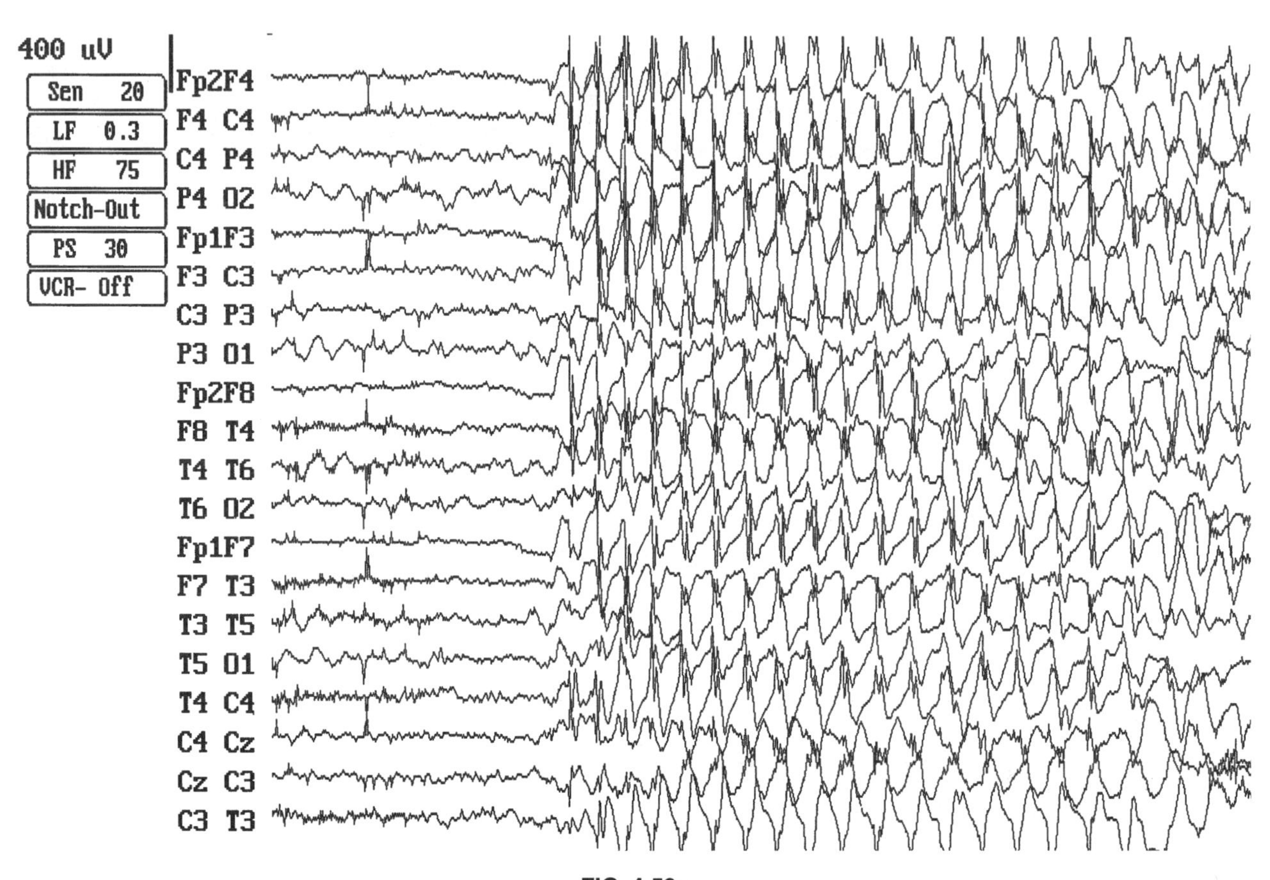
400 uV
Sen 20
LF 0.3
HF 75
Notch-Out
PS 30
VCR- Off
Fp2F4
F4 C4
C4 P4
P4 O2
Fp1F3
F3 C3
C3 P3
P3 O1
Fp2F8
F8 T4
T4 T6
T6 O2
Fp1F7
F7 T3
T3 T5
T5 O1
T4 C4
C4 Cz
Cz C3
C3 T3

FIG. 4-59c

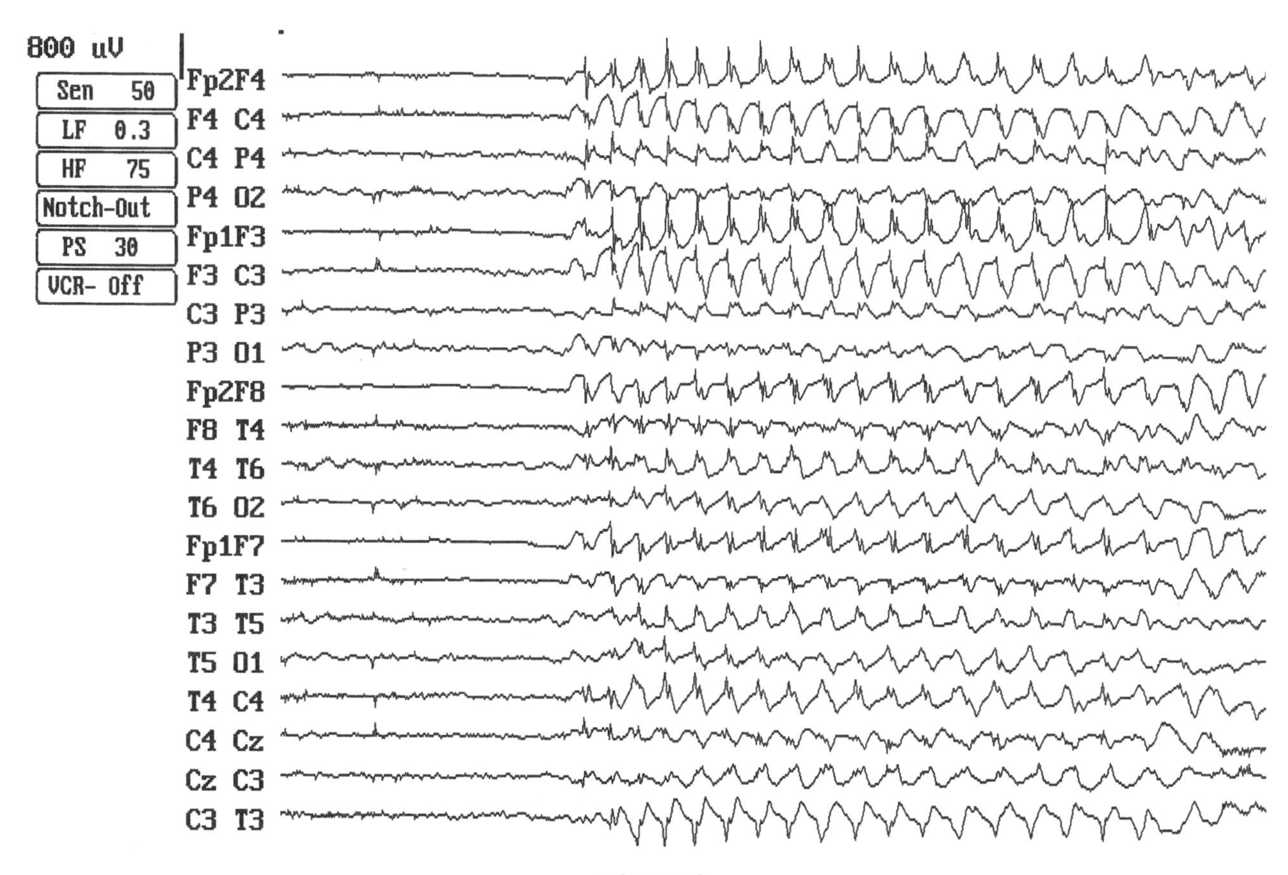
800 uV
Sen 50
LF 0.3
HF 75
Notch-Out
PS 30
VCR- Off
Fp2F4
F4 C4
C4 P4
P4 O2
Fp1F3
F3 C3
C3 P3
P3 O1
Fp2F8
F8 T4
T4 T6
T6 O2
Fp1F7
F7 T3
T3 T5
T5 O1
T4 C4
C4 Cz
Cz C3
C3 T3

FIG. 4-59d

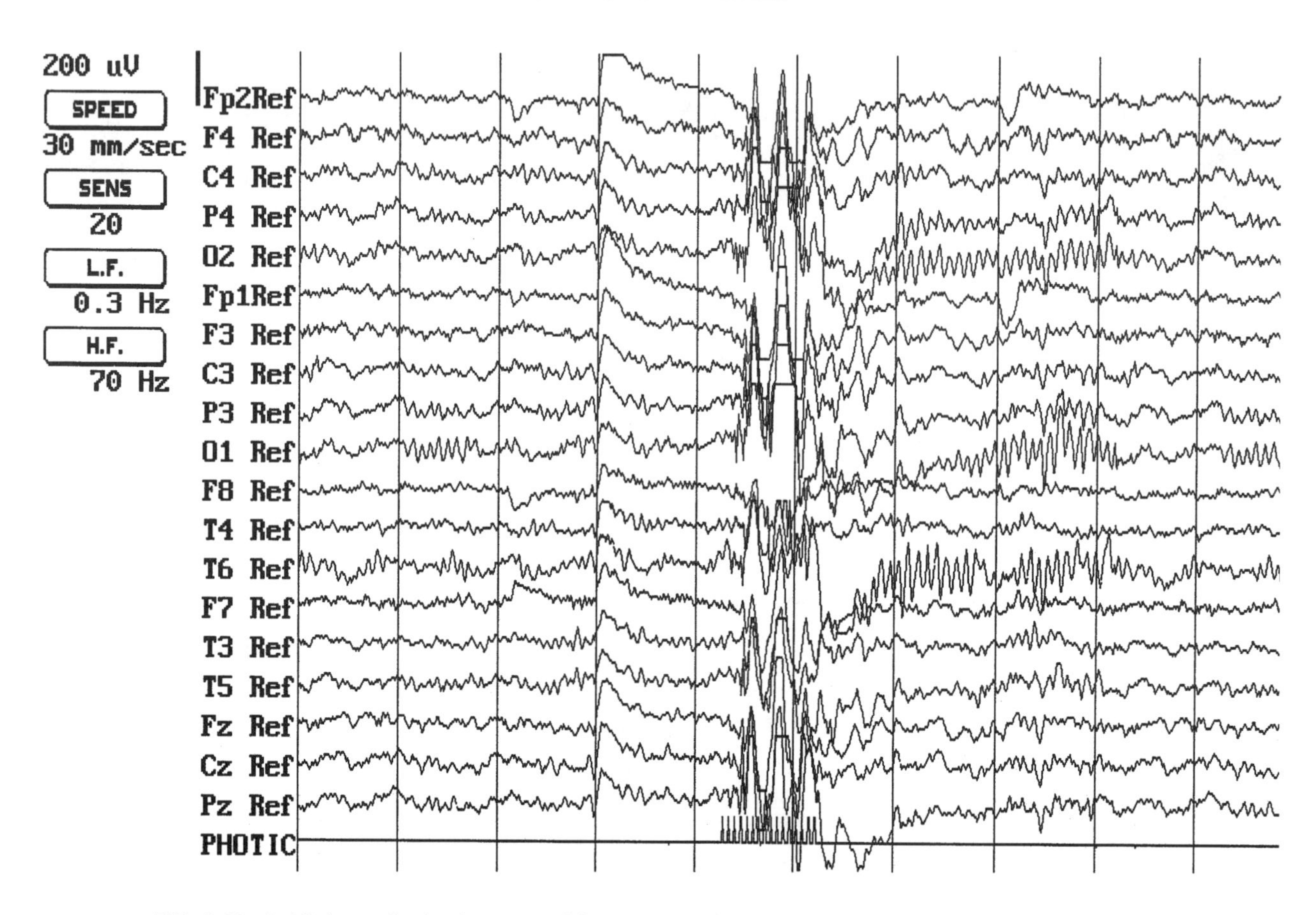

FIG. 4-60a,b High amplitude photoconvulsive response is seen on run 1, with PS of 30 and 60 mm/s.

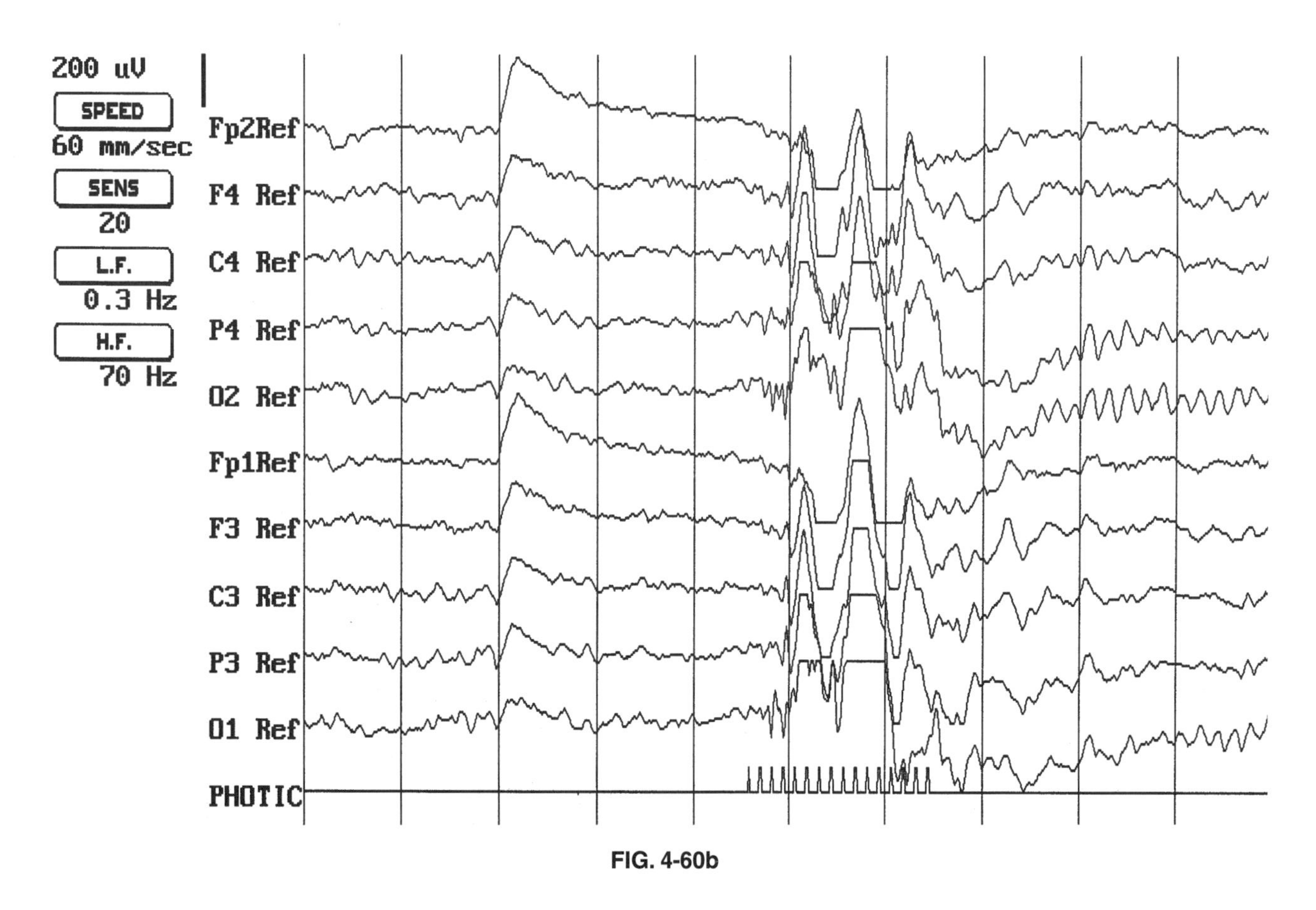
200 uV
SPEED
60 mm/sec
SENS
20
L.F.
0.3 Hz
H.F.
70 Hz
Fp2Ref
F4 Ref
C4 Ref
P4 Ref
O2 Ref
Fp1Ref
F3 Ref
C3 Ref
P3 Ref
O1 Ref
PHOTIC

FIG. 4-60b

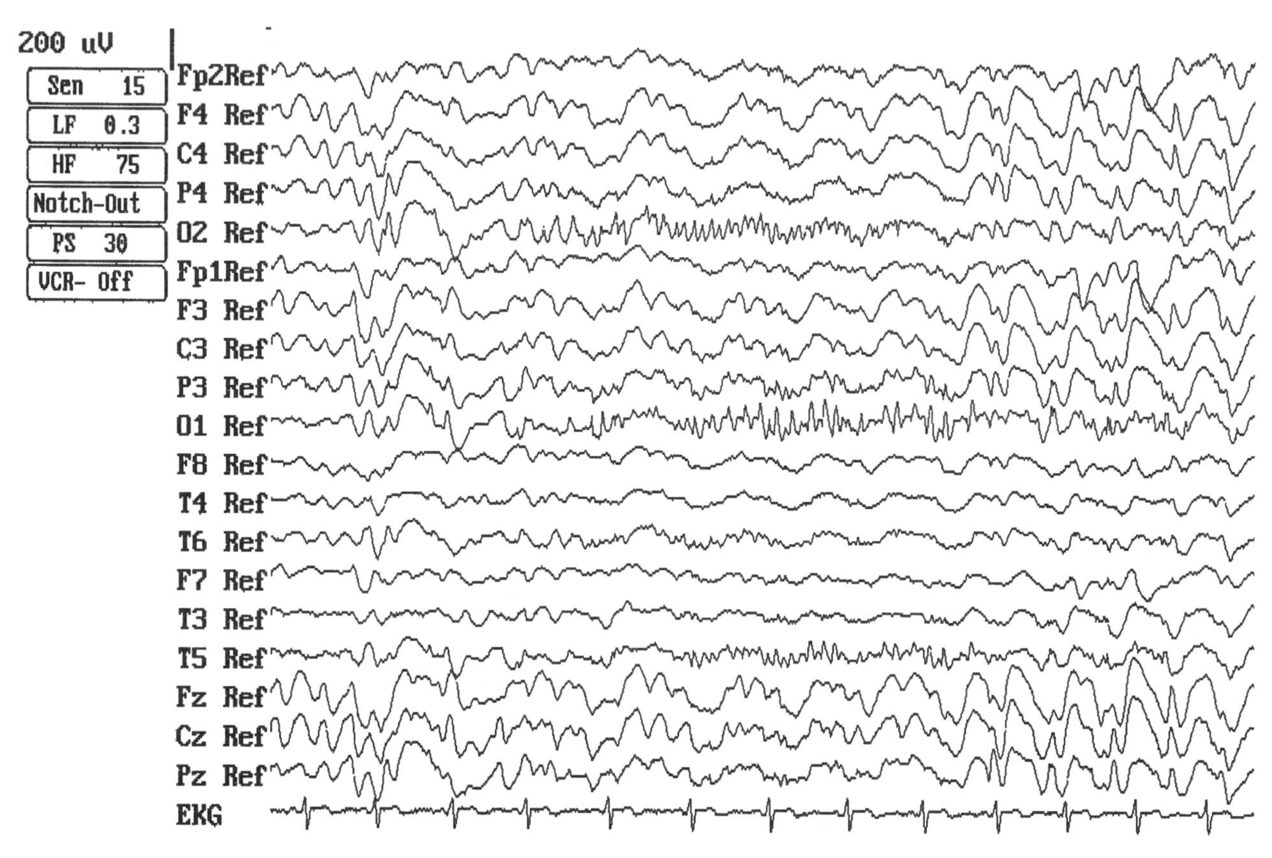

FIG. 4-61a,b A bioccipital seizure is seen on run 1, and is seen better on run 4 as a posterior halo.

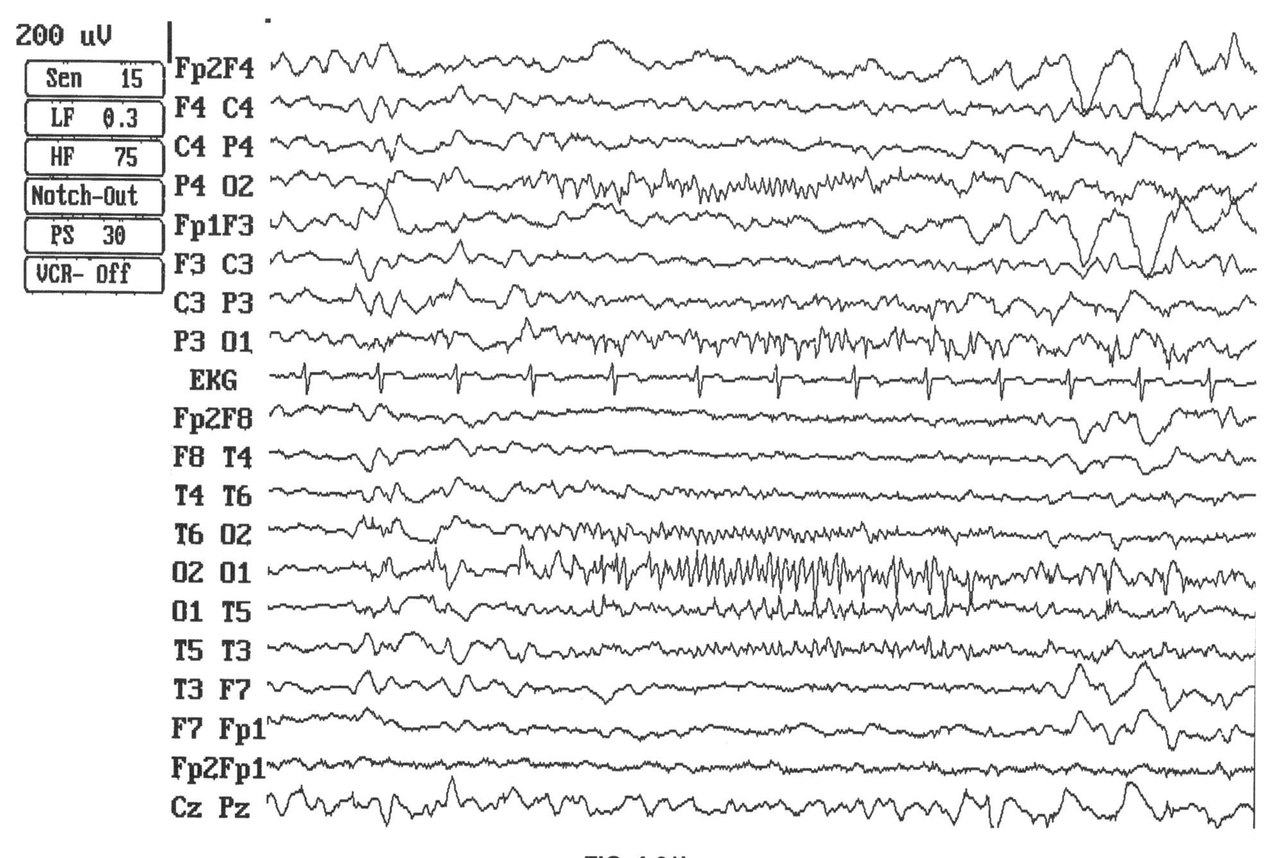
200 uV
Sen 15
LF 0.3
HF 75
Notch-Out
PS 30
VCR- Off
Fp2F4
F4 C4
C4 P4
P4 O2
Fp1F3
F3 C3
C3 P3
P3 O1
EKG
Fp2F8
F8 T4
T4 T6
T6 O2
O2 O1
O1 T5
T5 T3
T3 F7
F7 Fp1
Fp2Fp1
Cz Pz

FIG. 4-61b

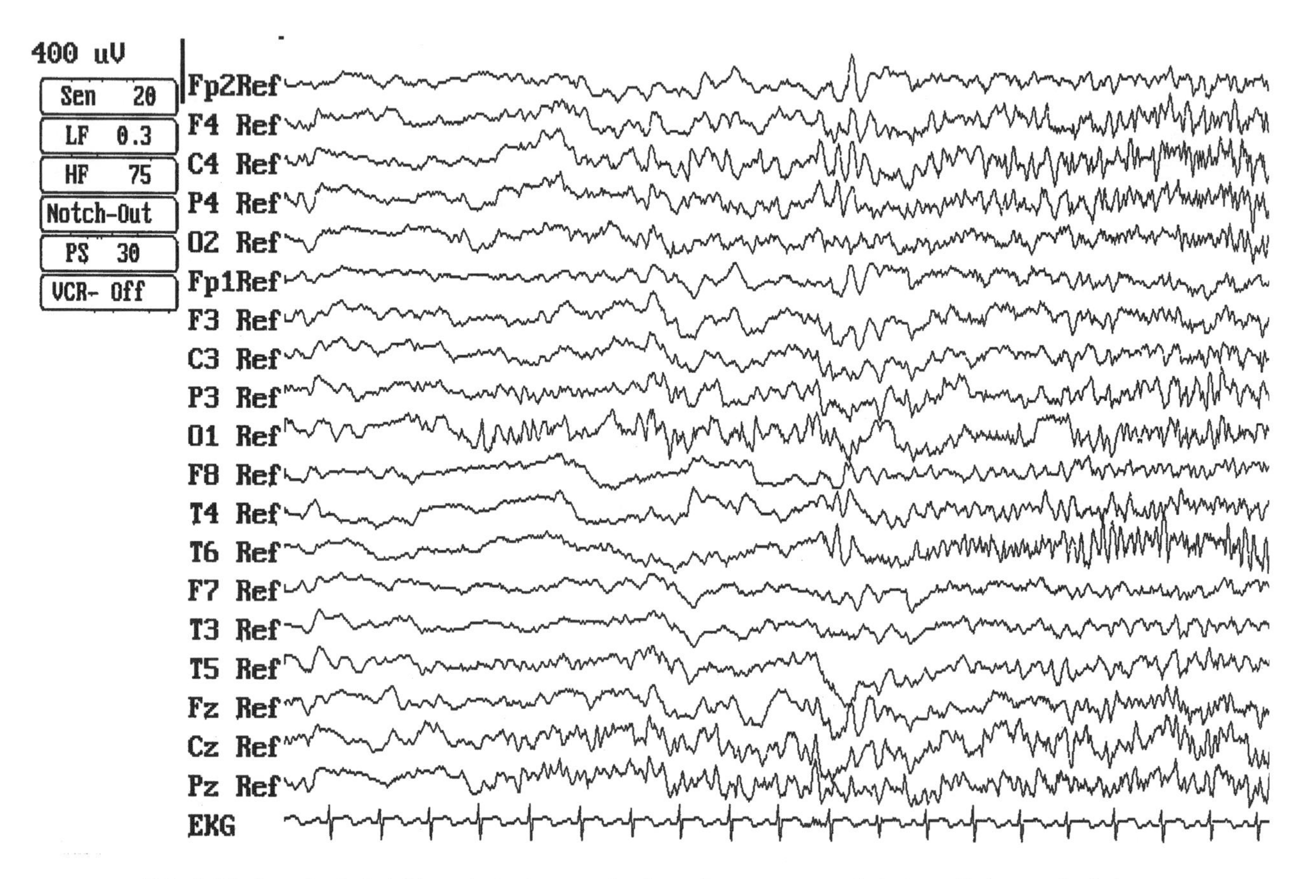

FIG. 4-62a,b,c,d,e,f A right posterior temporal seizure is seen on run 1, but run 2 shows nicely how the posterior temporal-parietal seizure involved the central region.

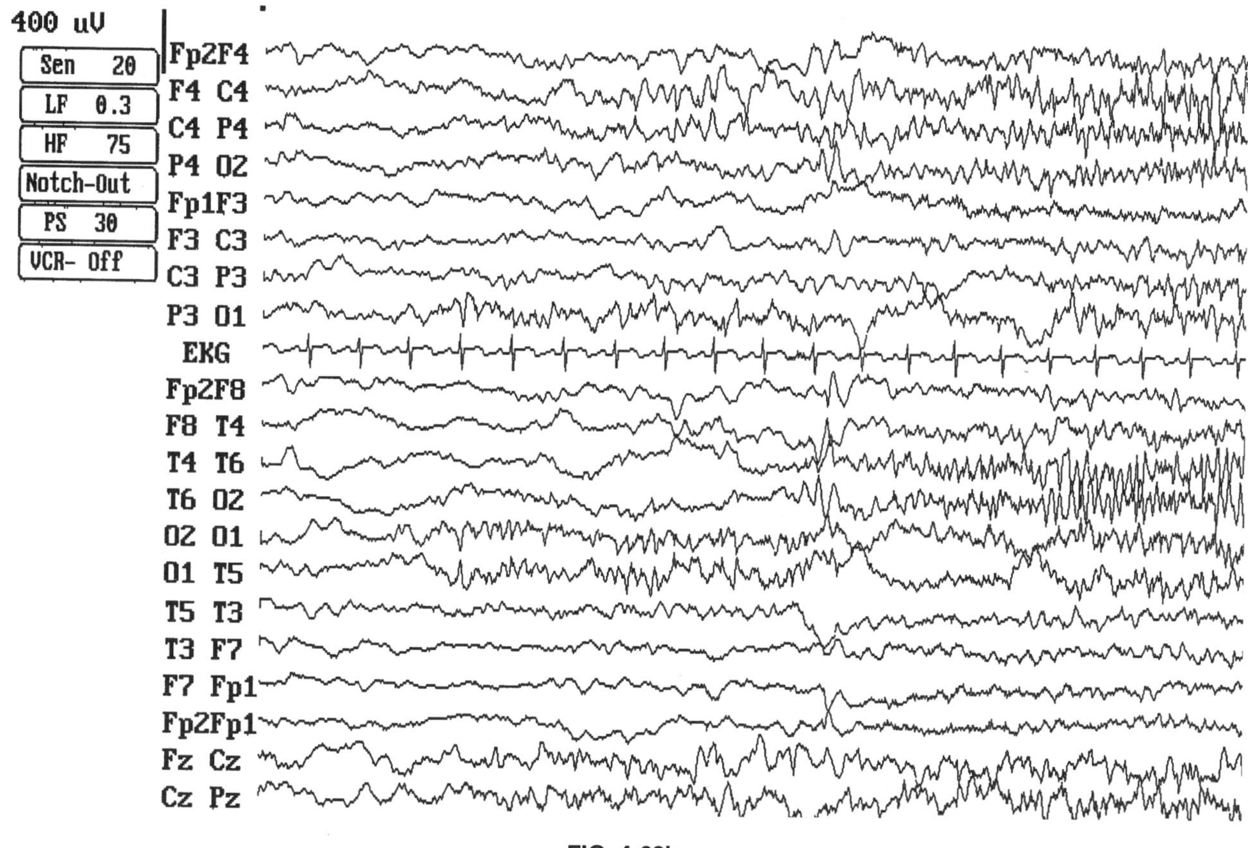
400 uV
Sen 20
LF 0.3
HF 75
Notch-Out
PS 30
VCR- Off
Fp2F4
F4 C4
C4 P4
P4 O2
Fp1F3
F3 C3
C3 P3
P3 O1
EKG
Fp2F8
F8 T4
T4 T6
T6 O2
O2 O1
O1 T5
T5 T3
T3 F7
F7 Fp1
Fp2Fp1
Fz Cz
Cz Pz

FIG. 4-62b

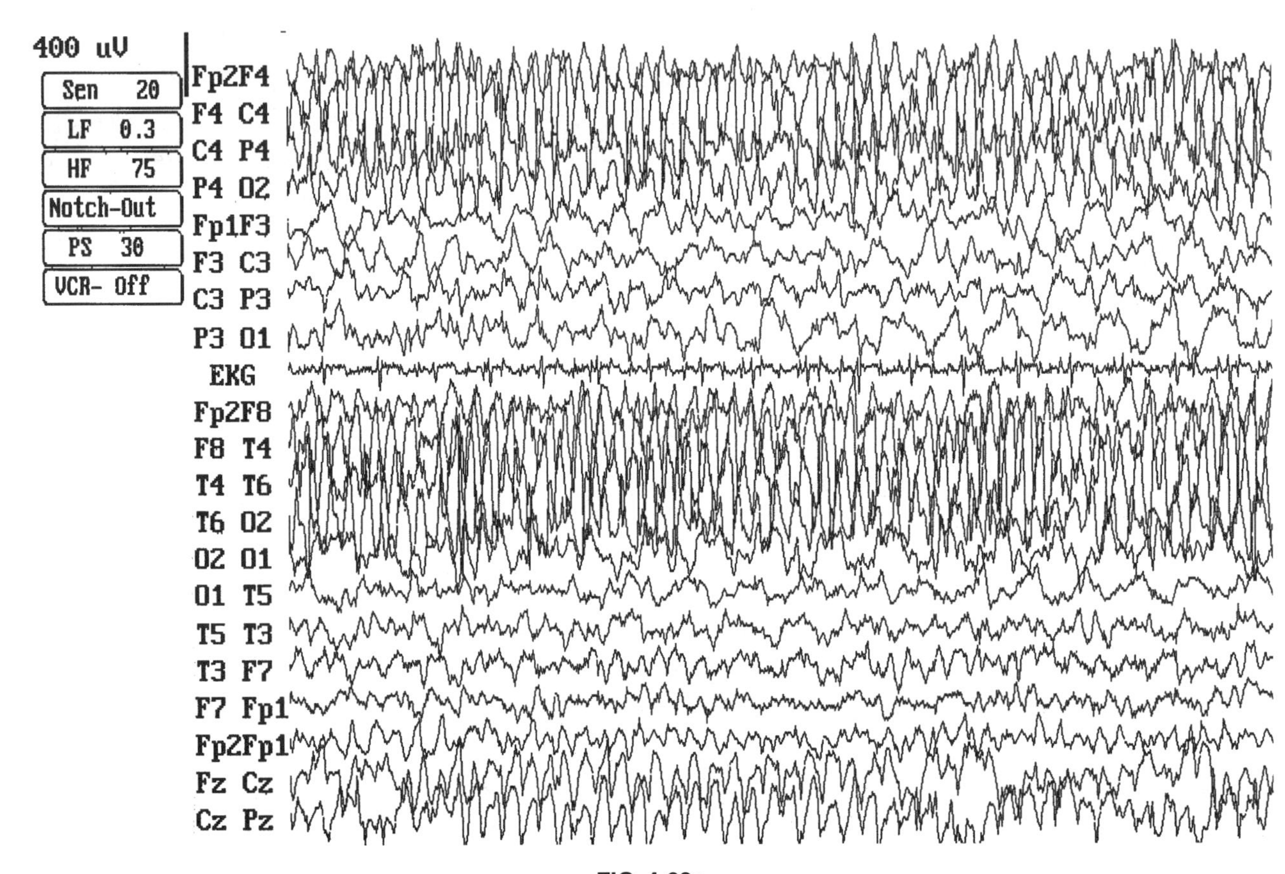
400 uV
Sen 20
LF 0.3
HF 75
Notch-Out
PS 30
VCR- Off
Fp2F4
F4 C4
C4 P4
P4 O2
Fp1F3
F3 C3
C3 P3
P3 O1
EKG
Fp2F8
F8 T4
T4 T6
T6 O2
O2 O1
O1 T5
T5 T3
T3 F7
F7 Fp1
Fp2Fp1
Fz Cz
Cz Pz

FIG. 4-62c

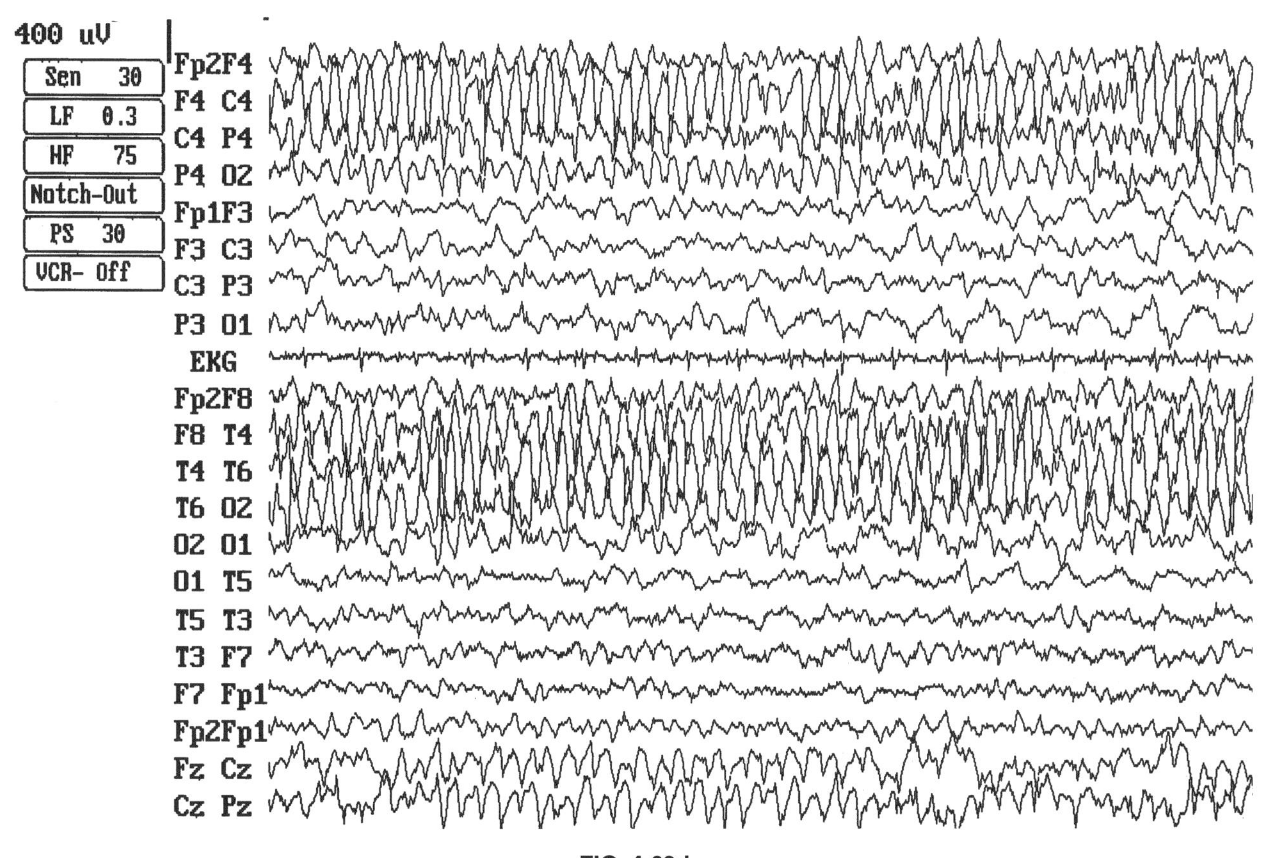
400 uV
Sen 30
LF 0.3
HF 75
Notch-Out
PS 30
VCR- Off
Fp2F4
F4 C4
C4 P4
P4 O2
Fp1F3
F3 C3
C3 P3
P3 O1
EKG
Fp2F8
F8 T4
T4 T6
T6 O2
O2 O1
O1 T5
T5 T3
T3 F7
F7 Fp1
Fp2Fp1
Fz Cz
Cz Pz

FIG. 4-62d

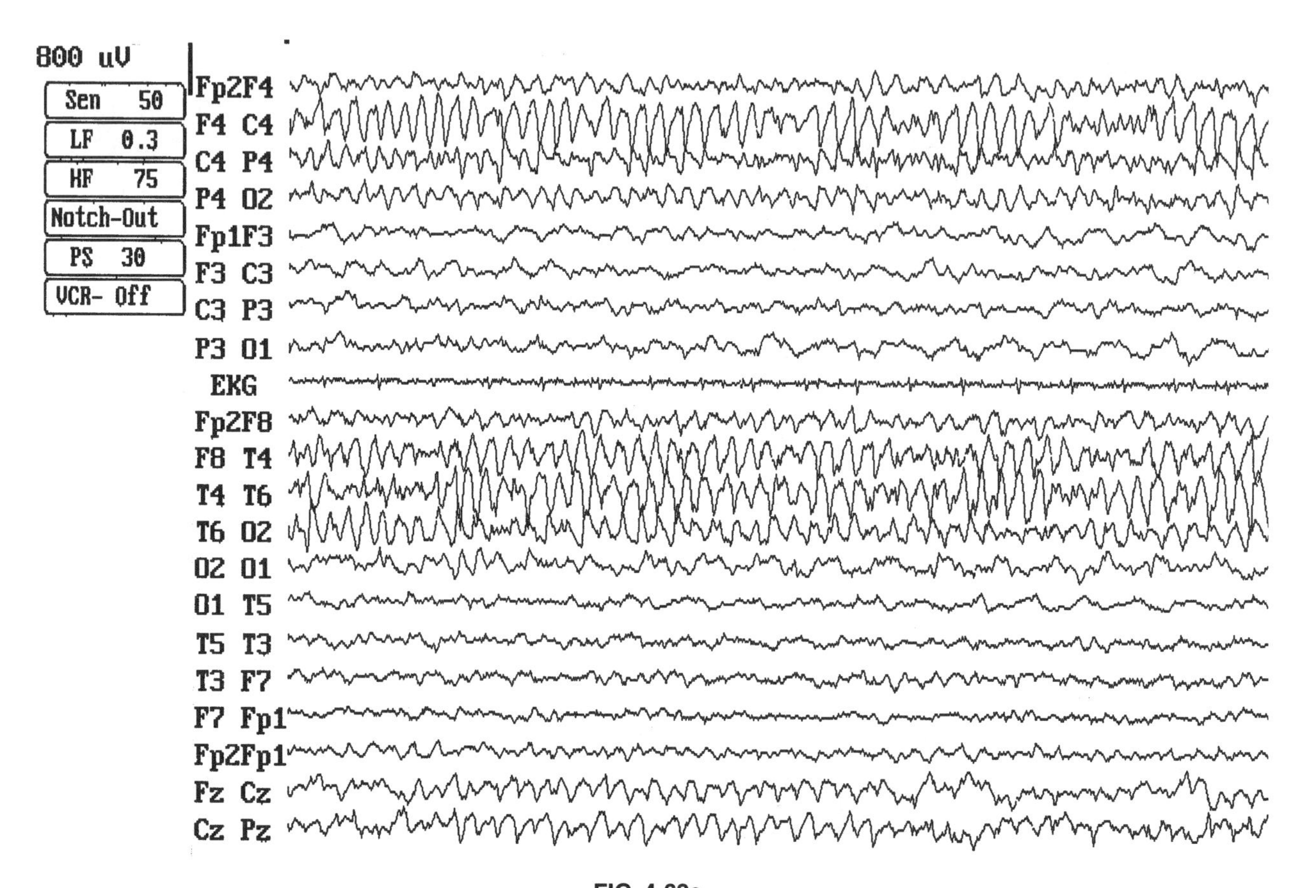
800 uV
Sen 50
LF 0.3
HF 75
Notch-Out
PS 30
VCR- Off
Fp2F4
F4 C4
C4 P4
P4 O2
Fp1F3
F3 C3
C3 P3
P3 O1
EKG
Fp2F8
F8 T4
T4 T6
T6 O2
O2 O1
O1 T5
T5 T3
T3 F7
F7 Fp1
Fp2Fp1
Fz Cz
Cz Pz

FIG. 4-62e

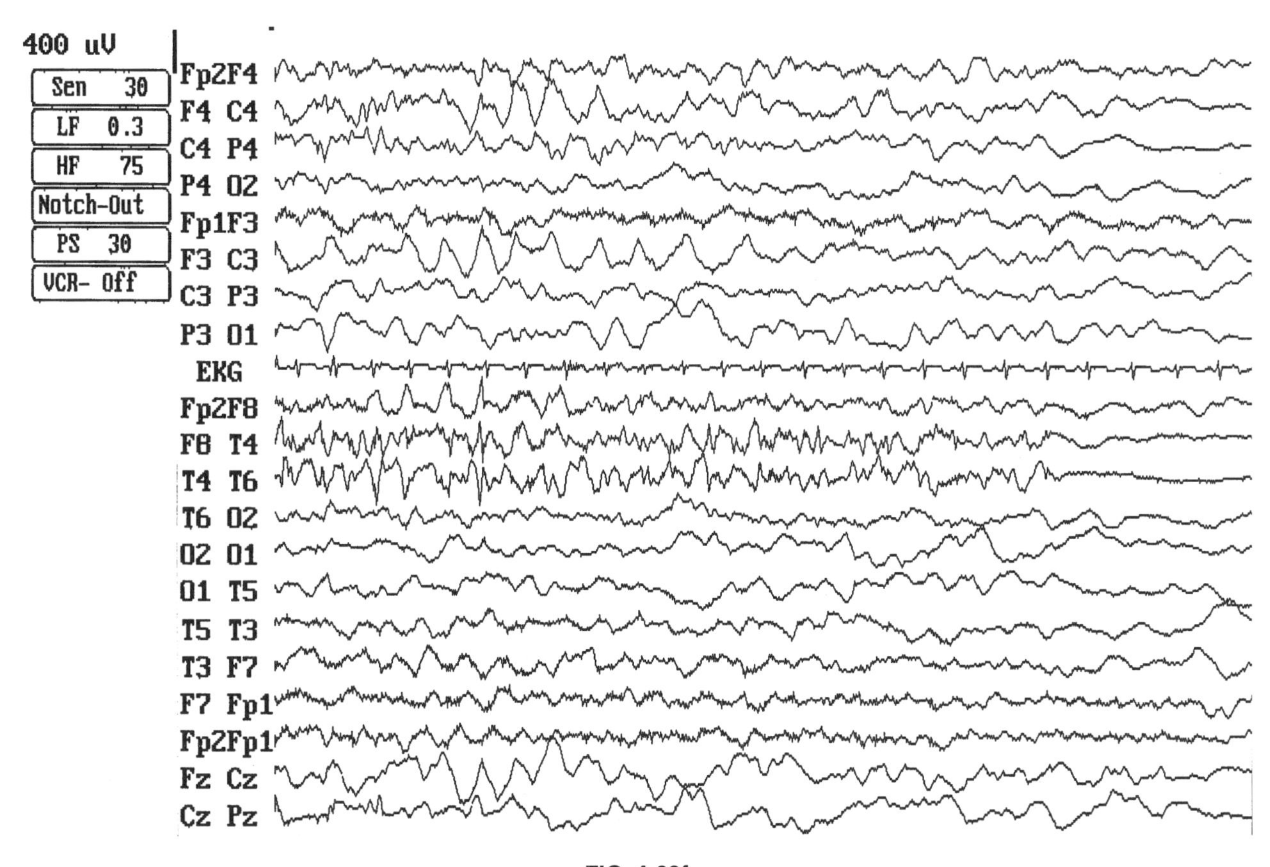
400 uV
Sen 30
LF 0.3
HF 75
Notch-Out
PS 30
VCR- Off
Fp2F4
F4 C4
C4 P4
P4 O2
Fp1F3
F3 C3
C3 P3
P3 O1
EKG
Fp2F8
F8 T4
T4 T6
T6 O2
O2 O1
O1 T5
T5 T3
T3 F7
F7 Fp1
Fp2Fp1
Fz Cz
Cz Pz

FIG. 4-62f

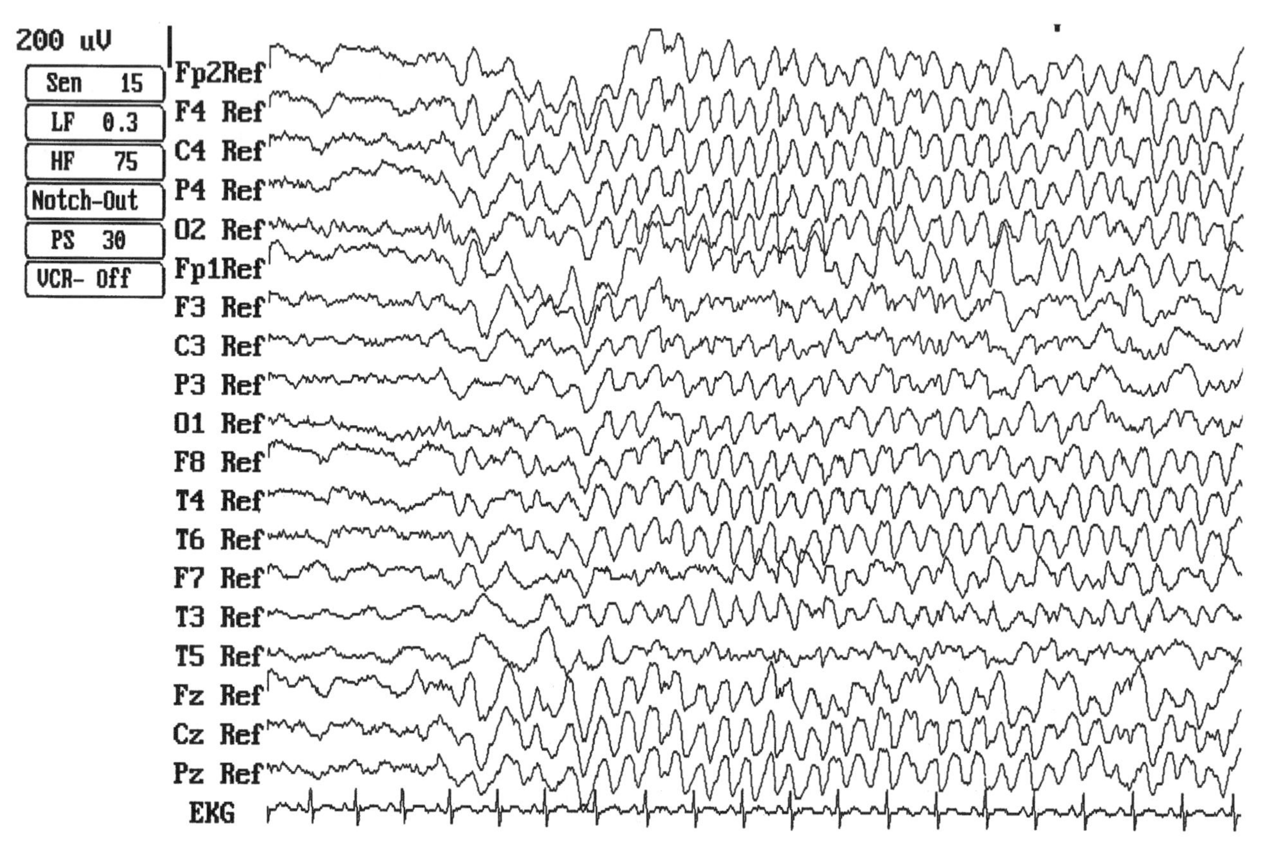

FIG. 4-63a,b,c,d A left temporal seizure with ear contamination is seen. Run 1 with A1+A2 reference shows diffuse slowing, maximal on the right. Run 2 clarifies a left temporal-central discharge, which is optimally displayed using O2 reference, while PS = 15 provides another perspective of the same data as in (c).

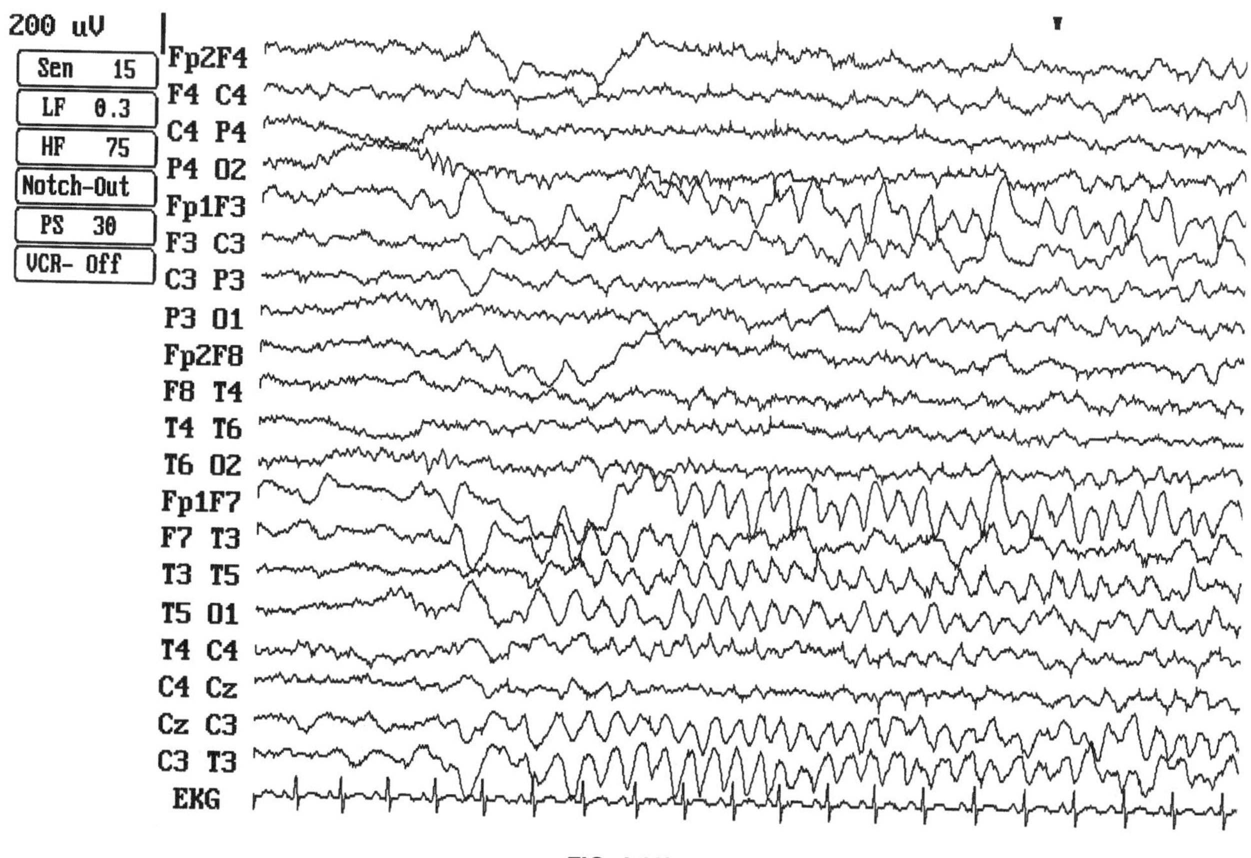
200 uV
Sen 15
LF 0.3
HF 75
Notch-Out
PS 30
VCR- Off
Fp2F4
F4 C4
C4 P4
P4 O2
Fp1F3
F3 C3
C3 P3
P3 O1
Fp2F8
F8 T4
T4 T6
T6 O2
Fp1F7
F7 T3
T3 T5
T5 O1
T4 C4
C4 Cz
Cz C3
C3 T3
EKG

FIG. 4-63b

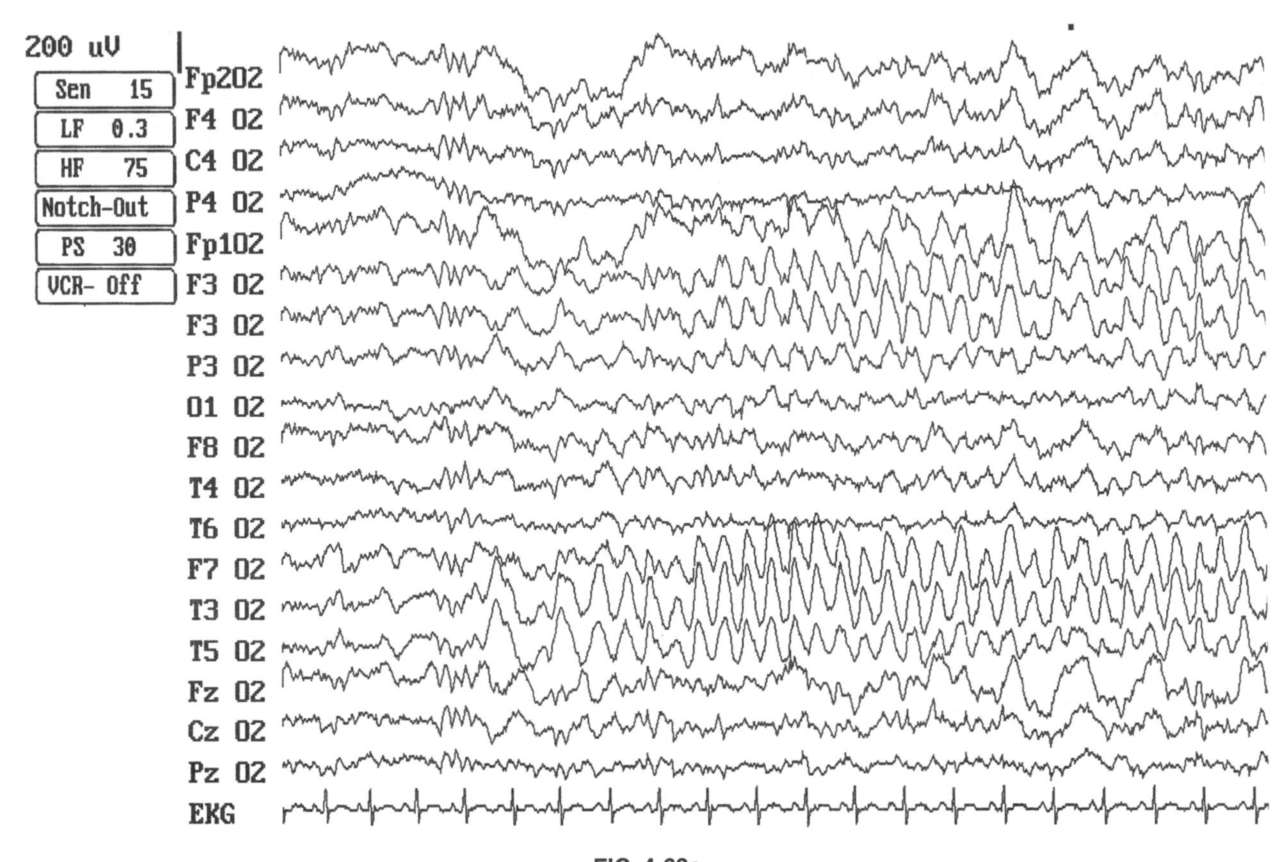
200 uV
Sen 15
LF 0.3
HF 75
Notch-Out
PS 30
VCR- Off
Fp2O2
F4 O2
C4 O2
P4 O2
Fp1O2
F3 O2
F3 O2
P3 O2
O1 O2
F8 O2
T4 O2
T6 O2
F7 O2
T3 O2
T5 O2
Fz O2
Cz O2
Pz O2
EKG

FIG. 4-63c

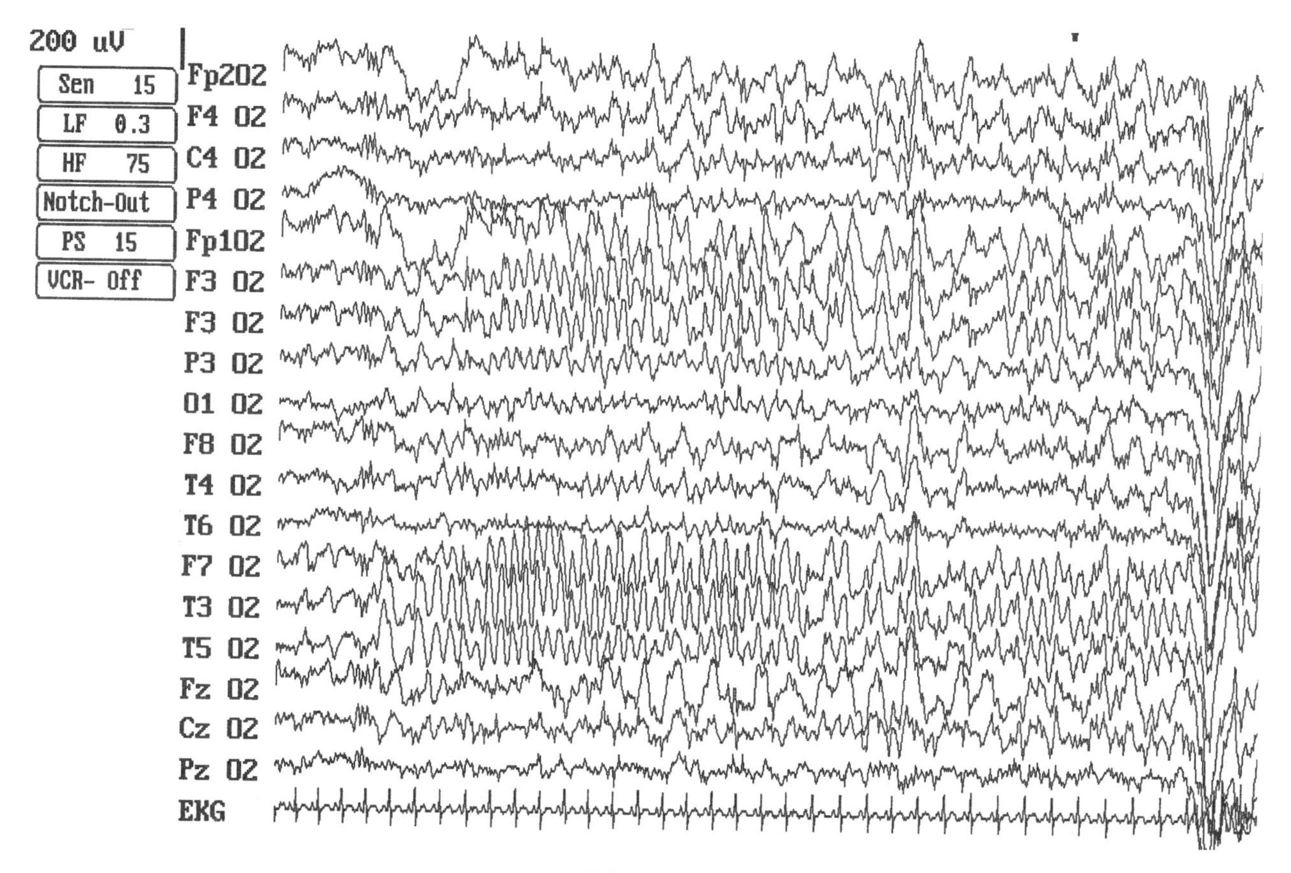
200 uV
Sen 15
LF 0.3
HF 75
Notch-Out
PS 15
VCR- Off
Fp2O2
F4 O2
C4 O2
P4 O2
Fp1O2
F3 O2
F3 O2
P3 O2
O1 O2
F8 O2
T4 O2
T6 O2
F7 O2
T3 O2
T5 O2
Fz O2
Cz O2
Pz O2
EKG

FIG. 4-63d

CLARIFICATION OF FINDINGS

Clarification of Morphology

FIG. 4-64a,b,c,d A generalized spike and wave fragment is seen on run 1. Run 2 suggests more right hemispheric discharge, while run 3 shows mainly frontal localization. PS = 60 is shown for comparison.
FIG. 4-65a,b,c In run 1 an apparent focal theta with sharp contour at T4 is seen near the middle of the page. Runs 2 and 3 clarified the nonepileptiform nature of this transient.
FIG. 4-66a,b Apparent persistent rhythmic focal slowing at T6 is seen on run 3 (cancellation), but on run 1 it is diffuse and there is lower amplitude at left temporal. The pattern is that of delta with broad field.
FIG. 4-67a,b,c Run 2 shows a spike at T4-T6 single deflection, while run 4 shows a definite T6-O2 spike. Run 1 confirmed this latter location.
FIG. 4-68a,b,c Run 2 shows a spike with phase reversal at F4, while run 3 shows a bifrontal location. This is confirmed on run 1.
FIG. 4-69a,b Run 1 with linked cheek reference shows diffuse suppression of background prior to seizure (note the preceding high voltage spiking on the left). The same montage with a slow paper speed enhanced the flattening of preictal background (note the ictal onset at the right of the figure).

Ambiguous normality

FIG. 4-70a,b A questionable T6 sharp wave is seen on run 2 at the middle of the page. Run 1 not confirmatory, showing the previous sharp phase reversal to be an idiosyncrasy of the alpha waveform, producing sharp slopes on subtraction (subtraction artifact).
FIG. 4-71a,b Run 1 shows a T6 delta wave, which gives a sharp phase reversal at T6 on run 3. Clearly, this is another subtraction artifact.
FIG. 4-72a,b Run 1 (middle of page) shows a sharply contoured wave maximal at Pz/P3, which, on reflection, has benign features. Run 2 shows nothing of note.
FIG. 4-73a,b Single sharp deflections are seen on run 2 at F3-C3, but not seen on run 1. Again, this is a subtraction artifact.
FIG. 4-74a,b A sharp wave at T4-T6 is seen at the middle of the page on run 2, but is not seen on run 1. This is also a subtraction artifact.
FIG. 4-75a,b Multiple tiny P3 sharp waveforms are seen on run 1, but are not seen on run 2. It is likely they are not significant.
FIG. 4-76a,b Run 2 shows multiple sharp-looking waves, none overtly epileptiform though worrisome (an example of so-called "spiky but normal EEG"). Run 1 shows the reason: profuse fast activity in the background causes multiple subtraction artifacts mimicking sharp transients.
FIG. 4-77a,b,c Run 2 shows a clear spike at F4/C4, but run 1 is nonconfirmatory. Closer inspection of the parasagittal channels of run 1 reveals the origin of the spike (the C4-F4 derivation at bottom shows the subtraction effect).

Missed Abnormality or Misinterpretation Because of Montage

FIG. 4-78a,b,c A sharp wave at C3 (middle of page) is seen clearly on run 2, much less obviously on run 3, and poorly on run 1 (though the waveform is present, it is hidden among others of higher amplitude activity).
FIG. 4-79a,b,c A right anterior quadrant spike is seen on run 1 (middle of page). Run 3 shows anterior temporal localization, but nothing is seen on run 2.
FIG. 4-80a,b Run 2 shows a spike at T5-O1 also involving C3, as well as a smaller spike at C4/F4. Due to the complex fields of both discharges and, additionally, the low amplitude of the latter, run 1 does not display either in an optimal fashion.
FIG. 4-81a,b,c A diffuse sharp wave maximal over the left hemisphere is seen on run 1. Run 3 shows it only at the end of chain channels, while run 2 does not show any hint of it. Here another reference might be helpful.
FIG. 4-82a,b,c,d,e Run 2 shows a left central-temporal spike, maximal over C3/T3. Run 1 shows a complex field, with simultaneous positivities and negativities overlapping at various electrode positions. This is best displayed using the 8 channel, 60 mm/s (e) page.

Clarification of Morphology

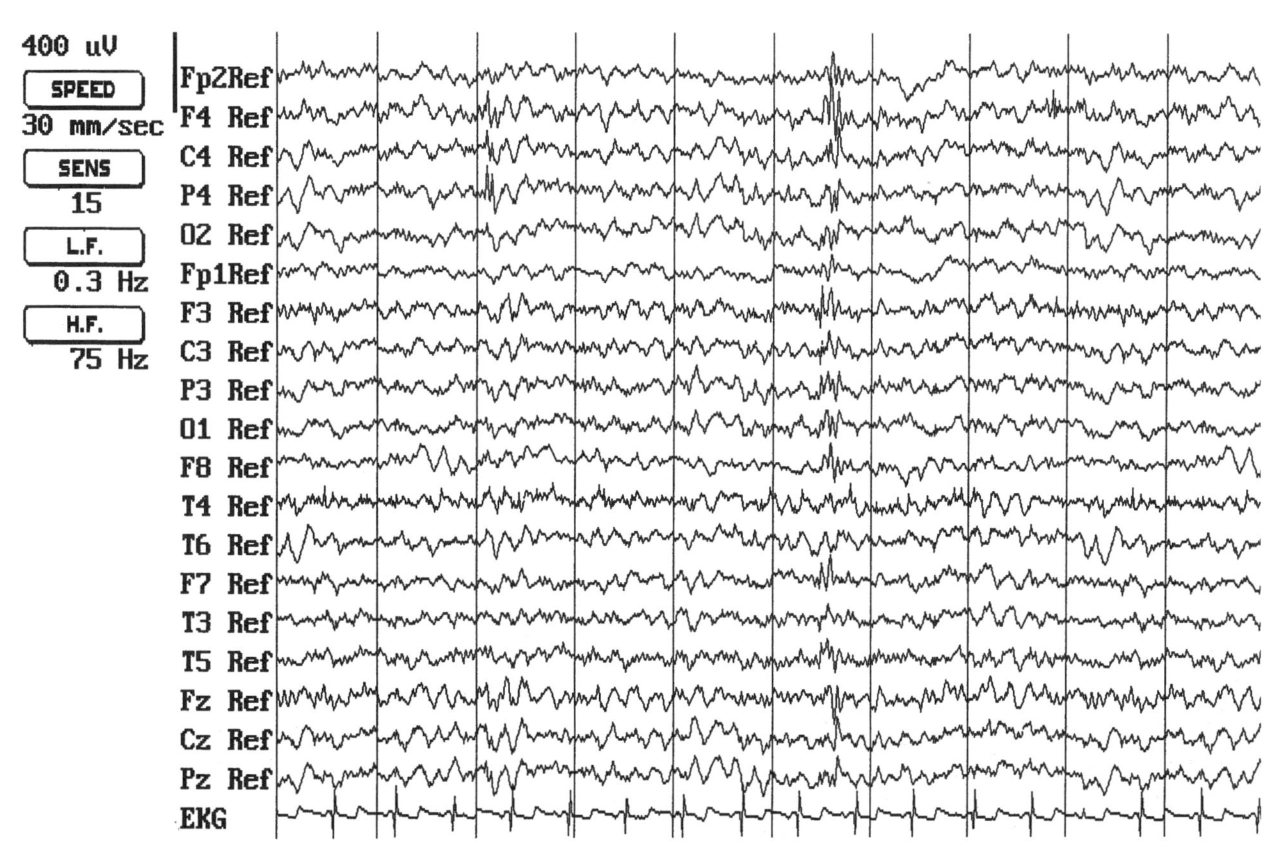

FIG. 4-64a,b,c,d A generalized spike and wave fragment is seen on run 1. Run 2 suggests more right hemispheric discharge, while run 3 shows mainly frontal localization. PS = 60 is shown for comparison.

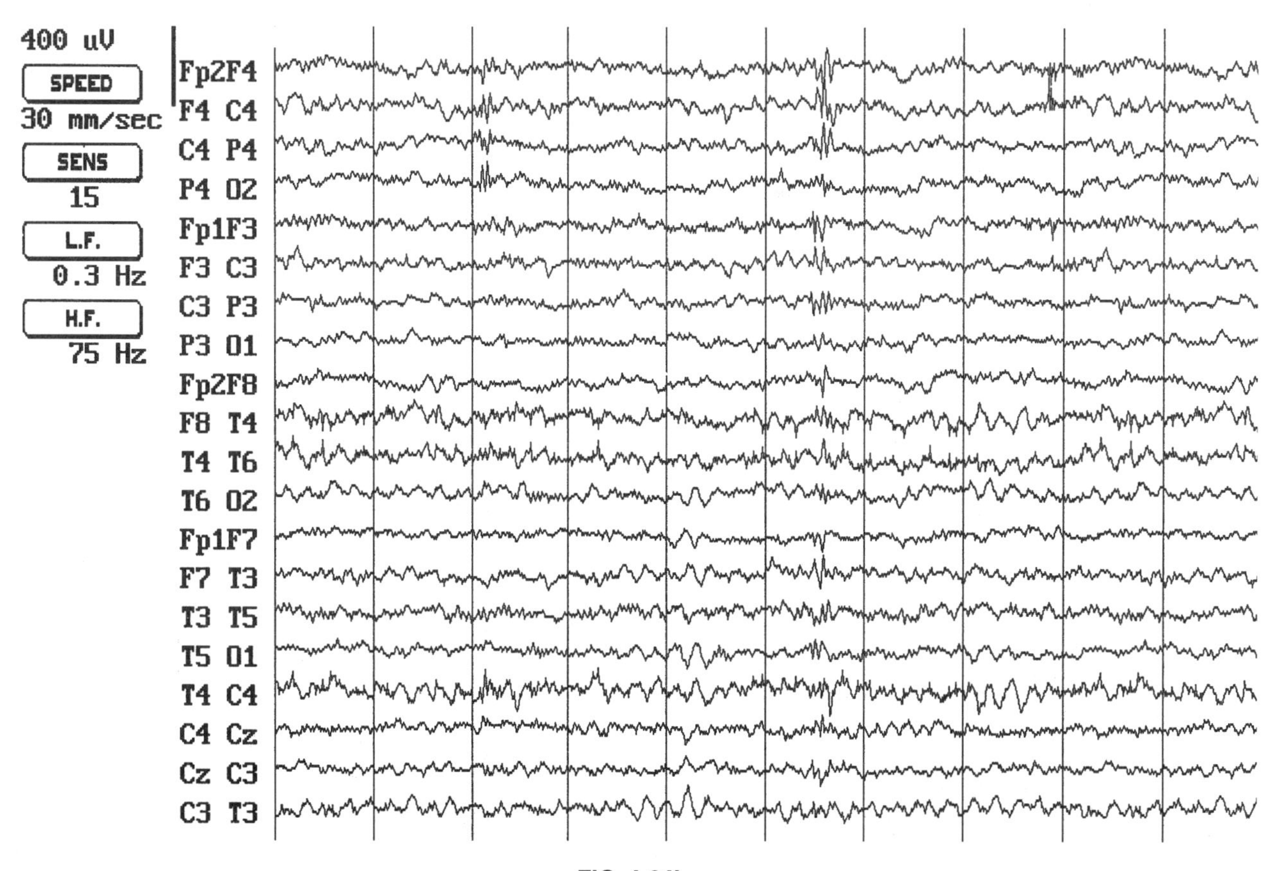
400 uV
SPEED
30 mm/sec
SENS
15
L.F.
0.3 Hz
H.F.
75 Hz
Fp2F4
F4 C4
C4 P4
P4 O2
Fp1F3
F3 C3
C3 P3
P3 O1
Fp2F8
F8 T4
T4 T6
T6 O2
Fp1F7
F7 T3
T3 T5
T5 O1
T4 C4
C4 Cz
Cz C3
C3 T3

FIG. 4-64b

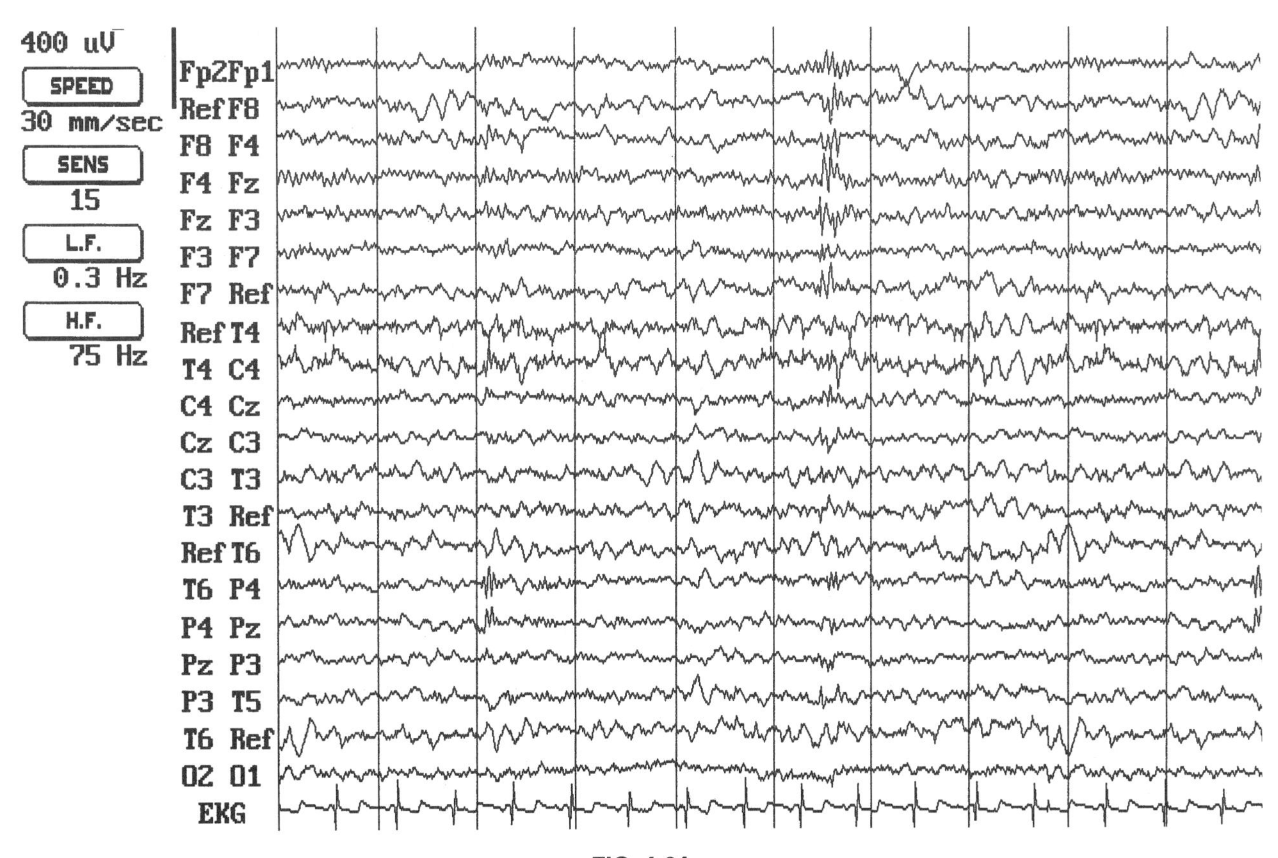
400 uV
SPEED
30 mm/sec
SENS
15
L.F.
0.3 Hz
H.F.
75 Hz
Fp2Fp1
Ref F8
F8 F4
F4 Fz
Fz F3
F3 F7
F7 Ref
Ref T4
T4 C4
C4 Cz
Cz C3
C3 T3
T3 Ref
Ref T6
T6 P4
P4 Pz
Pz P3
P3 T5
T6 Ref
O2 O1
EKG

FIG. 4-64c

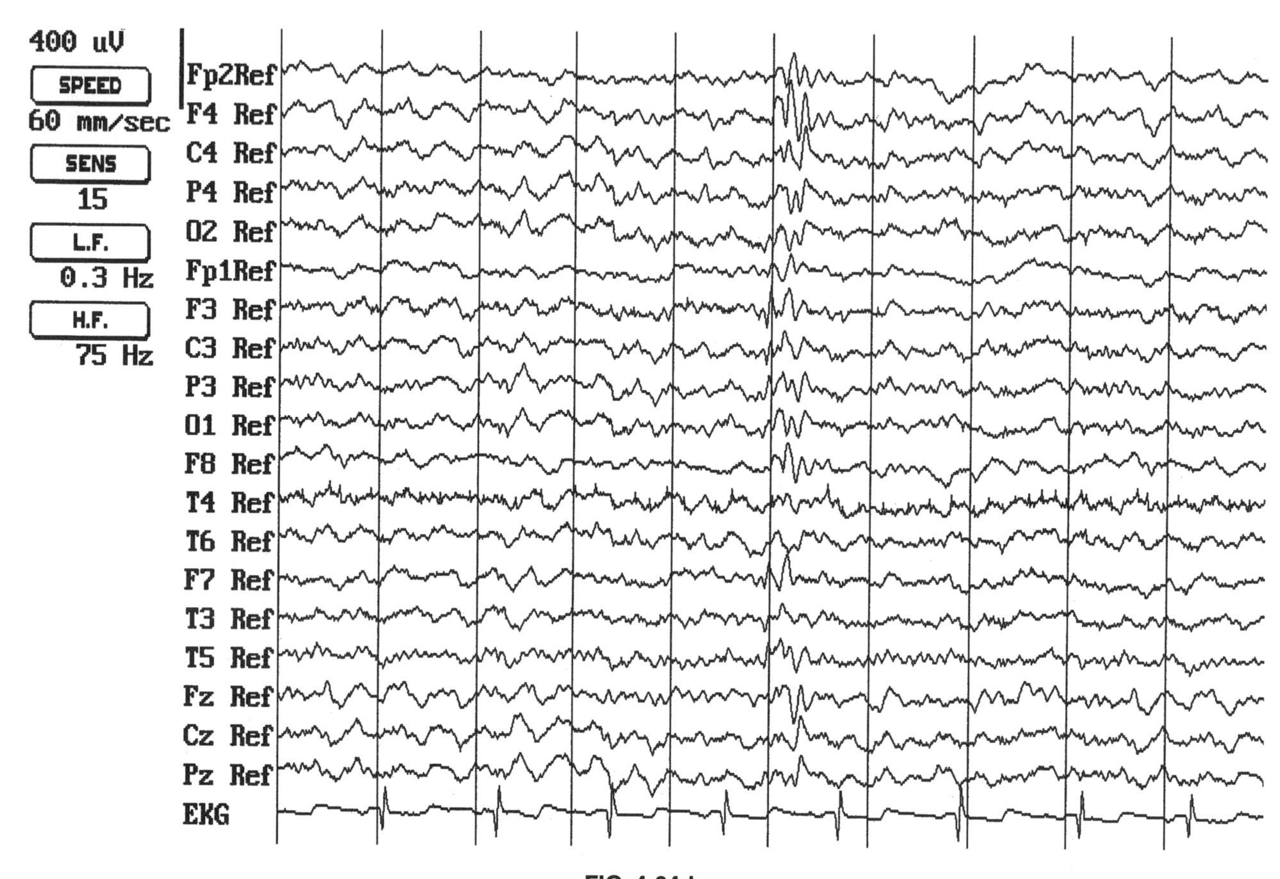
400 uV
SPEED
60 mm/sec
SENS
15
L.F.
0.3 Hz
H.F.
75 Hz
Fp2Ref
F4 Ref
C4 Ref
P4 Ref
O2 Ref
Fp1Ref
F3 Ref
C3 Ref
P3 Ref
O1 Ref
F8 Ref
T4 Ref
T6 Ref
F7 Ref
T3 Ref
T5 Ref
Fz Ref
Cz Ref
Pz Ref
EKG

FIG. 4-64d

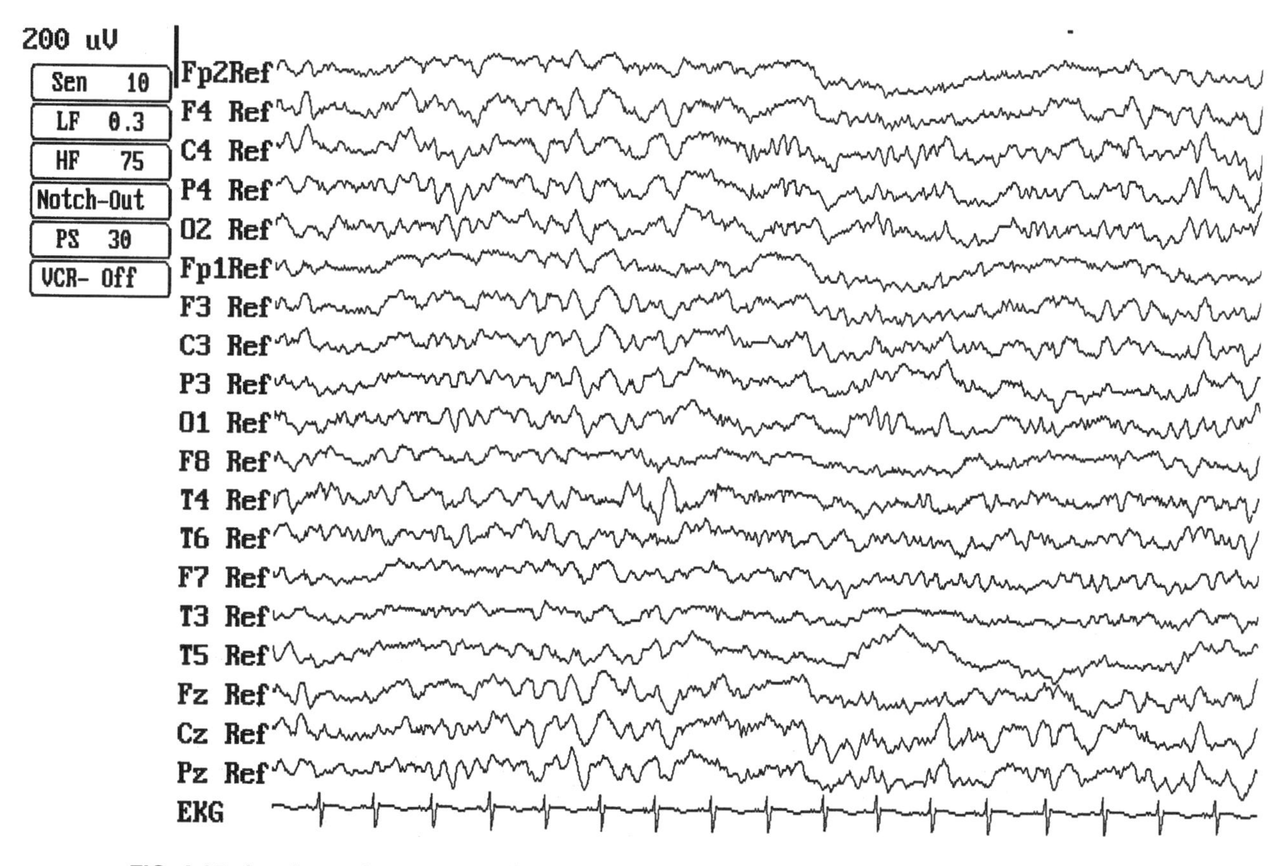

FIG. 4-65a,b,c In run 1 an apparent focal theta with sharp contour at T4 is seen near the middle of the page. Runs 2 and 3 clarified the non-epileptiform nature of this transient.

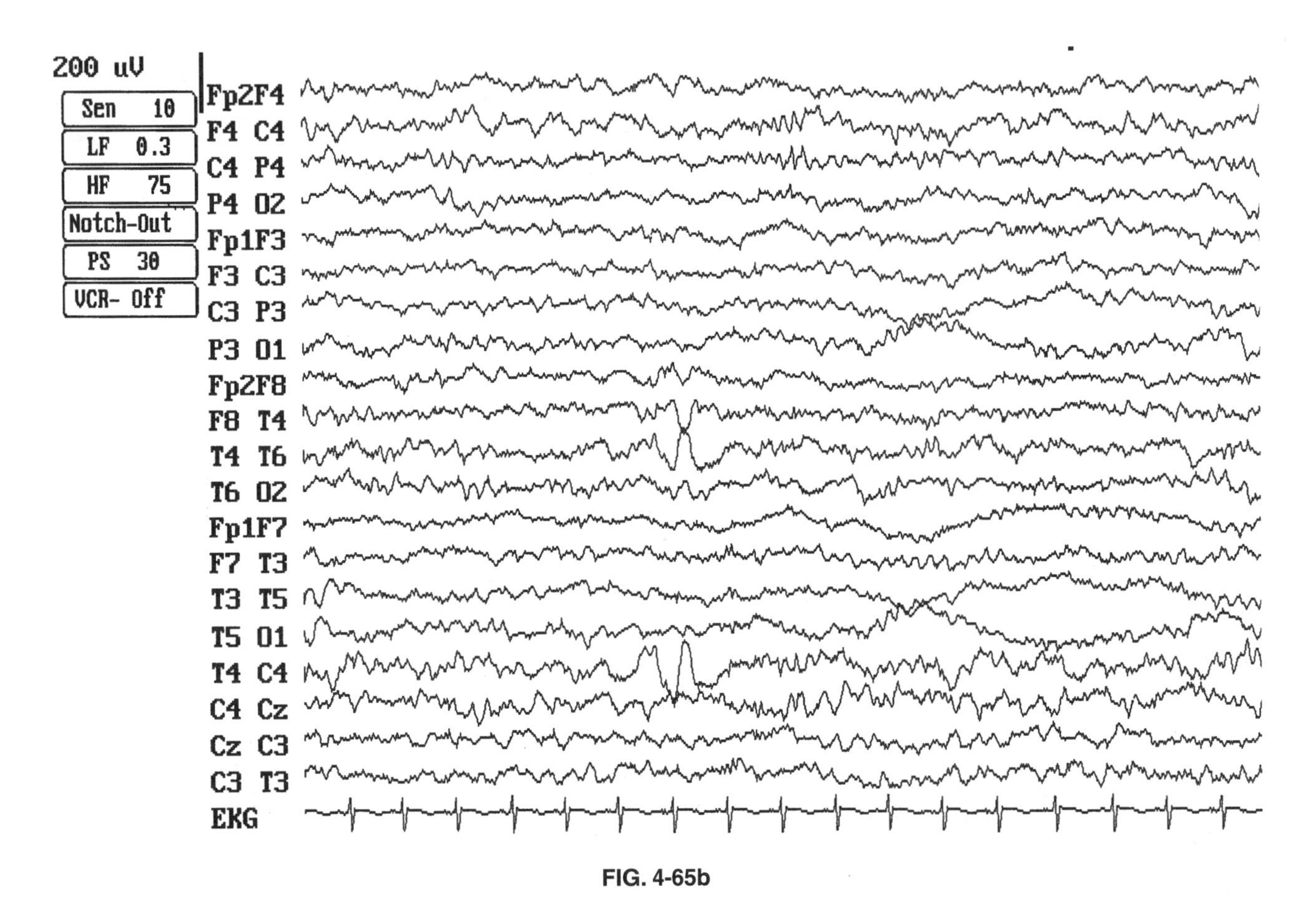
200 uV
Sen 10
LF 0.3
HF 75
Notch-Out
PS 30
VCR- Off
Fp2F4
F4 C4
C4 P4
P4 O2
Fp1F3
F3 C3
C3 P3
P3 O1
Fp2F8
F8 T4
T4 T6
T6 O2
Fp1F7
F7 T3
T3 T5
T5 O1
T4 C4
C4 Cz
Cz C3
C3 T3
EKG

FIG. 4-65b

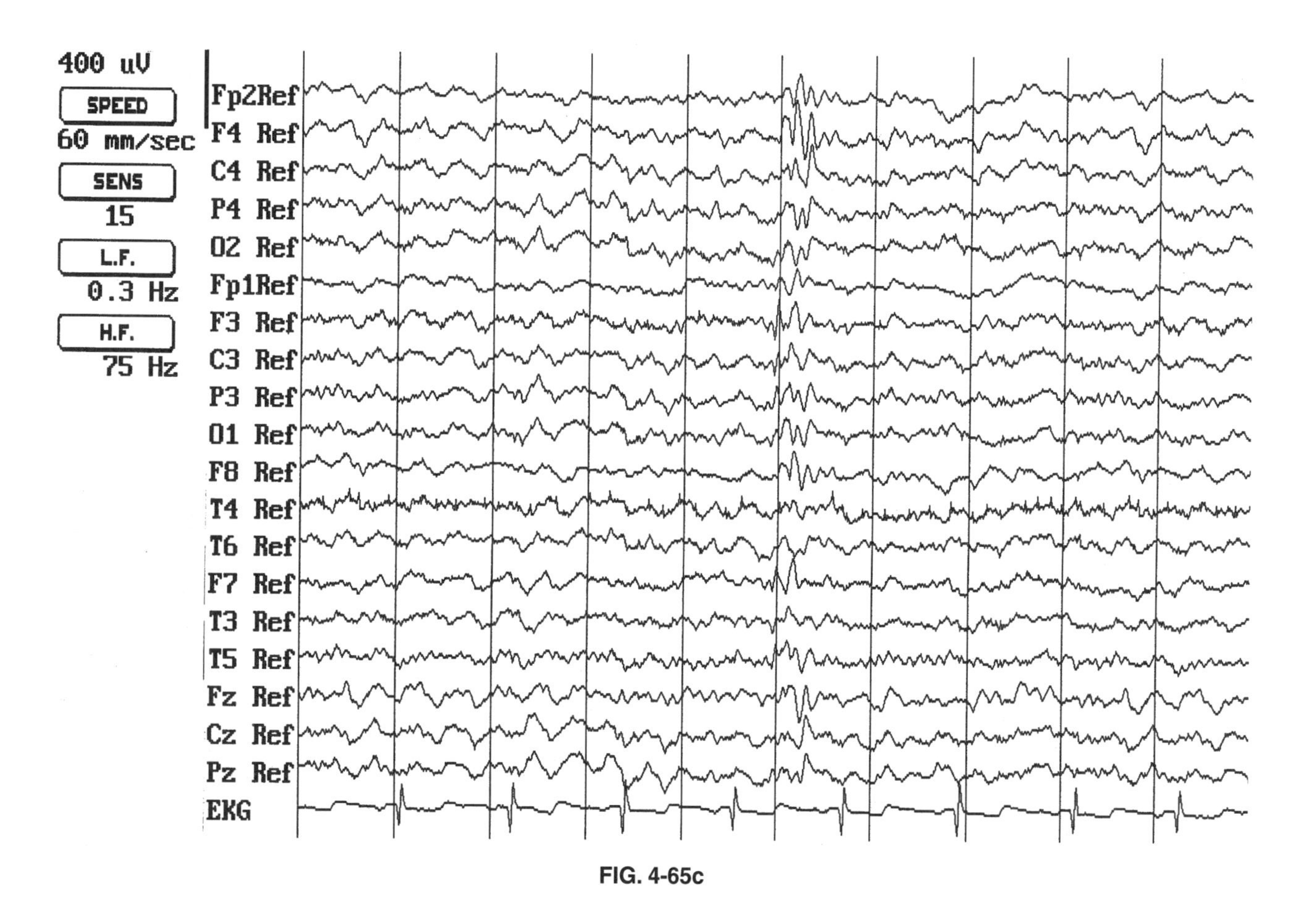
400 uV
SPEED
60 mm/sec
SENS
15
L.F.
0.3 Hz
H.F.
75 Hz
Fp2Ref
F4 Ref
C4 Ref
P4 Ref
O2 Ref
Fp1Ref
F3 Ref
C3 Ref
P3 Ref
O1 Ref
F8 Ref
T4 Ref
T6 Ref
F7 Ref
T3 Ref
T5 Ref
Fz Ref
Cz Ref
Pz Ref
EKG

FIG. 4-65c

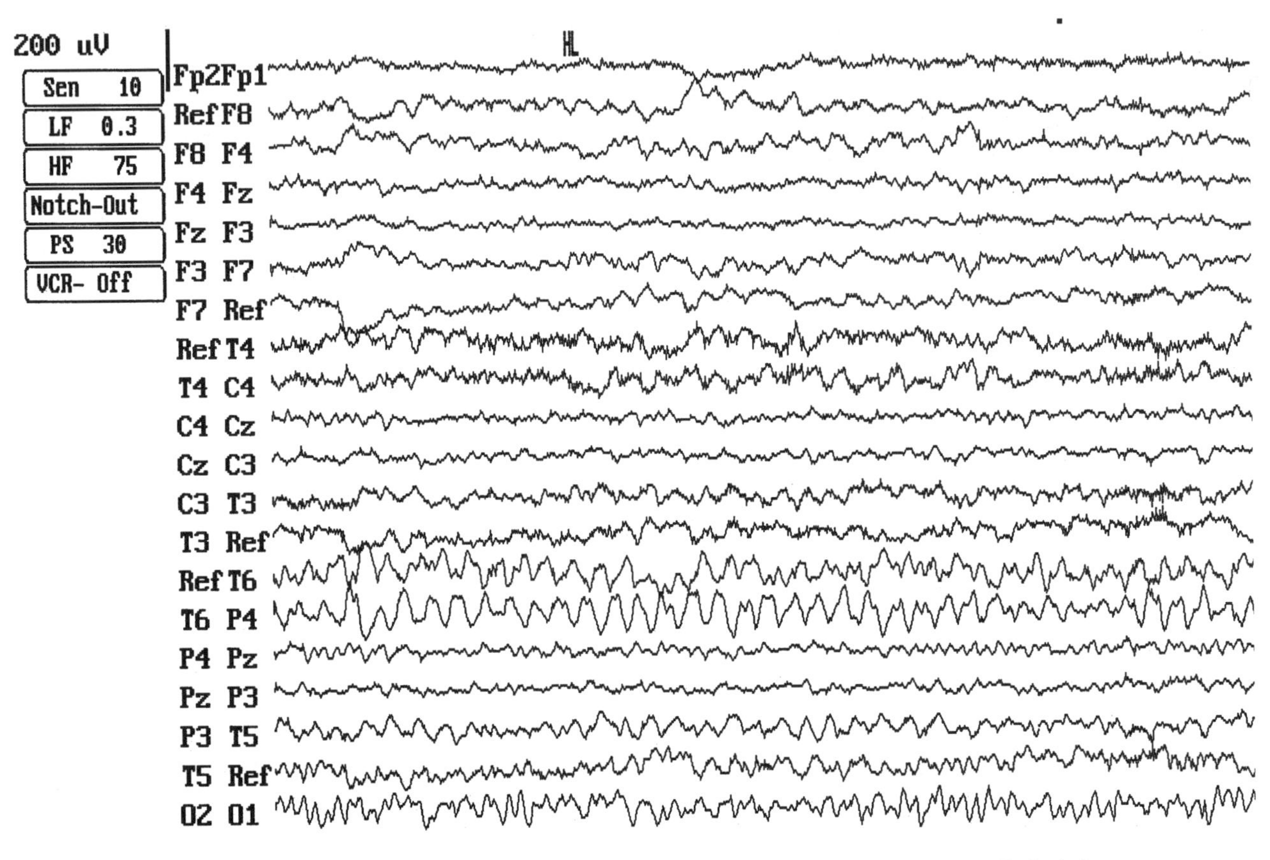

FIG. 4-66a,b Apparent persistent rhythmic focal slowing at T6 is seen on run 3 (cancellation), but on run 1 it is diffuse and there is lower amplitude at left temporal. The pattern is that of delta with broad field.

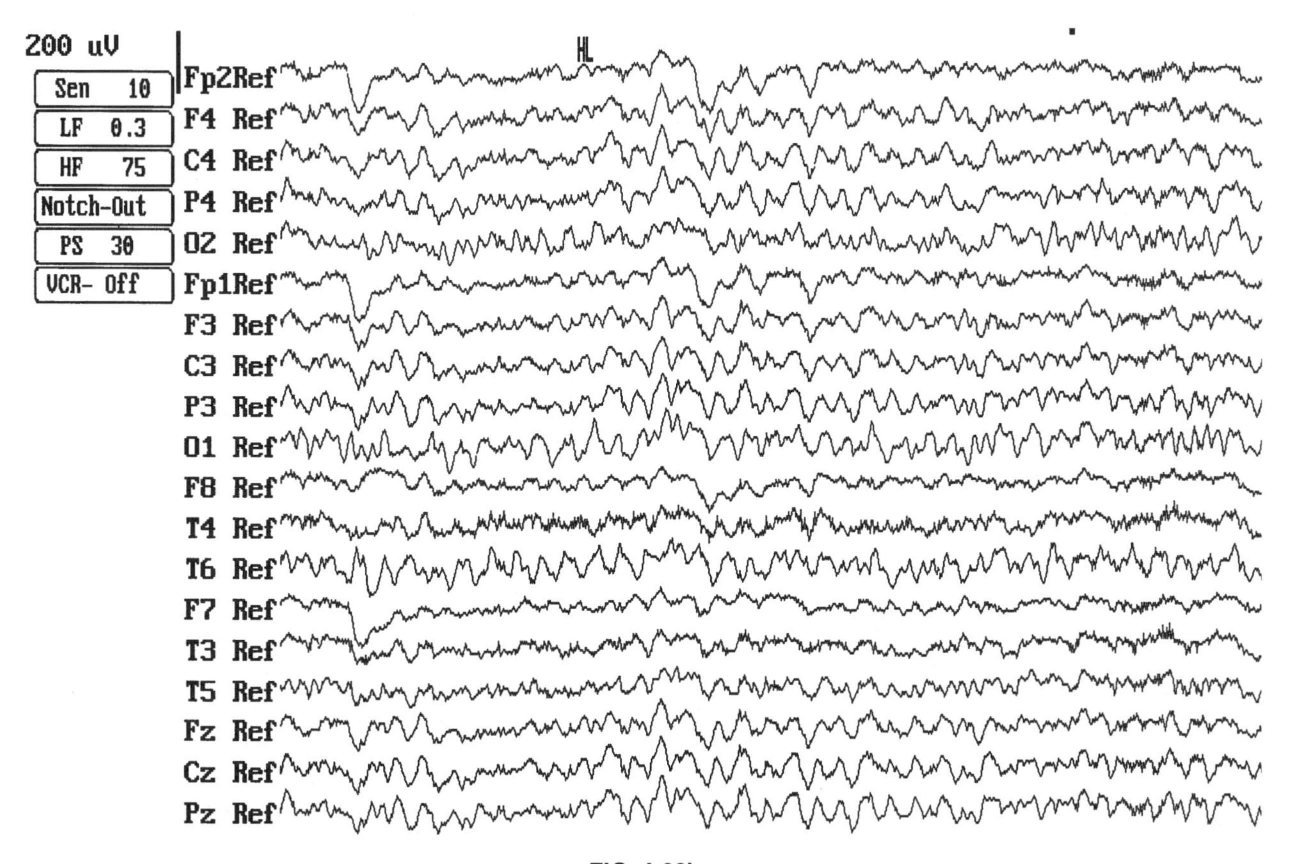
200 uV
Sen 10
LF 0.3
HF 75
Notch-Out
PS 30
VCR- Off
HL
Fp2Ref
F4 Ref
C4 Ref
P4 Ref
O2 Ref
Fp1Ref
F3 Ref
C3 Ref
P3 Ref
O1 Ref
F8 Ref
T4 Ref
T6 Ref
F7 Ref
T3 Ref
T5 Ref
Fz Ref
Cz Ref
Pz Ref

FIG. 4-66b

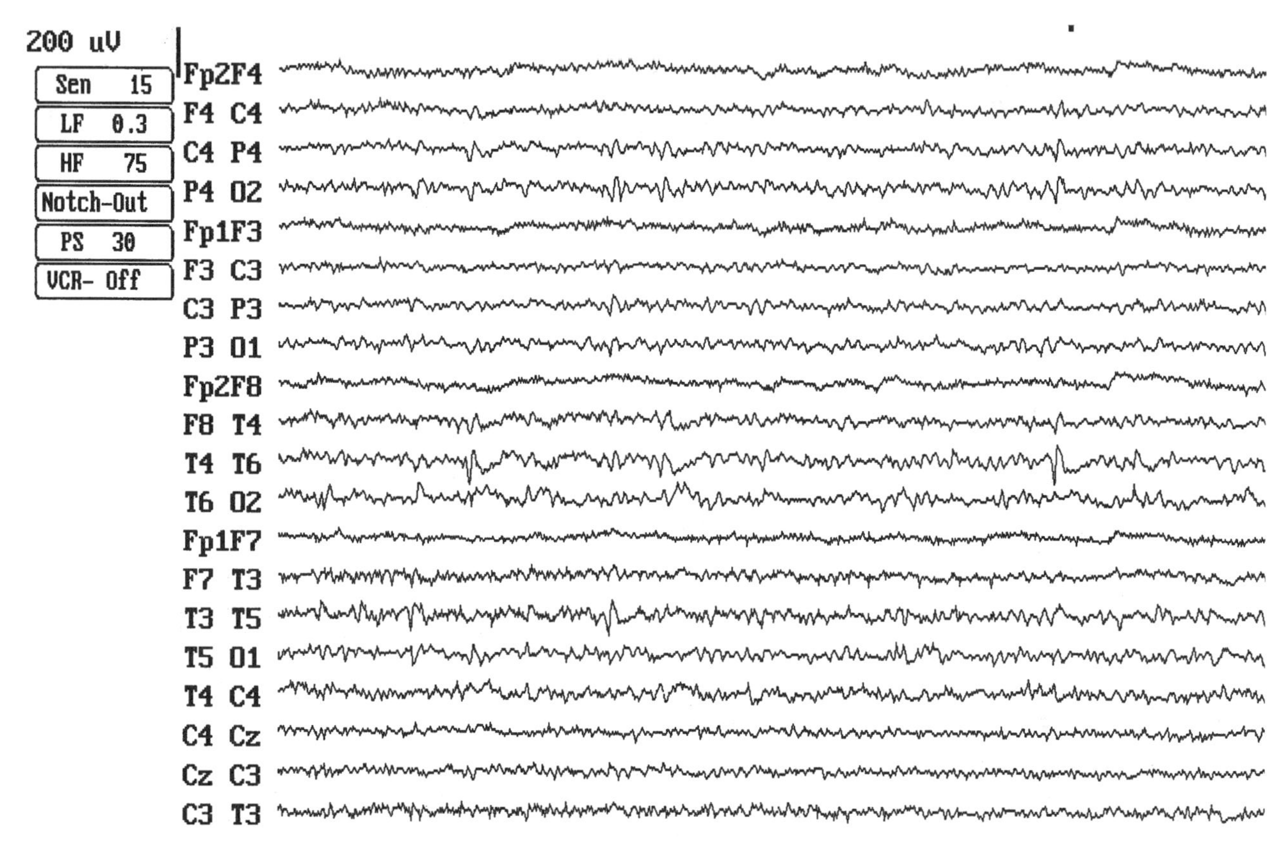

FIG. 4-67a,b,c Run 2 shows a spike at T4-T6 single deflection, while run 4 shows a definite T6-O2 spike. Run 1 confirmed this latter location.

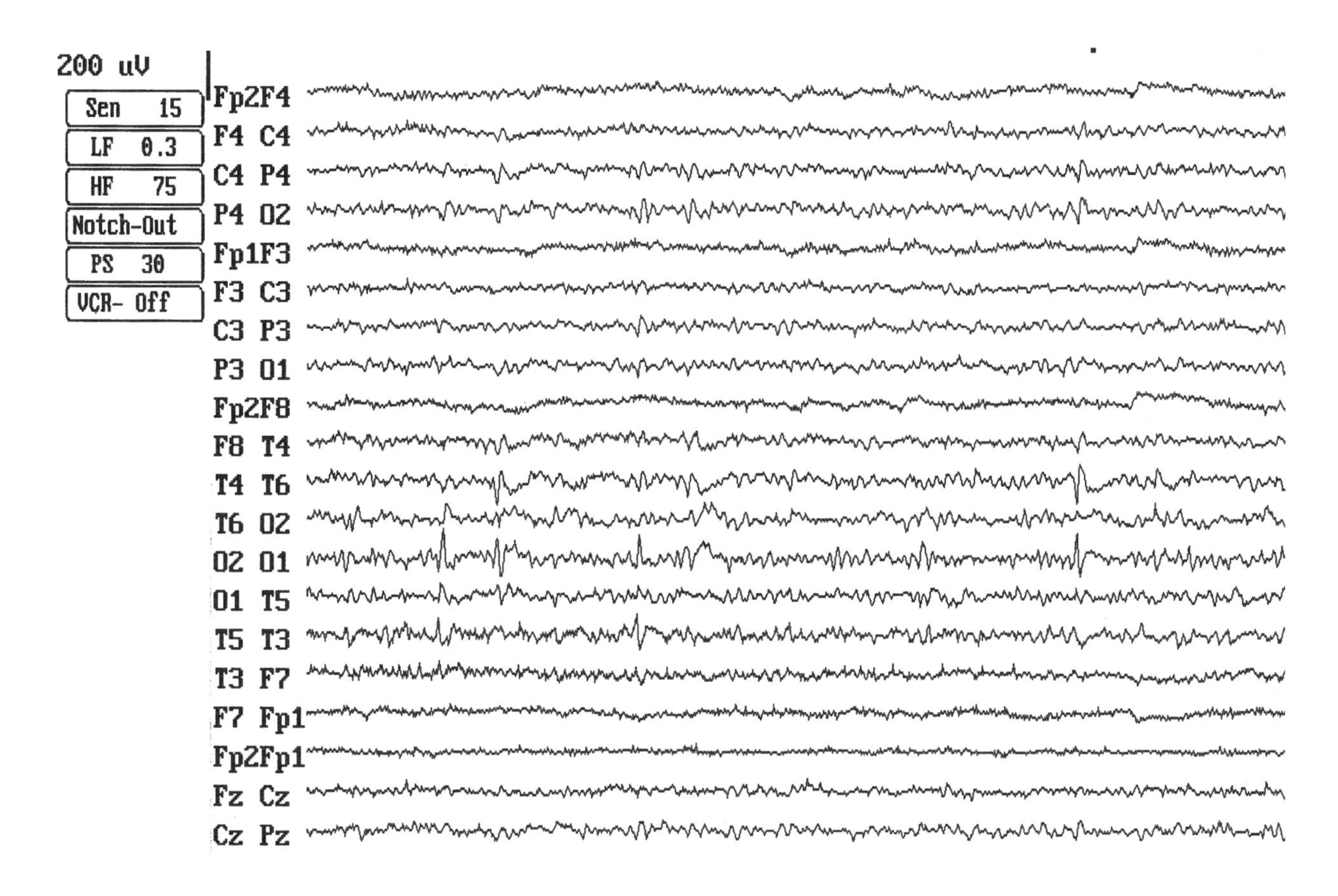
200 uV
Sen 15
LF 0.3
HF 75
Notch-Out
PS 30
VCR- Off
Fp2F4
F4 C4
C4 P4
P4 O2
Fp1F3
F3 C3
C3 P3
P3 O1
Fp2F8
F8 T4
T4 T6
T6 O2
O2 O1
O1 T5
T5 T3
T3 F7
F7 Fp1
Fp2Fp1
Fz Cz
Cz Pz

FIG. 4-67b

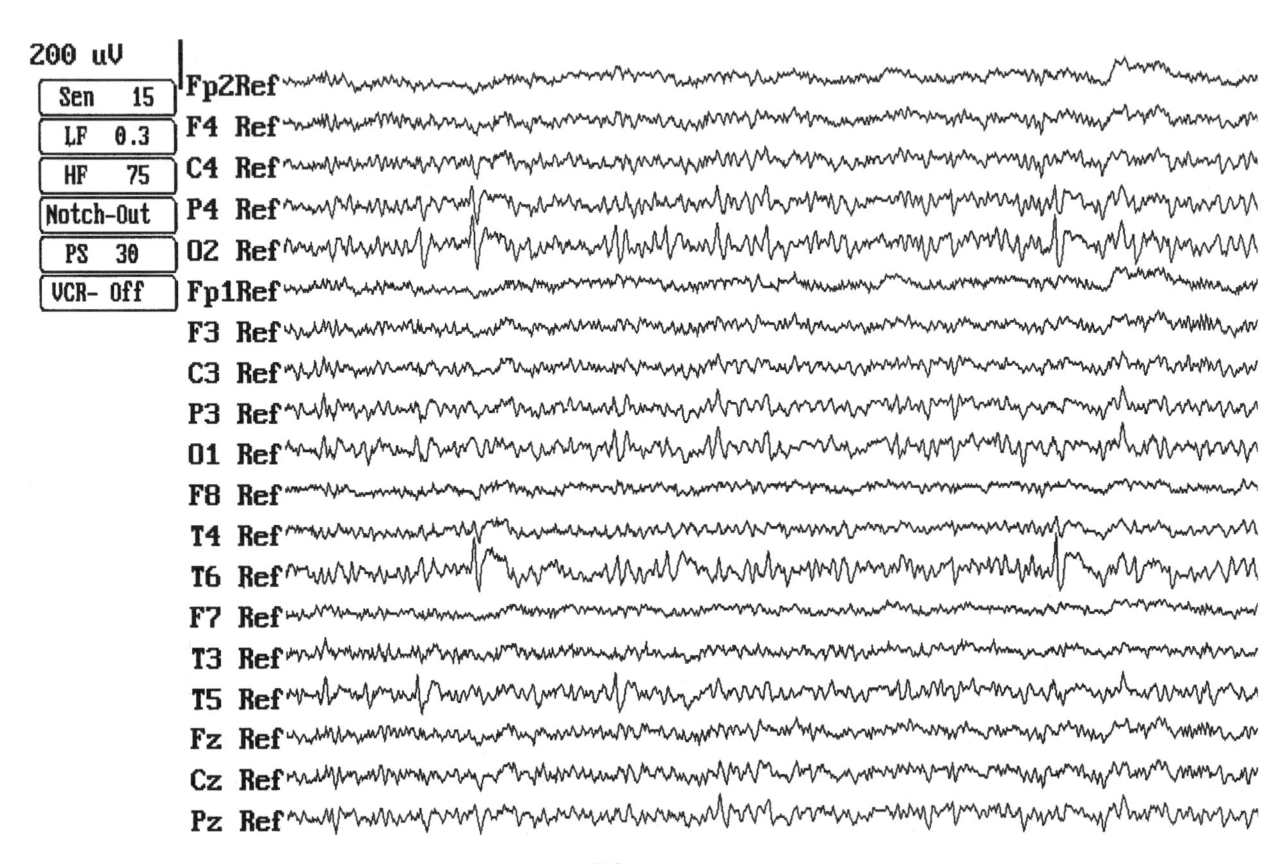
200 uV
Sen 15
LF 0.3
HF 75
Notch-Out
PS 30
VCR- Off
Fp2Ref
F4 Ref
C4 Ref
P4 Ref
O2 Ref
Fp1Ref
F3 Ref
C3 Ref
P3 Ref
O1 Ref
F8 Ref
T4 Ref
T6 Ref
F7 Ref
T3 Ref
T5 Ref
Fz Ref
Cz Ref
Pz Ref

FIG. 4-67c

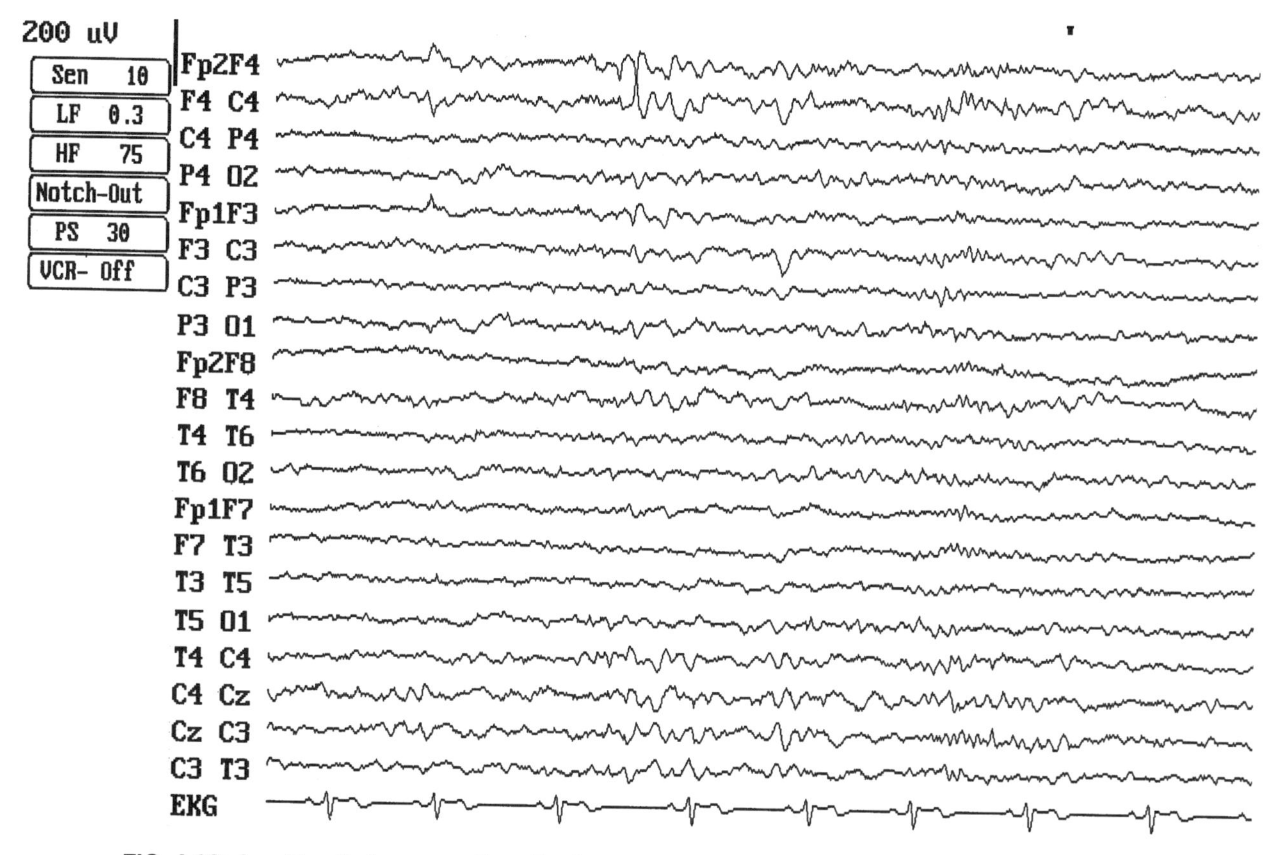

FIG. 4-68a,b,c Run 2 shows a spike with phase reversal at F4, while run 3 shows a bifrontal location. This is confirmed on run 1.

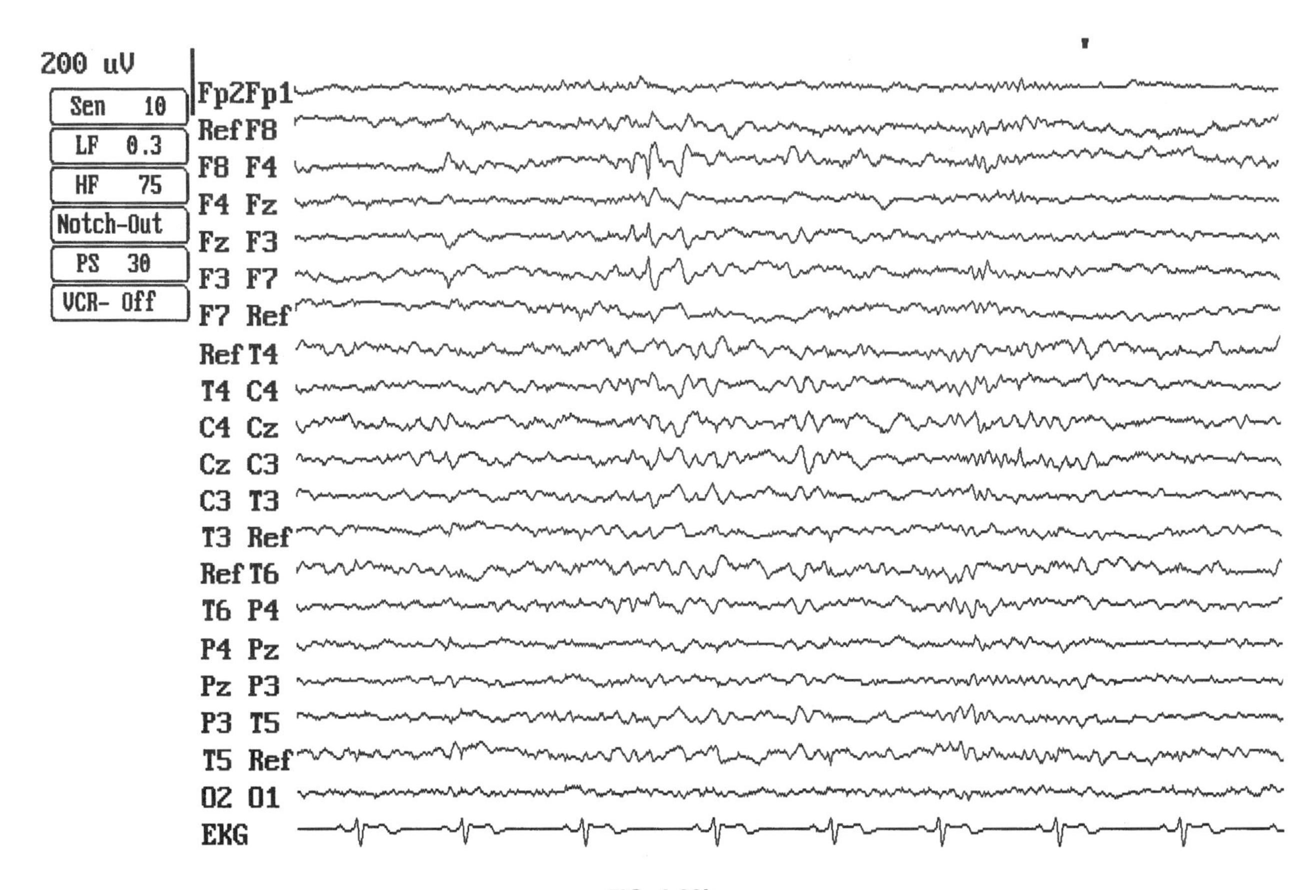
200 uV
Sen 10
LF 0.3
HF 75
Notch-Out
PS 30
VCR- Off
Fp2Fp1
Ref F8
F8 F4
F4 Fz
Fz F3
F3 F7
F7 Ref
Ref T4
T4 C4
C4 Cz
Cz C3
C3 T3
T3 Ref
Ref T6
T6 P4
P4 Pz
Pz P3
P3 T5
T5 Ref
O2 O1
EKG

FIG. 4-68b

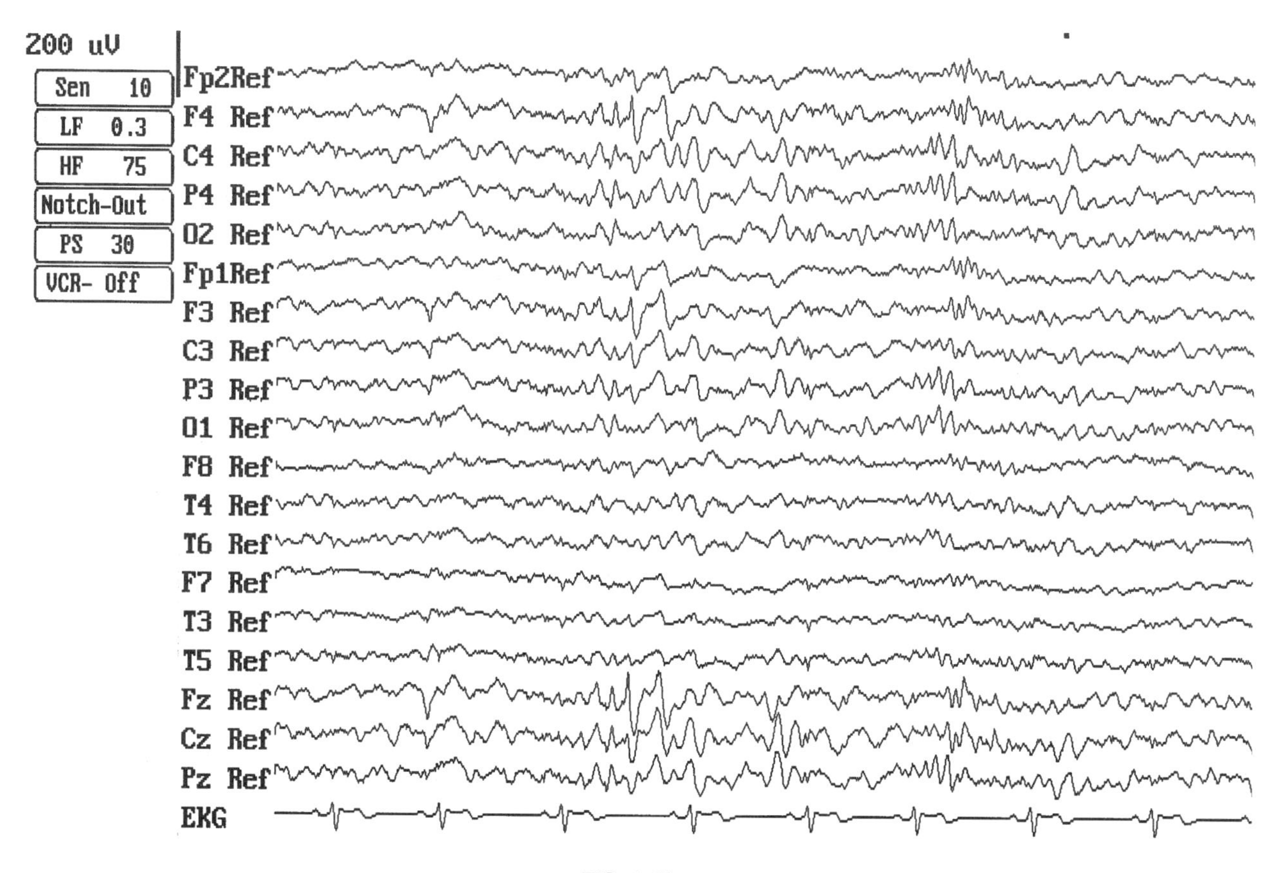
200 uV
Sen 10
LF 0.3
HF 75
Notch-Out
PS 30
VCR- Off
Fp2Ref
F4 Ref
C4 Ref
P4 Ref
O2 Ref
Fp1Ref
F3 Ref
C3 Ref
P3 Ref
O1 Ref
F8 Ref
T4 Ref
T6 Ref
F7 Ref
T3 Ref
T5 Ref
Fz Ref
Cz Ref
Pz Ref
EKG

FIG. 4-68c

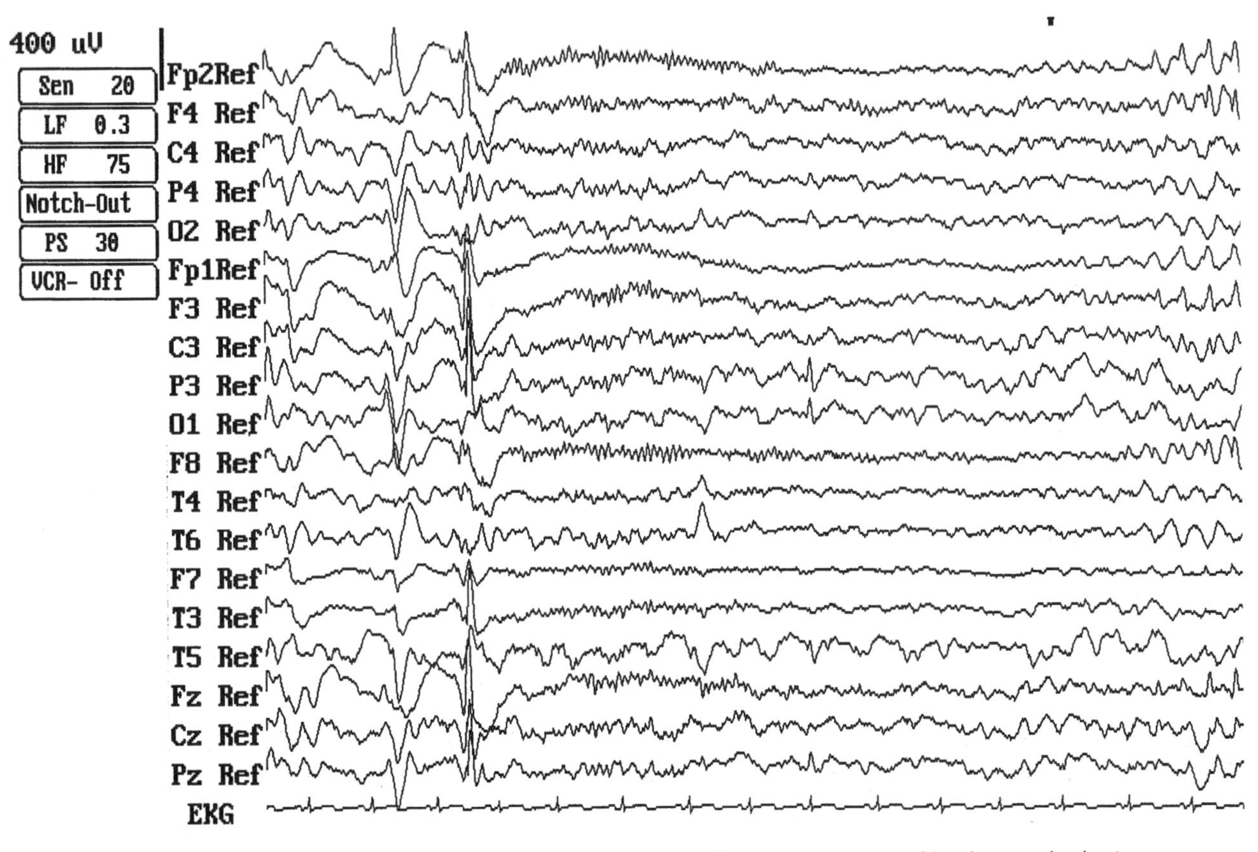

FIG. 4-69a,b Run 1 with linked cheek reference shows diffuse suppression of background prior to seizure (note the preceding high voltage spiking on the left). The same montage with a slow paper speed enhanced the flattening of preictal background (note the ictal onset at the right of the figure).

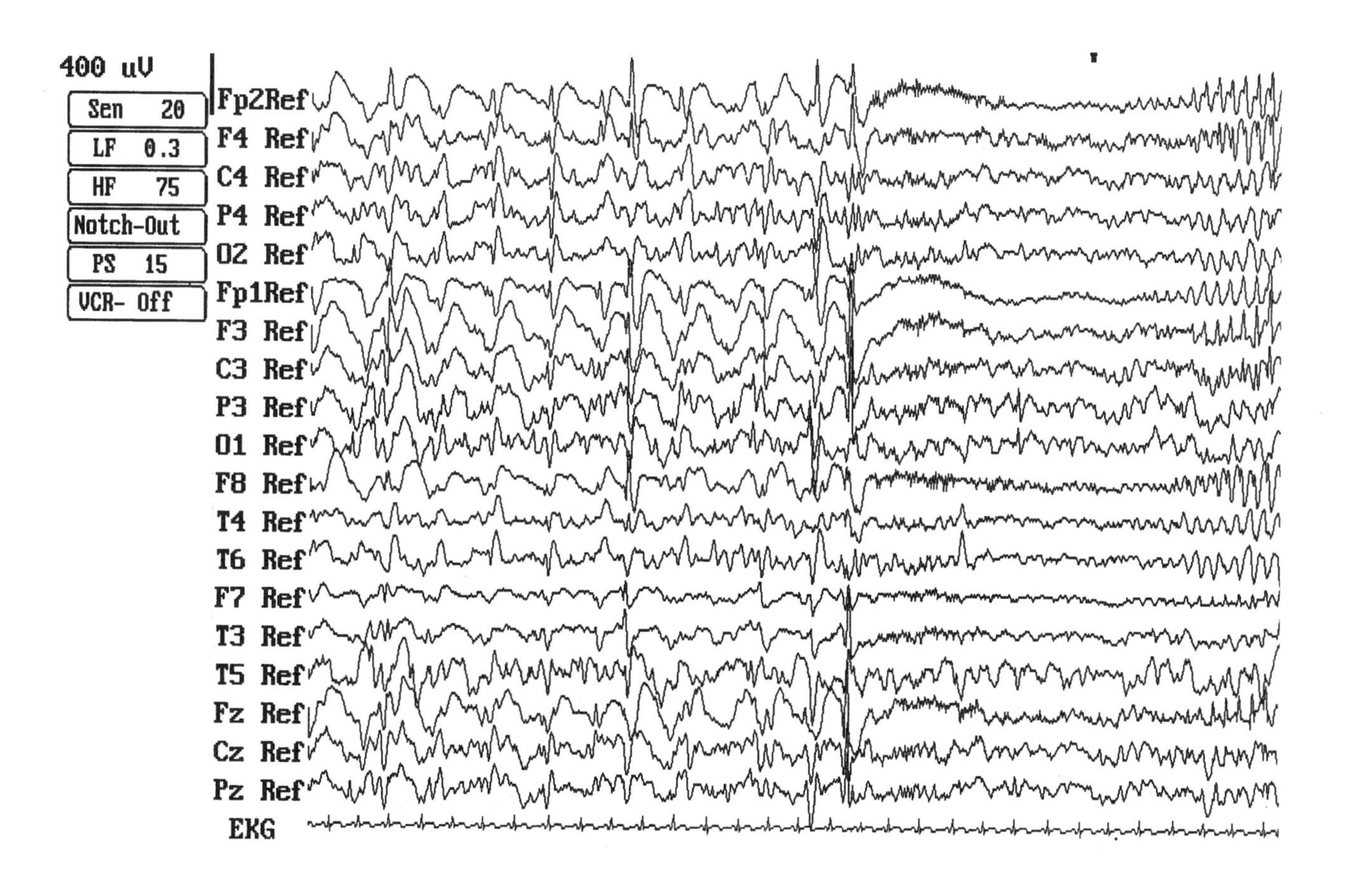
400 uV
Sen 20
LF 0.3
HF 75
Notch-Out
PS 15
VCR- Off
Fp2Ref
F4 Ref
C4 Ref
P4 Ref
O2 Ref
Fp1Ref
F3 Ref
C3 Ref
P3 Ref
O1 Ref
F8 Ref
T4 Ref
T6 Ref
F7 Ref
T3 Ref
T5 Ref
Fz Ref
Cz Ref
Pz Ref
EKG

FIG. 4-69b

Ambiguous normality

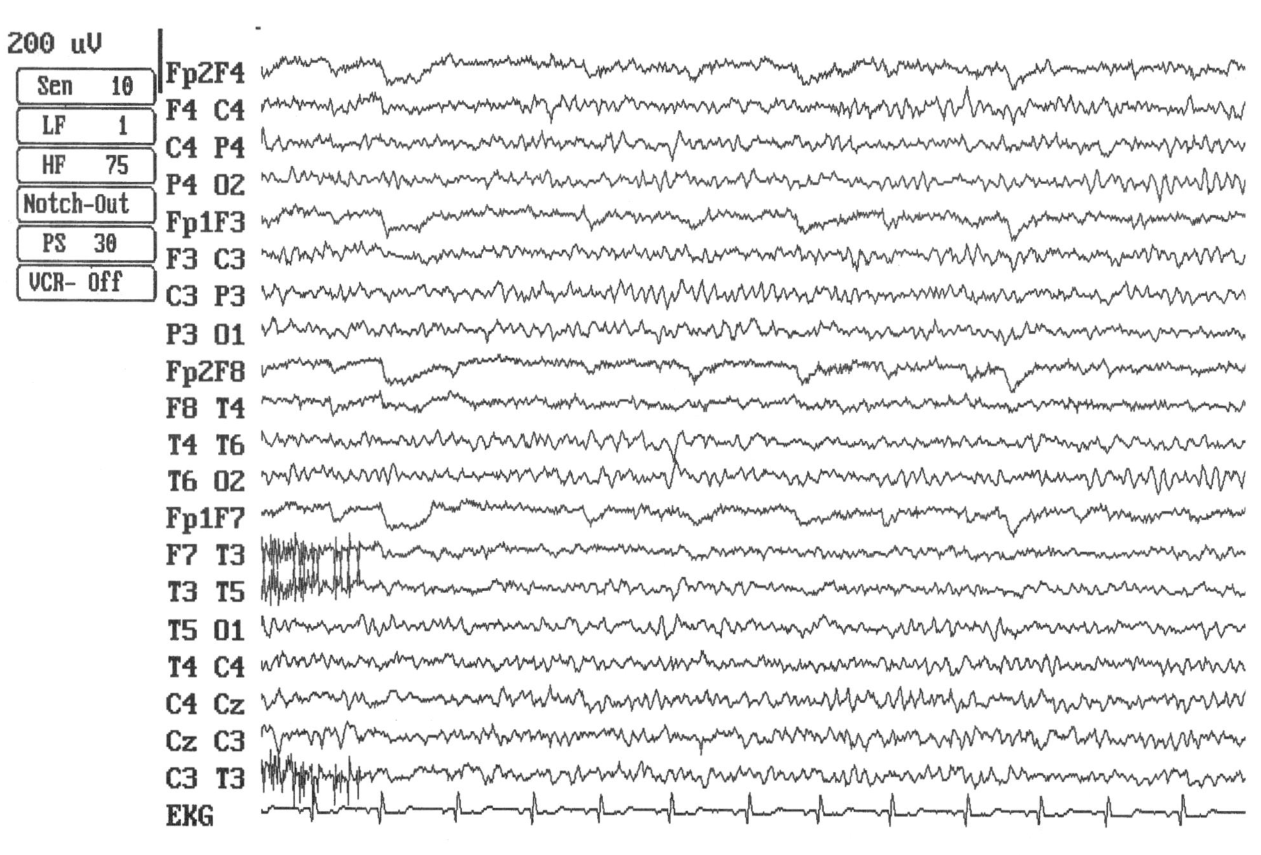

FIG. 4-70a,b A questionable T6 sharp wave is seen on run 2 at the middle of the page. Run 1 not confirmatory, showing the previous sharp phase reversal to be an idiosyncrasy of the alpha waveform, producing sharp slopes on subtraction (subtraction artifact).

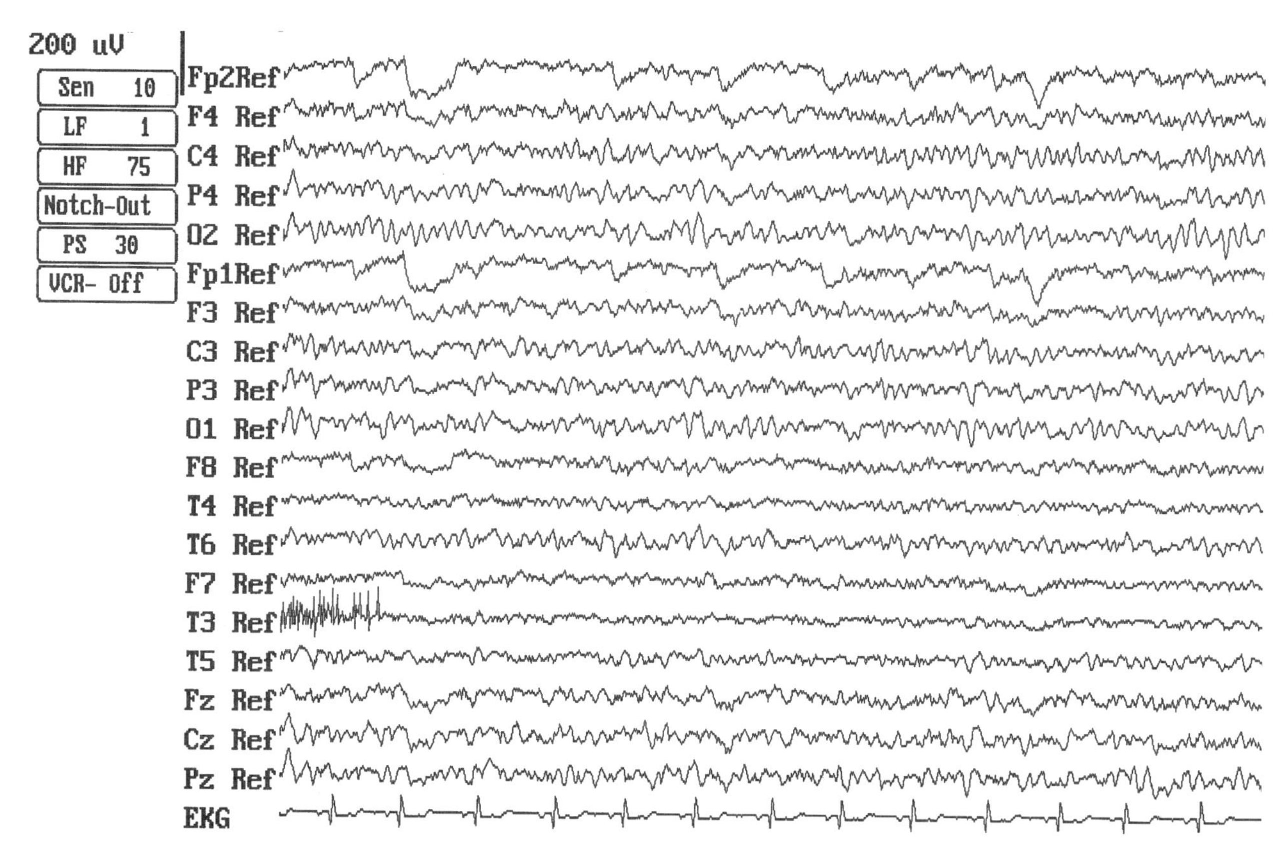
200 uV
Sen 10
LF 1
HF 75
Notch-Out
PS 30
VCR- Off
Fp2Ref
F4 Ref
C4 Ref
P4 Ref
O2 Ref
Fp1Ref
F3 Ref
C3 Ref
P3 Ref
O1 Ref
F8 Ref
T4 Ref
T6 Ref
F7 Ref
T3 Ref
T5 Ref
Fz Ref
Cz Ref
Pz Ref
EKG

FIG. 4-70b

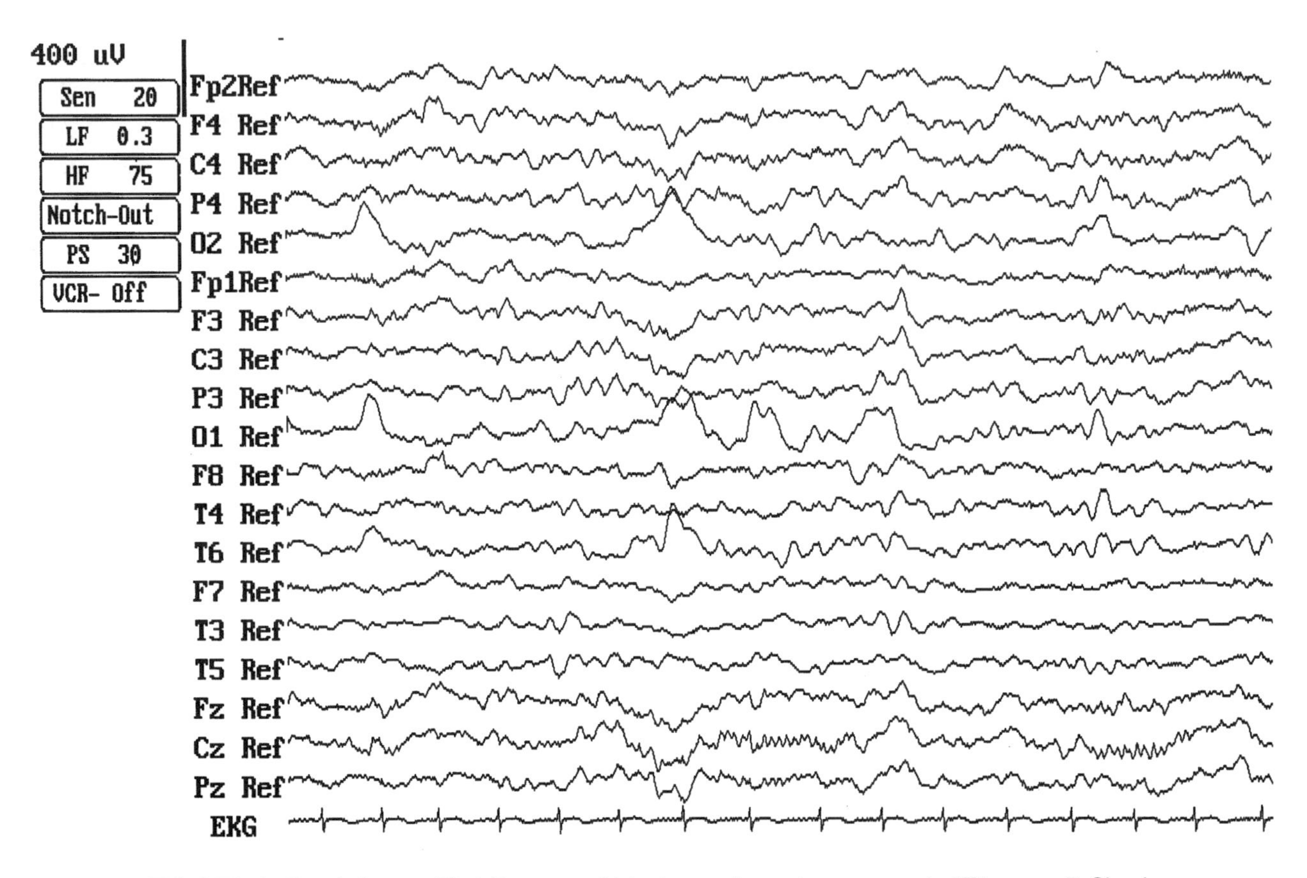

FIG. 4-71a,b Run 1 shows a T6 delta wave, which gives a sharp phase reversal at T6 on run 3. Clearly, this is another subtraction artifact.

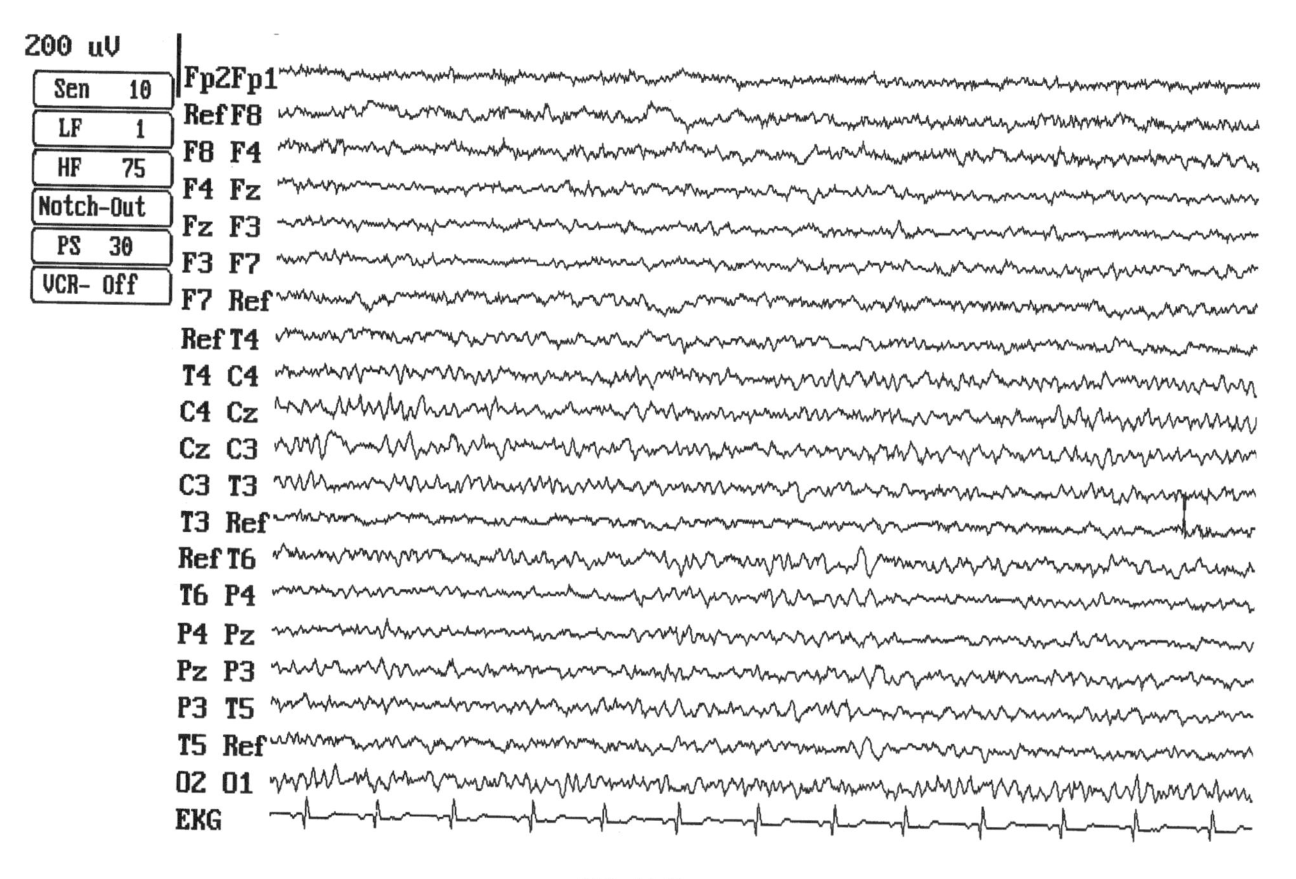
200 uV
Sen 10
LF 1
HF 75
Notch-Out
PS 30
VCR- Off
Fp2Fp1
Ref F8
F8 F4
F4 Fz
Fz F3
F3 F7
F7 Ref
Ref T4
T4 C4
C4 Cz
Cz C3
C3 T3
T3 Ref
Ref T6
T6 P4
P4 Pz
Pz P3
P3 T5
T5 Ref
O2 O1
EKG

FIG. 4-71b

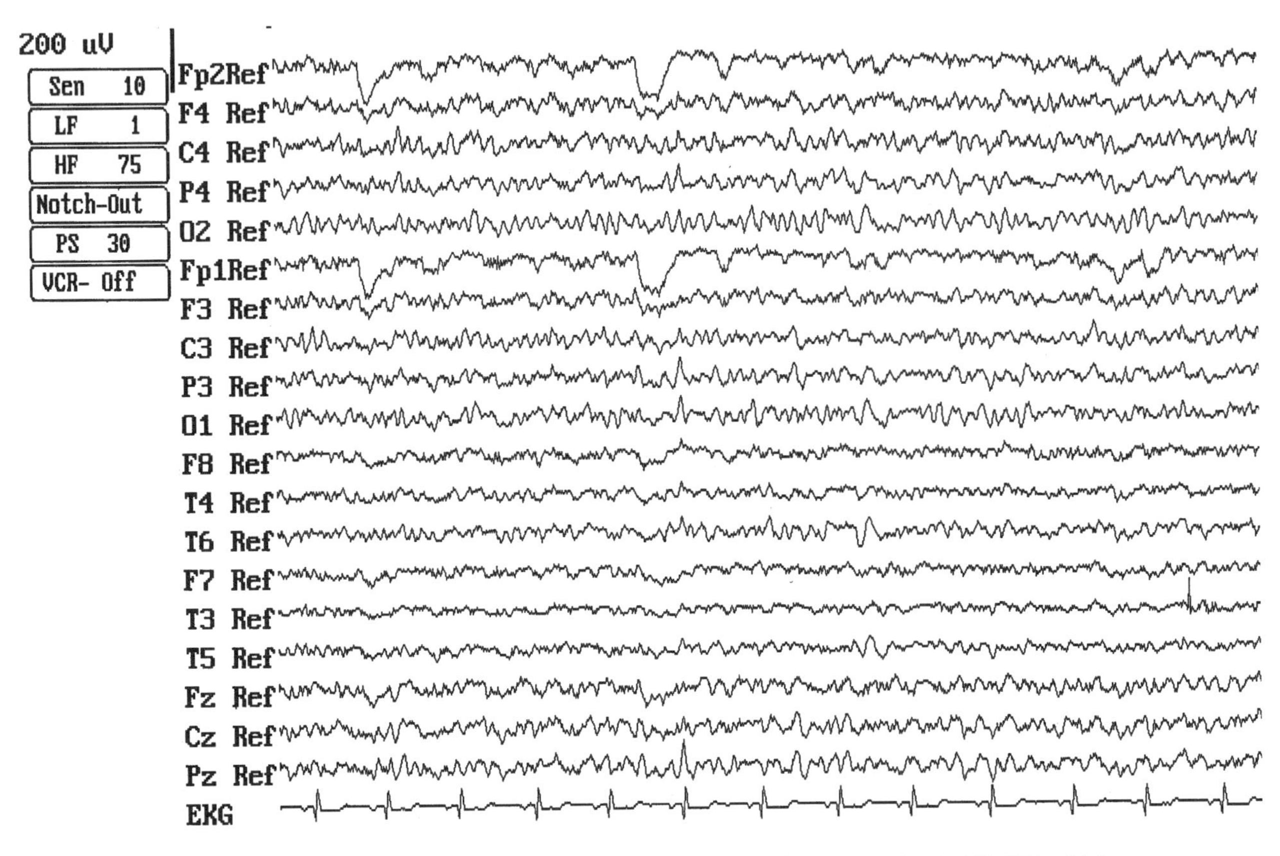

FIG. 4-72a,b Run 1 (middle of page) shows a sharply contoured wave maximal at Pz/P3, which, on reflection, has benign features. Run 2 shows nothing of note.

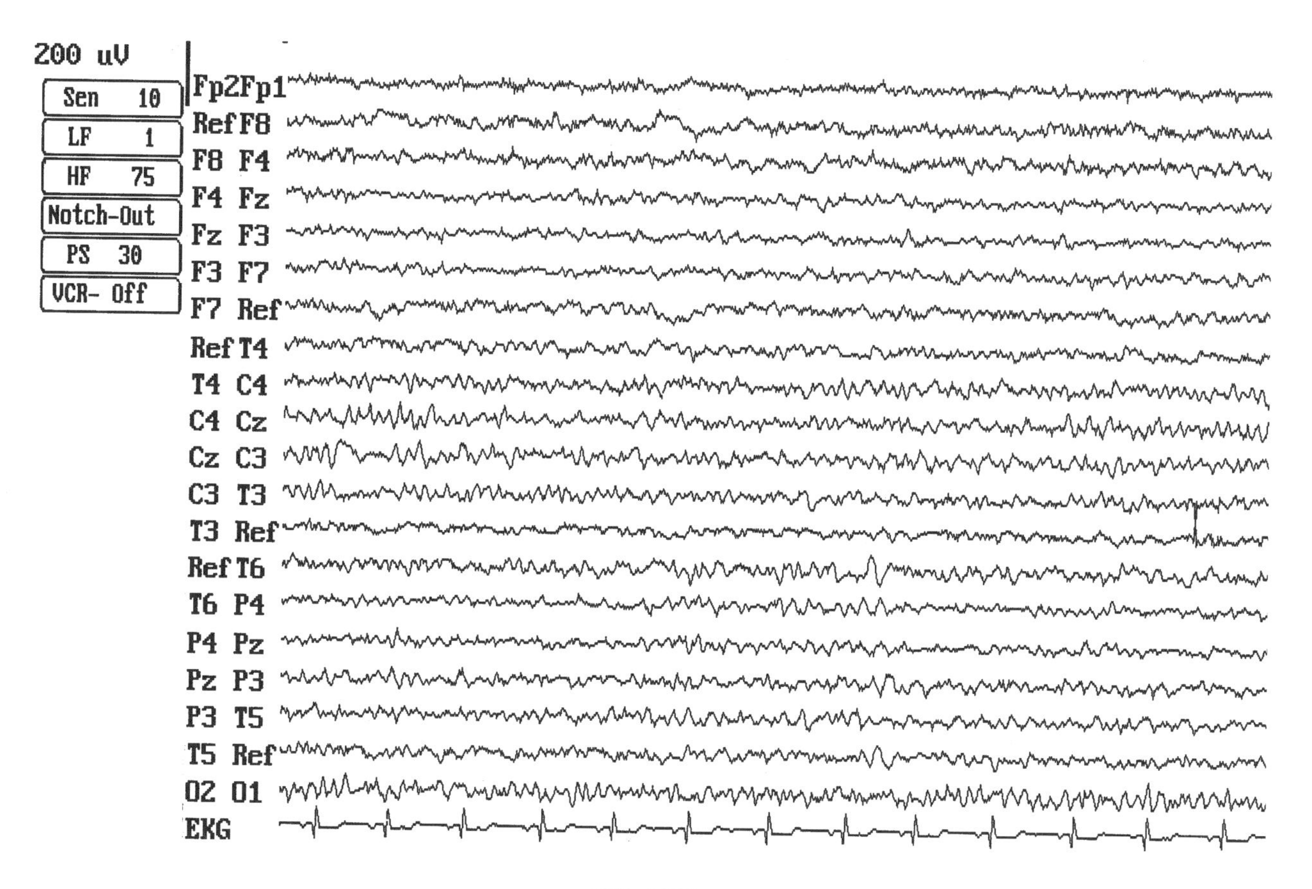
200 uV
Sen 10
LF 1
HF 75
Notch-Out
PS 30
VCR- Off
Fp2Fp1
Ref F8
F8 F4
F4 Fz
Fz F3
F3 F7
F7 Ref
Ref T4
T4 C4
C4 Cz
Cz C3
C3 T3
T3 Ref
Ref T6
T6 P4
P4 Pz
Pz P3
P3 T5
T5 Ref
O2 O1
EKG

FIG. 4-72b

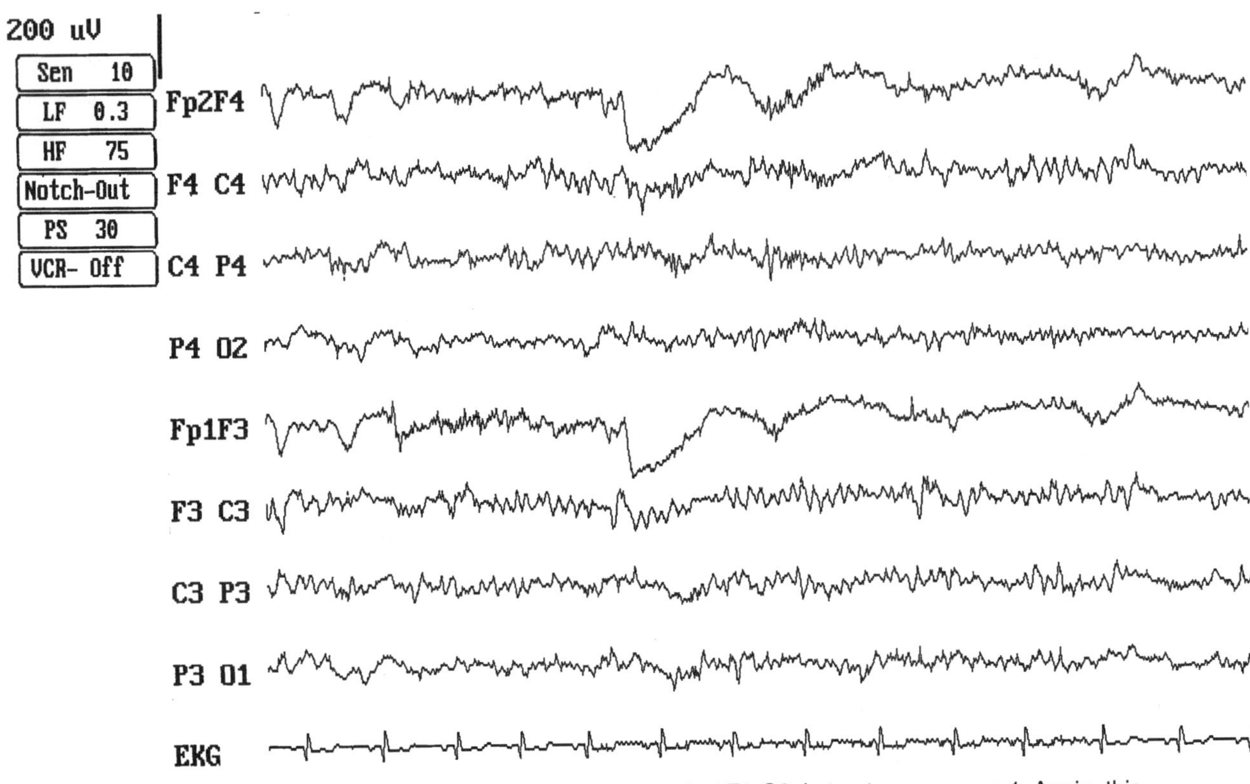

FIG. 4-73a,b Single sharp deflections are seen on run 2 at F3-C3, but not seen on run 1. Again, this is a subtraction artifact.

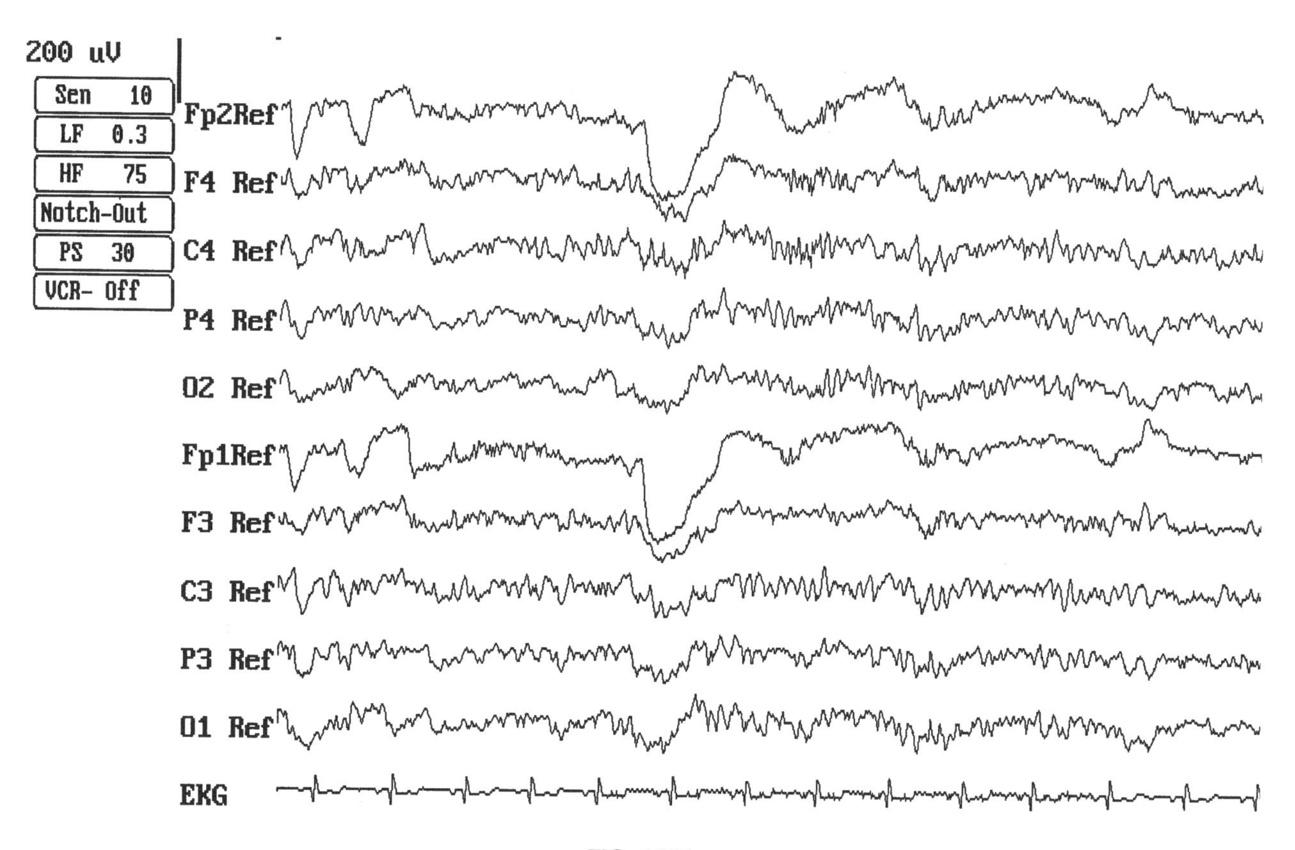
200 uV
Sen 10
LF 0.3
HF 75
Notch-Out
PS 30
VCR- Off
Fp2Ref
F4 Ref
C4 Ref
P4 Ref
O2 Ref
Fp1Ref
F3 Ref
C3 Ref
P3 Ref
O1 Ref
EKG

FIG. 4-73b

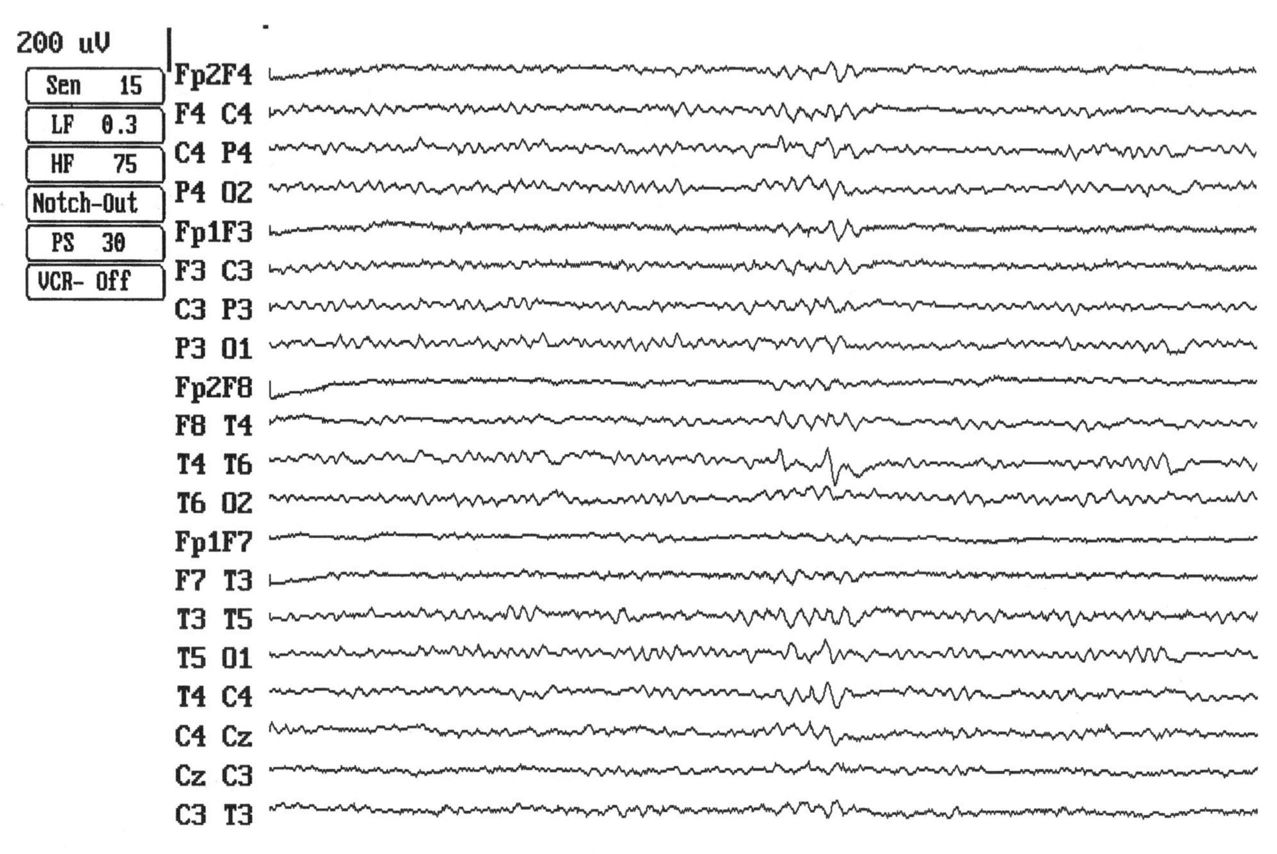

FIG. 4-74a,b A sharp wave at T4-T6 is seen at the middle of the page on run 2, but is not seen on run 1. This is also a subtraction artifact.

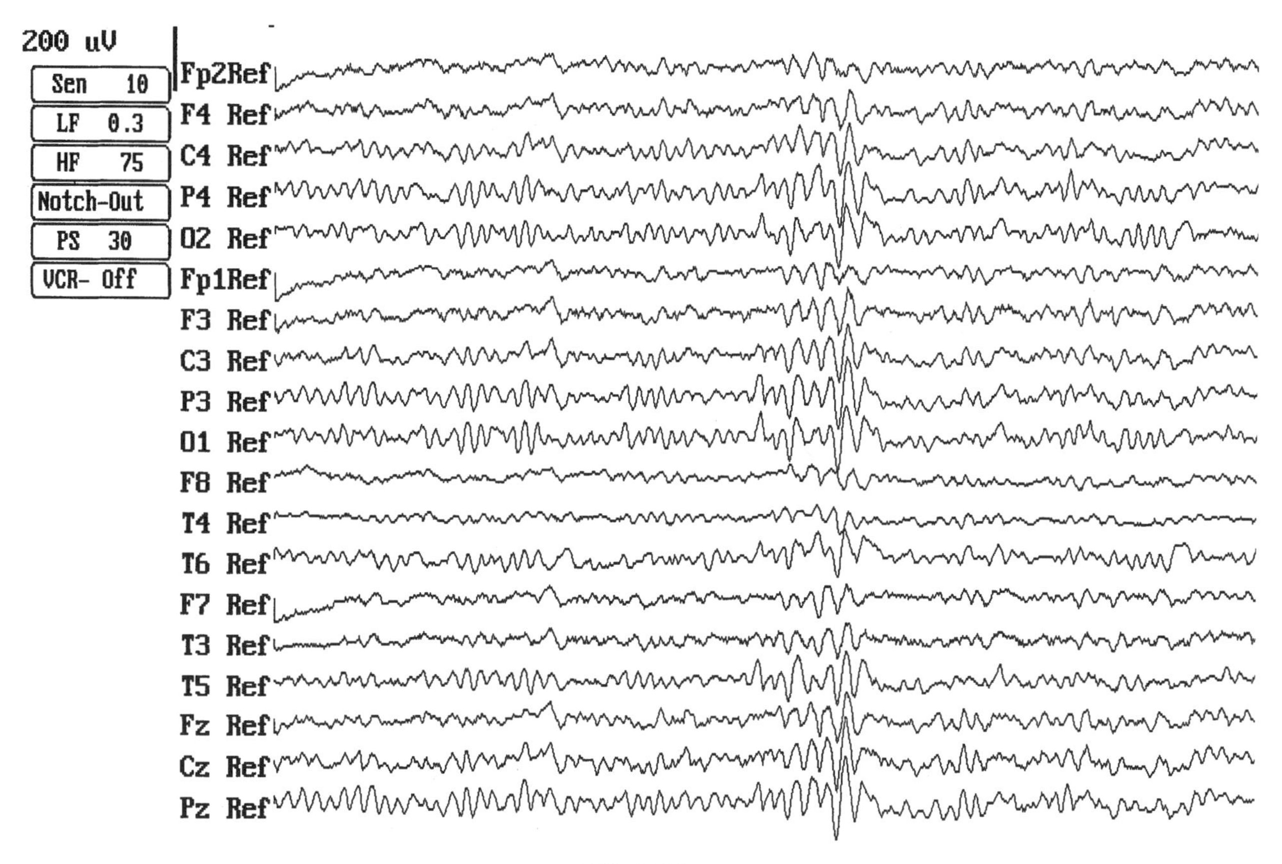
200 uV
Sen 10
LF 0.3
HF 75
Notch-Out
PS 30
VCR- Off
Fp2Ref
F4 Ref
C4 Ref
P4 Ref
O2 Ref
Fp1Ref
F3 Ref
C3 Ref
P3 Ref
O1 Ref
F8 Ref
T4 Ref
T6 Ref
F7 Ref
T3 Ref
T5 Ref
Fz Ref
Cz Ref
Pz Ref

FIG. 4-74b

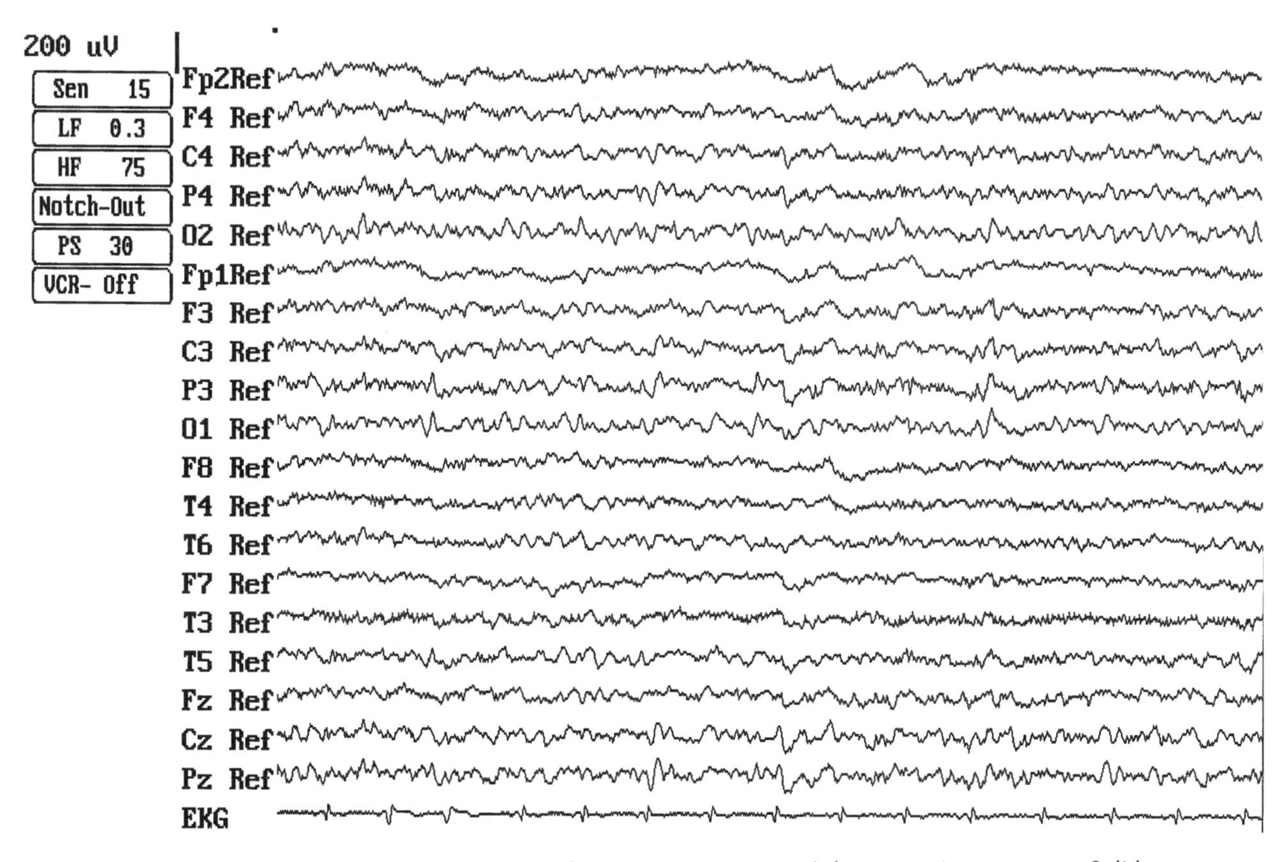

FIG. 4-75a,b Multiple tiny P3 sharp waveforms are seen on run 1, but are not seen on run 2. It is likely they are not significant.

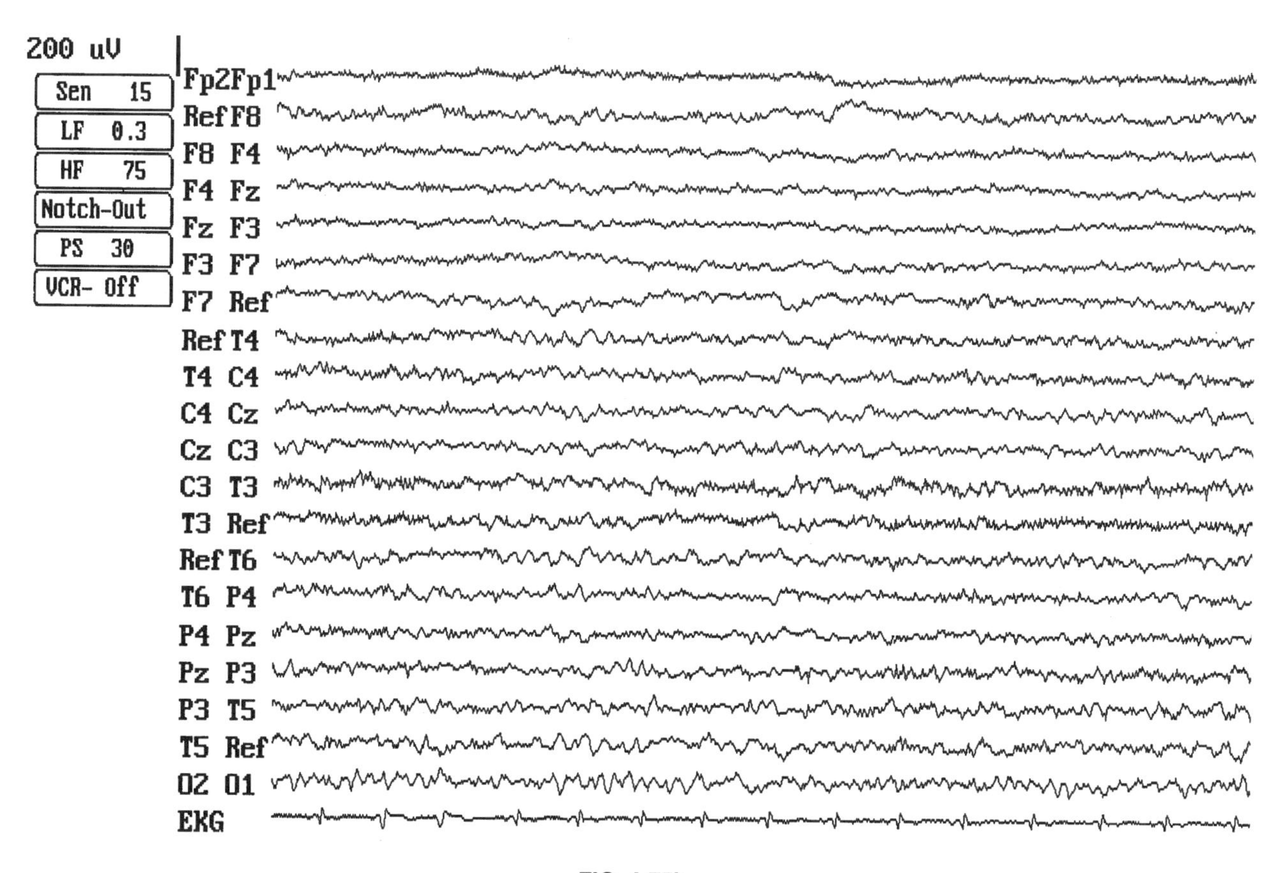
200 uV
Sen 15
LF 0.3
HF 75
Notch-Out
PS 30
VCR- Off
Fp2Fp1
Ref F8
F8 F4
F4 Fz
Fz F3
F3 F7
F7 Ref
Ref T4
T4 C4
C4 Cz
Cz C3
C3 T3
T3 Ref
Ref T6
T6 P4
P4 Pz
Pz P3
P3 T5
T5 Ref
O2 O1
EKG

FIG. 4-75b

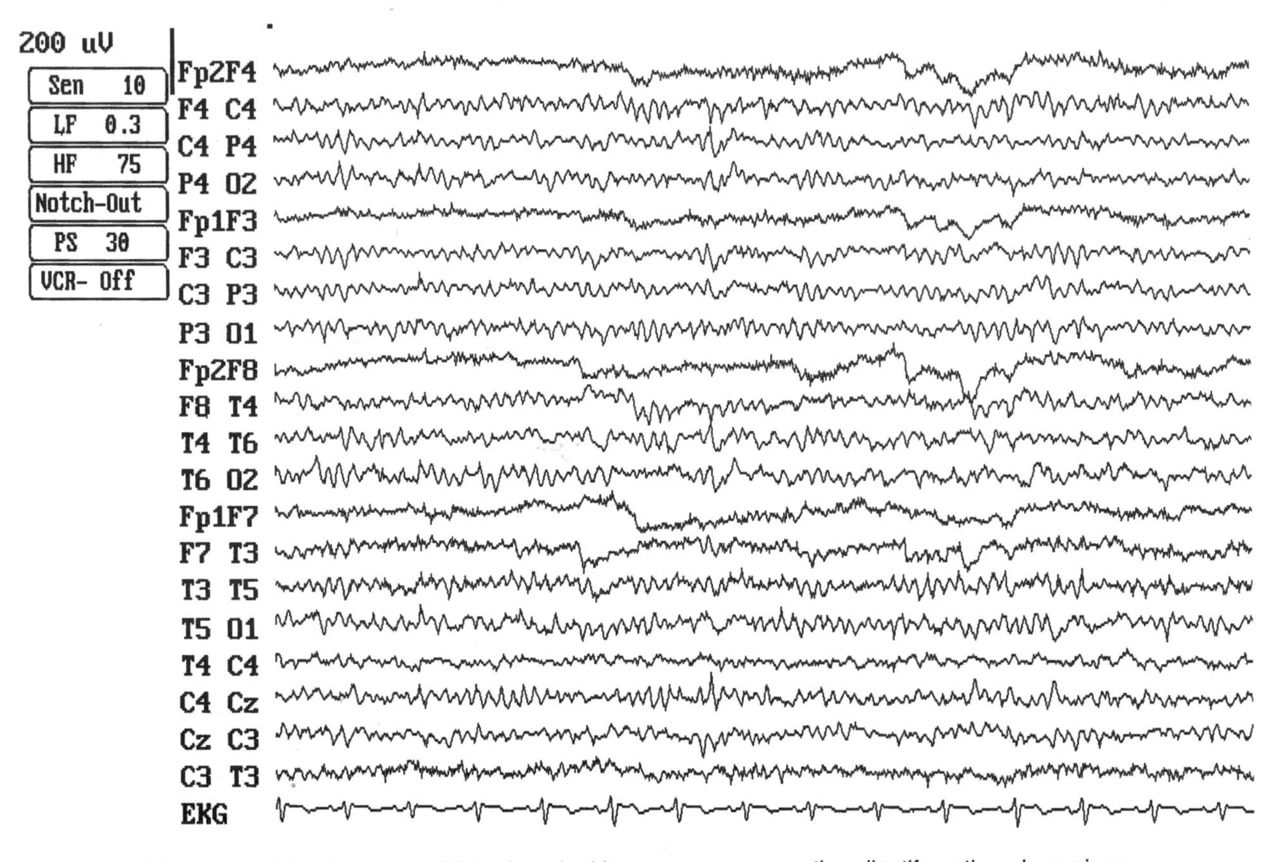

FIG. 4-76a,b Run 2 shows multiple sharp-looking waves, none overtly epileptiform though worrisome (an example of so-called "spiky but normal EEG"). Run 1 shows the reason: profuse fast activity in the background causes multiple subtraction artifacts mimicking sharp transients.

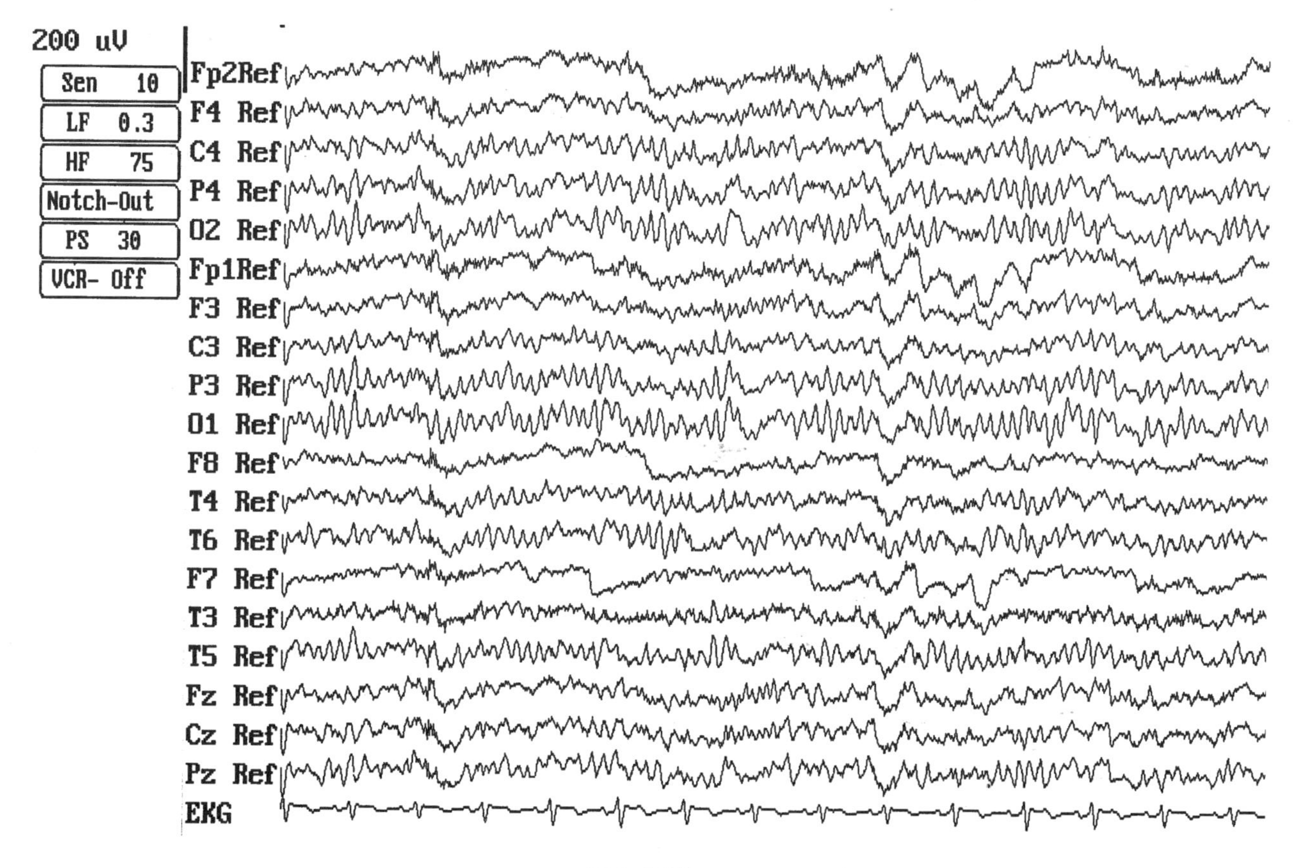
200 uV
Sen 10
LF 0.3
HF 75
Notch-Out
PS 30
VCR- Off
Fp2Ref
F4 Ref
C4 Ref
P4 Ref
O2 Ref
Fp1Ref
F3 Ref
C3 Ref
P3 Ref
O1 Ref
F8 Ref
T4 Ref
T6 Ref
F7 Ref
T3 Ref
T5 Ref
Fz Ref
Cz Ref
Pz Ref
EKG

FIG. 4-76b

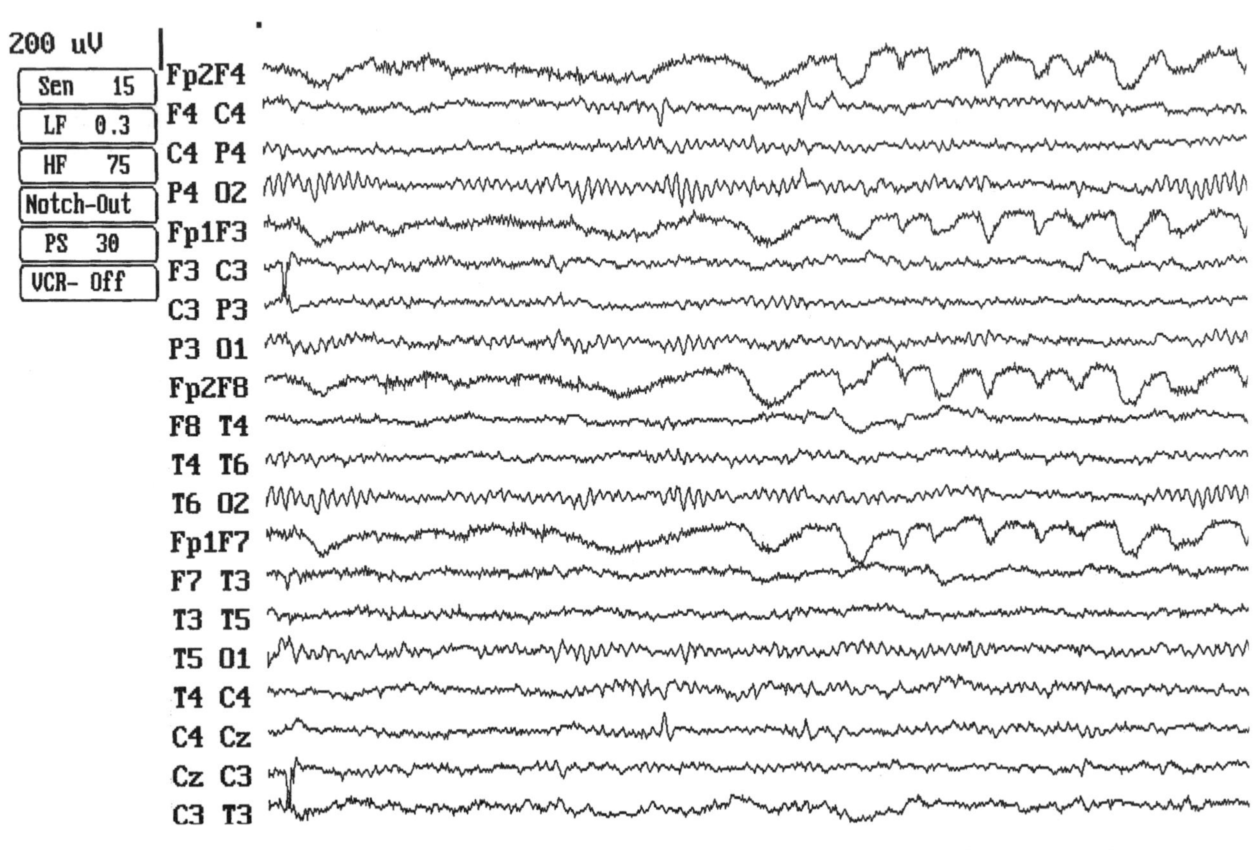

FIG. 4-77a,b,c Run 2 shows a clear spike at F4/C4, but run 1 is nonconfirmatory. Closer inspection of the parasagittal channels of run 1 reveals the origin of the spike (the C4-F4 derivation at bottom shows the subtraction effect).

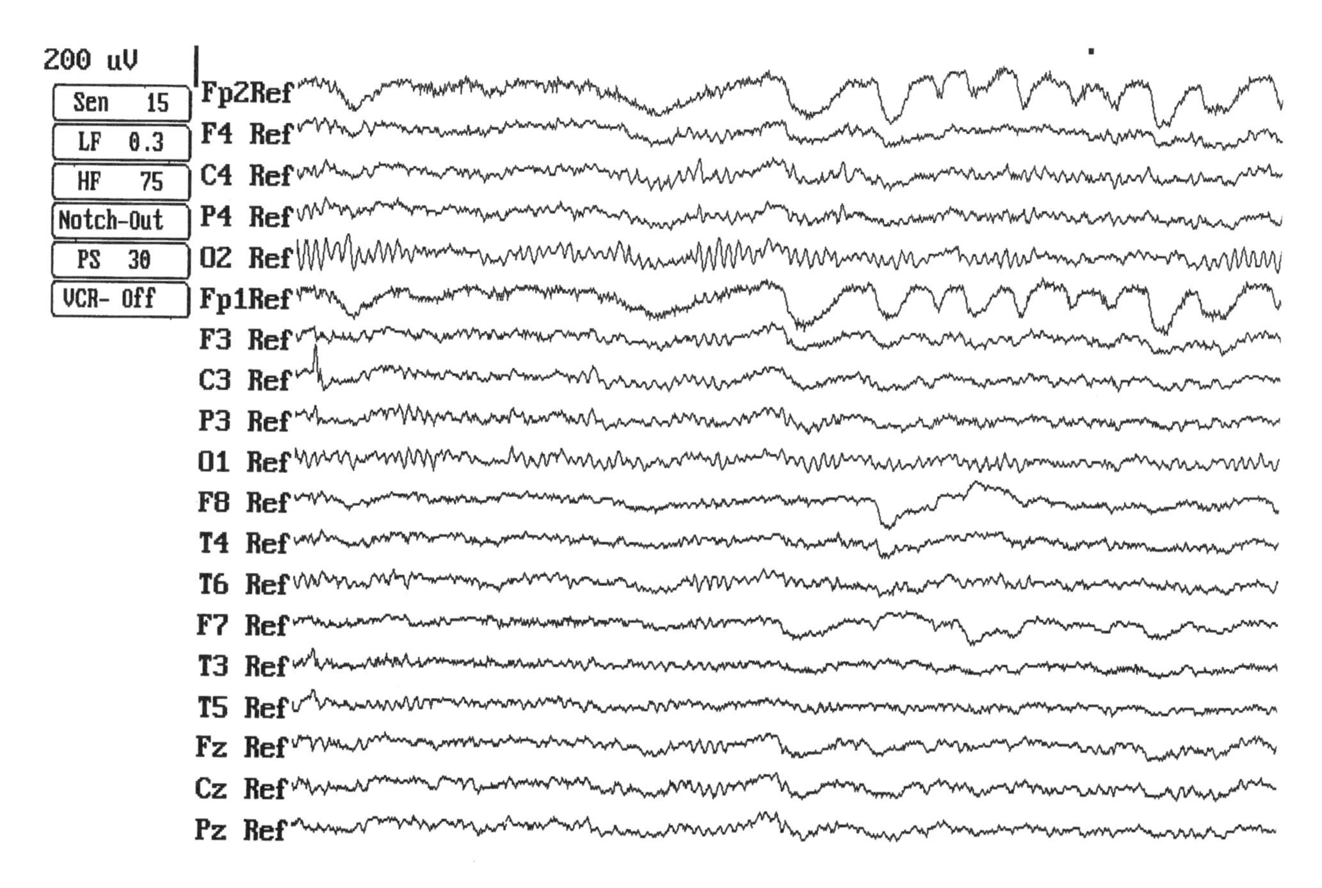
200 uV
Sen 15
LF 0.3
HF 75
Notch-Out
PS 30
VCR- Off
Fp2Ref
F4 Ref
C4 Ref
P4 Ref
O2 Ref
Fp1Ref
F3 Ref
C3 Ref
P3 Ref
O1 Ref
F8 Ref
T4 Ref
T6 Ref
F7 Ref
T3 Ref
T5 Ref
Fz Ref
Cz Ref
Pz Ref

FIG. 4-77b

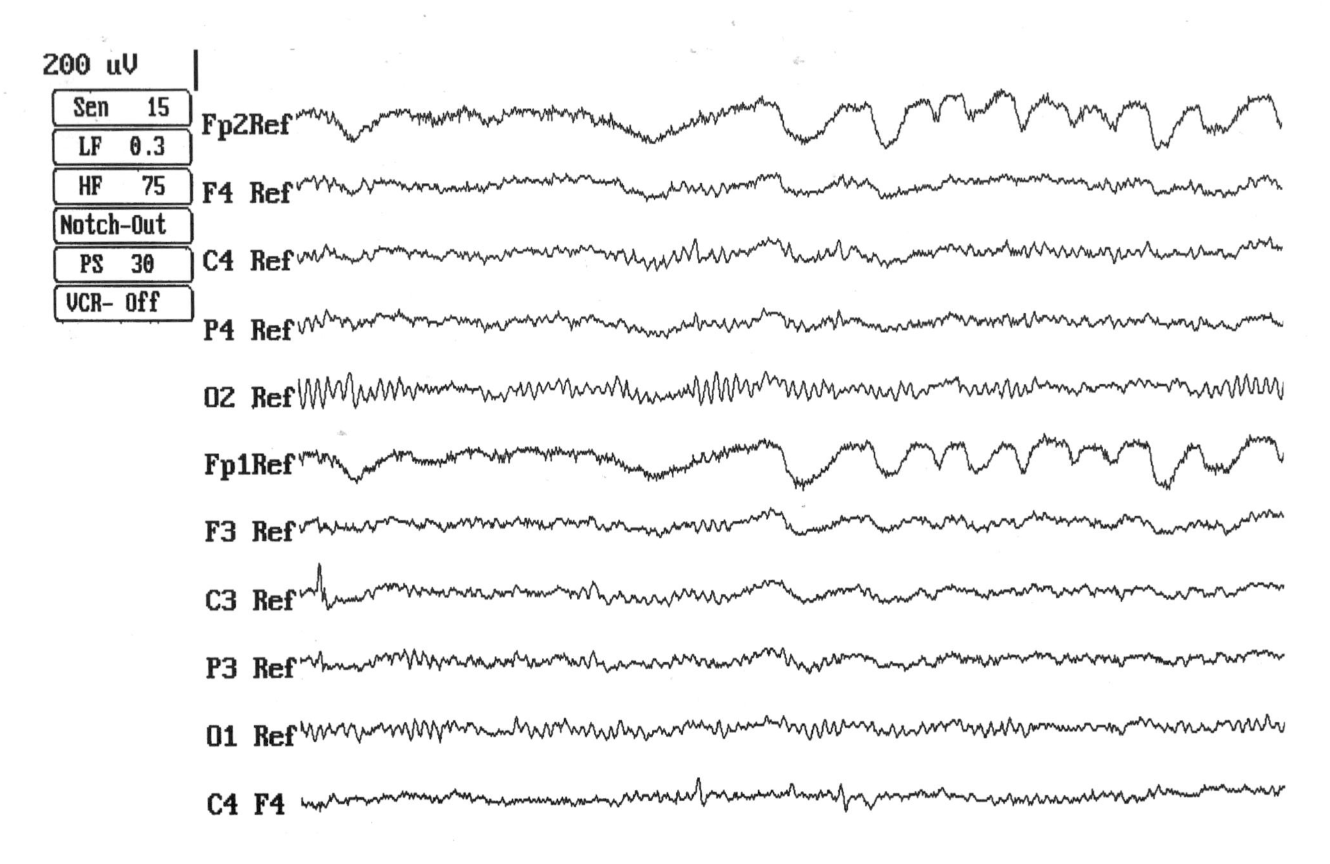
200 uV
Sen 15
LF 0.3
HF 75
Notch-Out
PS 30
VCR- Off
Fp2Ref
F4 Ref
C4 Ref
P4 Ref
O2 Ref
Fp1Ref
F3 Ref
C3 Ref
P3 Ref
O1 Ref
C4 F4

FIG. 4-77c

Missed Abnormality or Misinterpretation Because of Montage

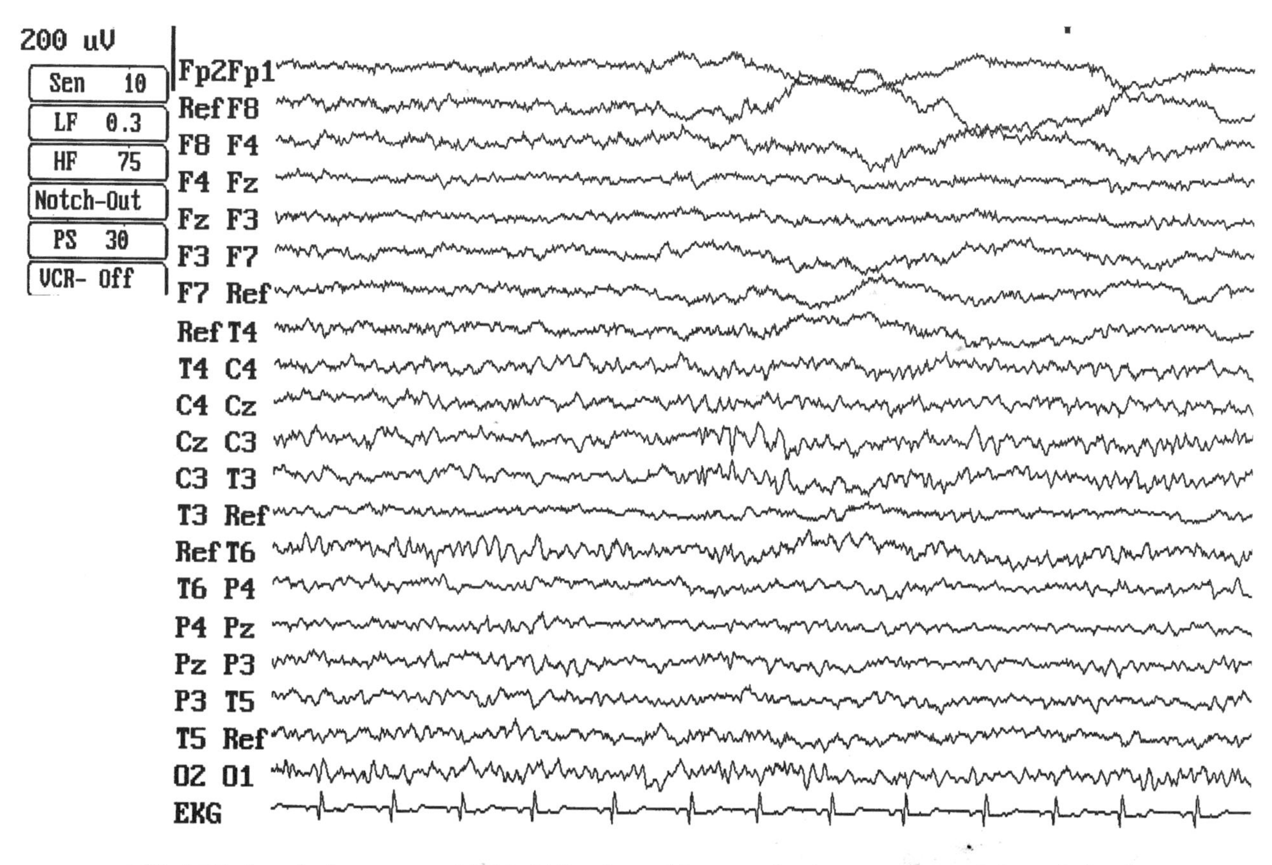

FIG. 4-78a,b,c A sharp wave at C3 (middle of page) is seen clearly on run 2, much less obviously on run 3, and poorly on run 1 (though the waveform is present, it is hidden among others of higher amplitude activity).

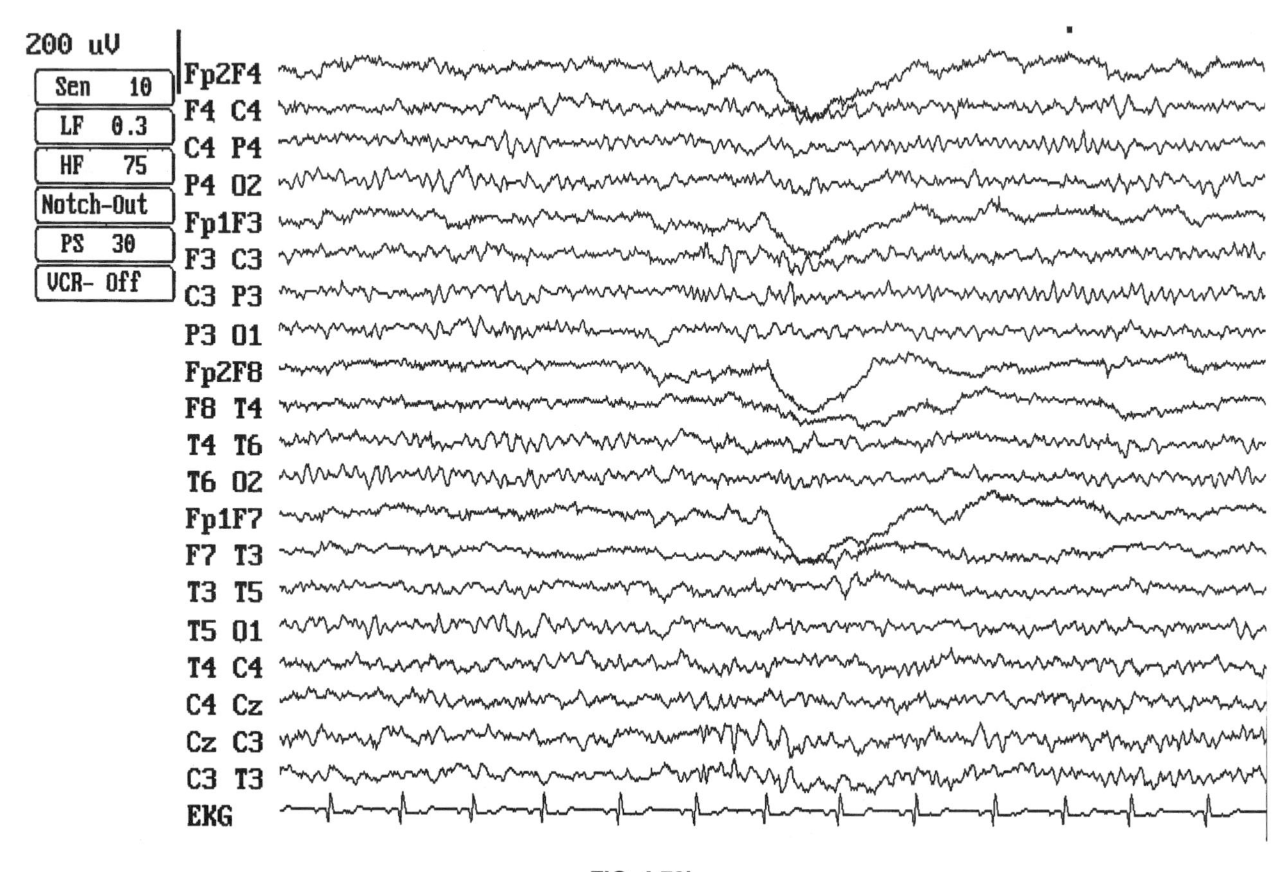
200 uV
Sen 10
LF 0.3
HF 75
Notch-Out
PS 30
VCR- Off
Fp2F4
F4 C4
C4 P4
P4 O2
Fp1F3
F3 C3
C3 P3
P3 O1
Fp2F8
F8 T4
T4 T6
T6 O2
Fp1F7
F7 T3
T3 T5
T5 O1
T4 C4
C4 Cz
Cz C3
C3 T3
EKG

FIG. 4-78b

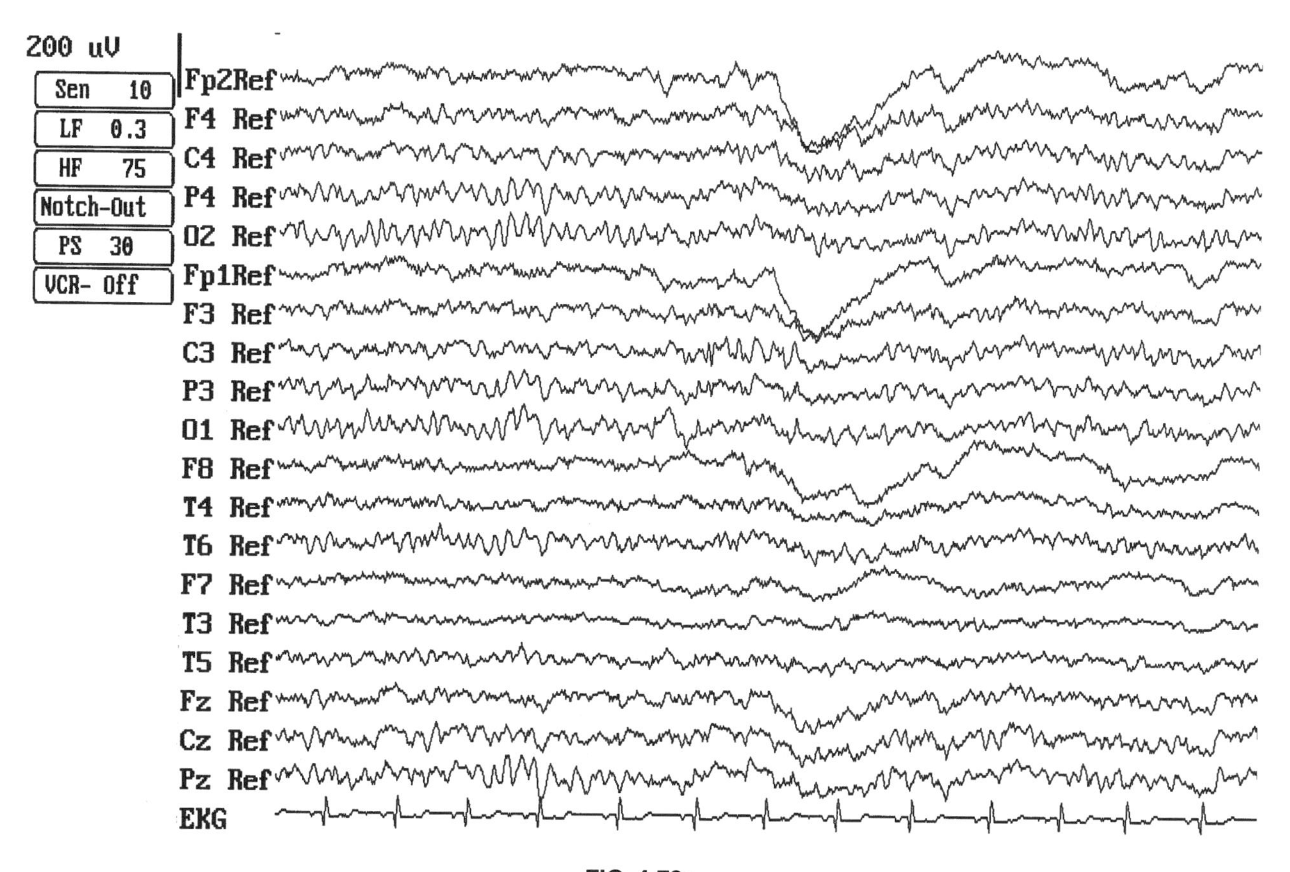
200 uV
Sen 10
LF 0.3
HF 75
Notch-Out
PS 30
VCR- Off
Fp2Ref
F4 Ref
C4 Ref
P4 Ref
O2 Ref
Fp1Ref
F3 Ref
C3 Ref
P3 Ref
O1 Ref
F8 Ref
T4 Ref
T6 Ref
F7 Ref
T3 Ref
T5 Ref
Fz Ref
Cz Ref
Pz Ref
EKG

FIG. 4-78c

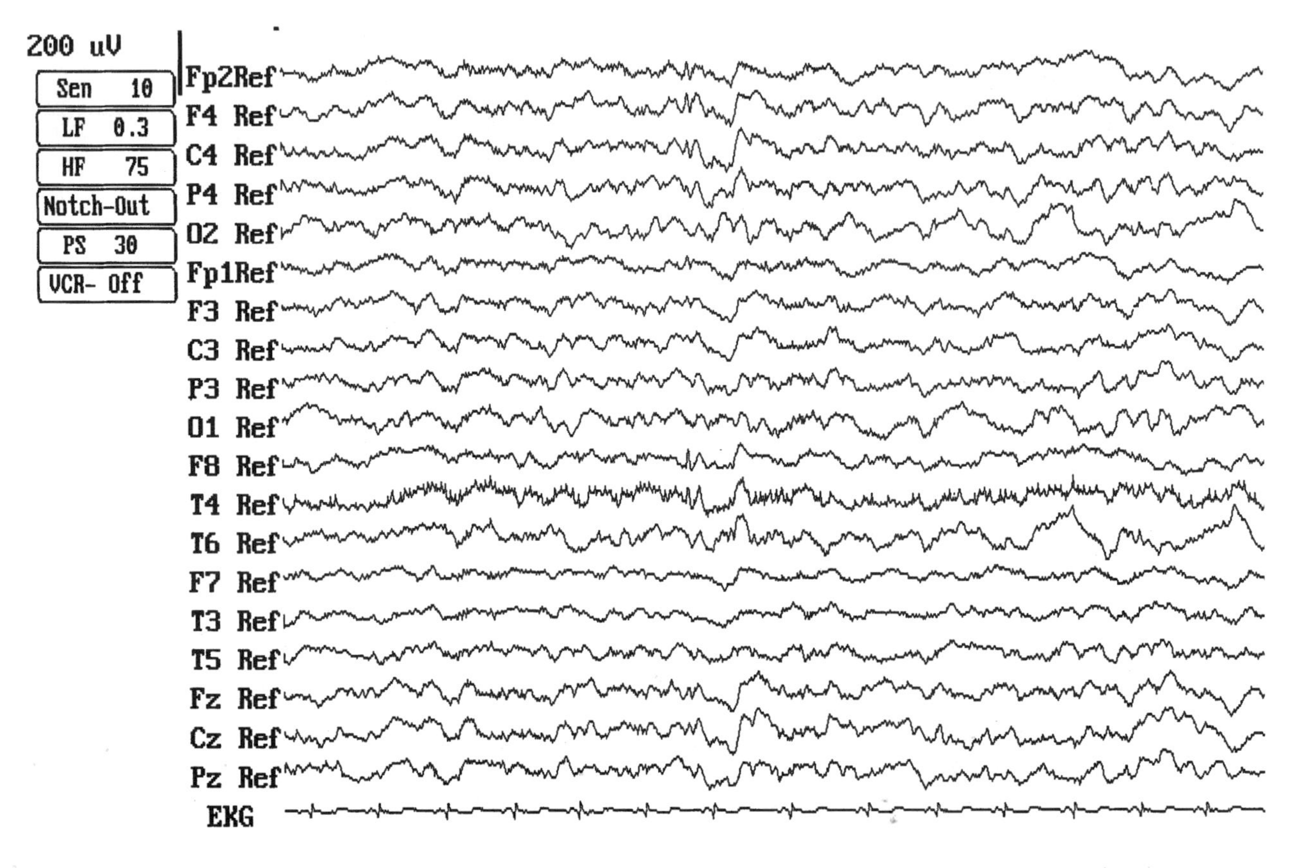

FIG. 4-79a,b,c A right anterior quadrant spike is seen on run 1 (middle of page). Run 3 shows anterior temporal localization, but nothing is seen on run 2.

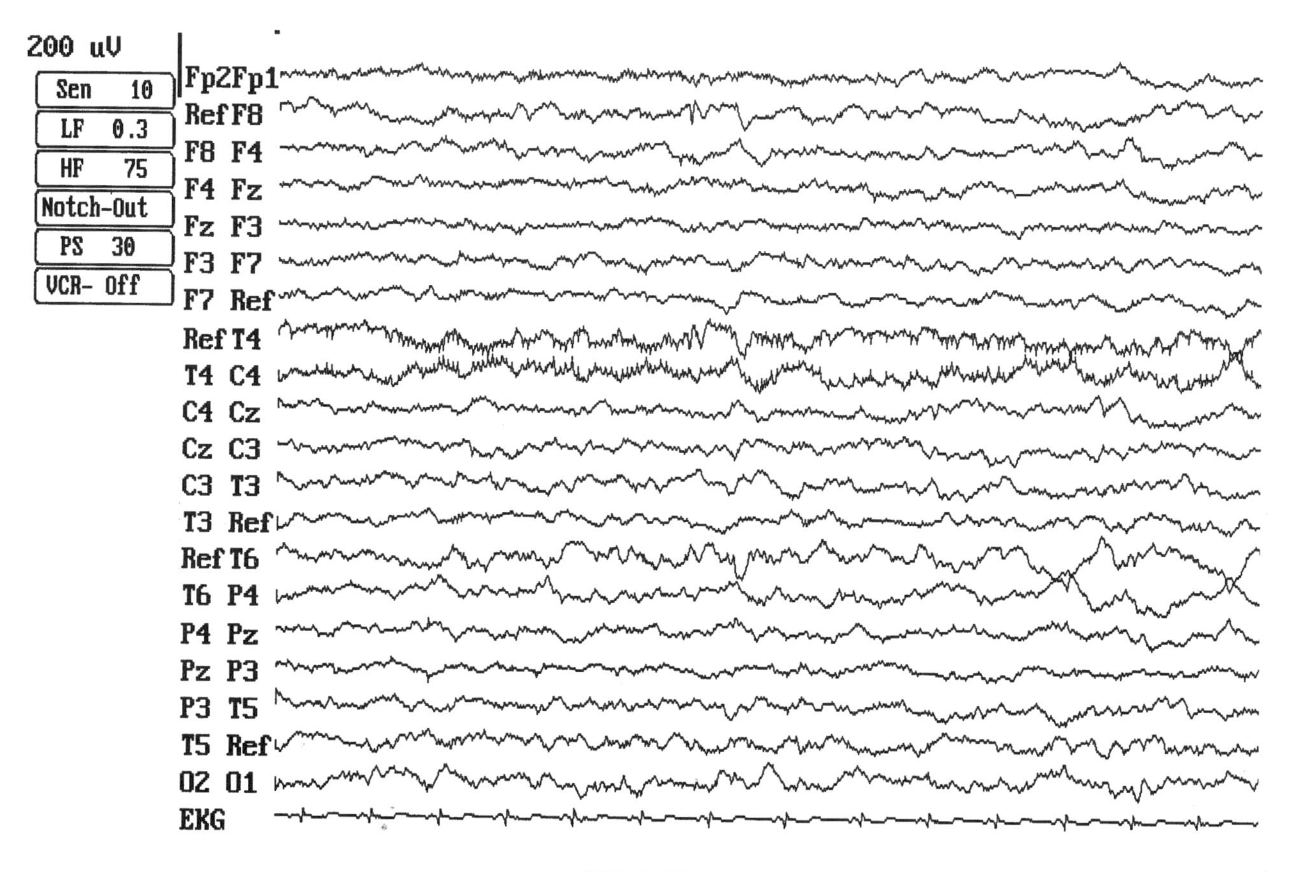
200 uV
Sen 10
LF 0.3
HF 75
Notch-Out
PS 30
VCR- Off
Fp2Fp1
Ref F8
F8 F4
F4 Fz
Fz F3
F3 F7
F7 Ref
Ref T4
T4 C4
C4 Cz
Cz C3
C3 T3
T3 Ref
Ref T6
T6 P4
P4 Pz
Pz P3
P3 T5
T5 Ref
O2 O1
EKG

FIG. 4-79b

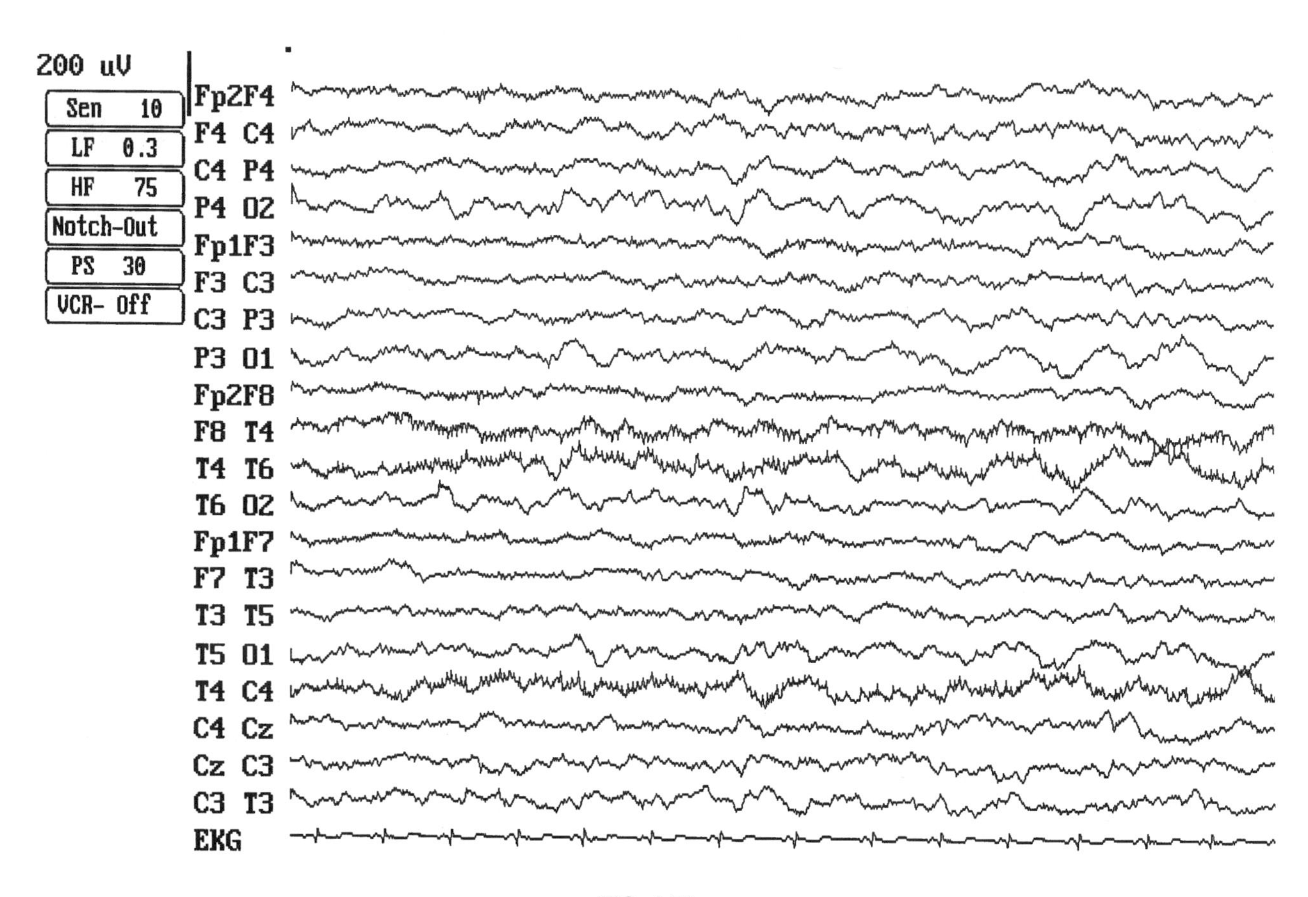
200 uV
Sen 10
LF 0.3
HF 75
Notch-Out
PS 30
VCR- Off
Fp2F4
F4 C4
C4 P4
P4 O2
Fp1F3
F3 C3
C3 P3
P3 O1
Fp2F8
F8 T4
T4 T6
T6 O2
Fp1F7
F7 T3
T3 T5
T5 O1
T4 C4
C4 Cz
Cz C3
C3 T3
EKG

FIG. 4-79c

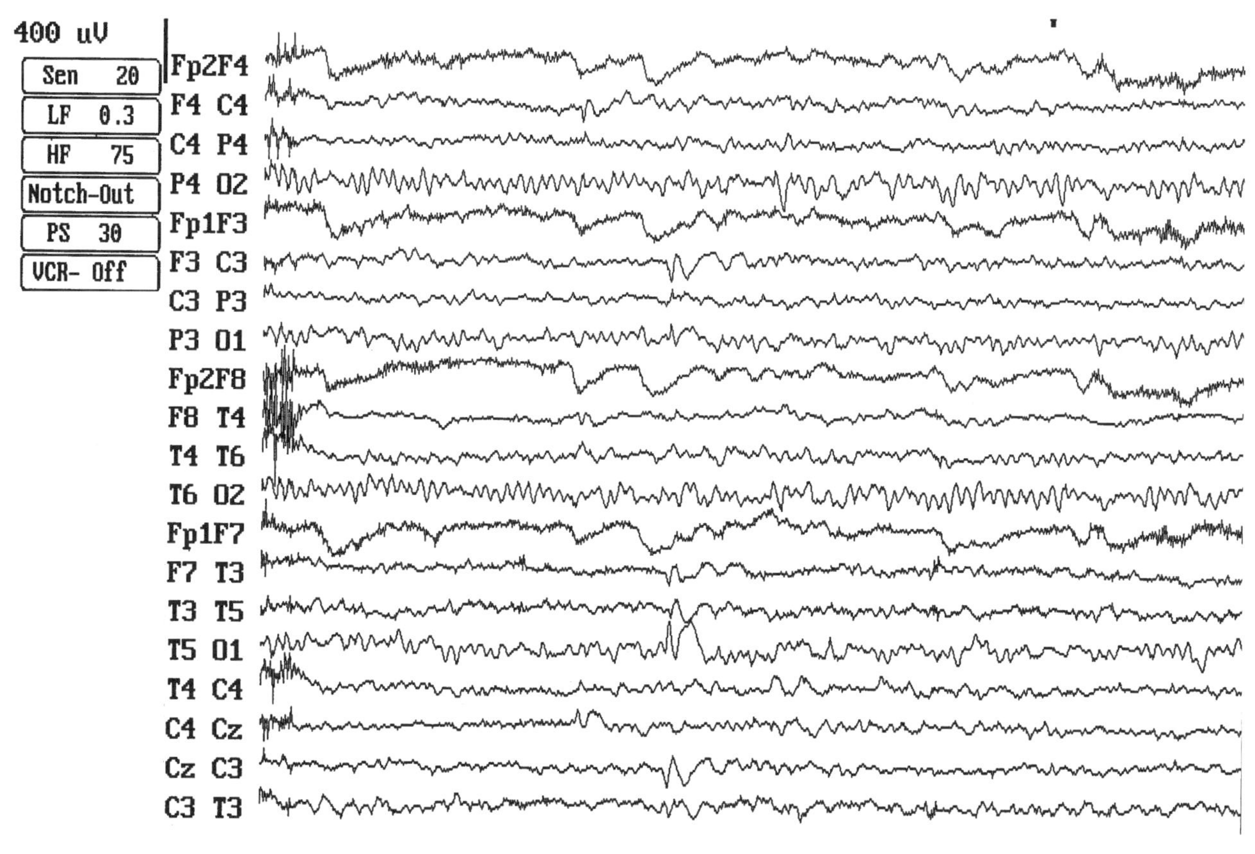

FIG. 4-80a,b Run 2 shows a spike at T5-O1 also involving C3, as well as a smaller spike at C4/F4. Due to the complex fields of both discharges and, additionally, the low amplitude of the latter, run 1 does not display either in an optimal fashion.

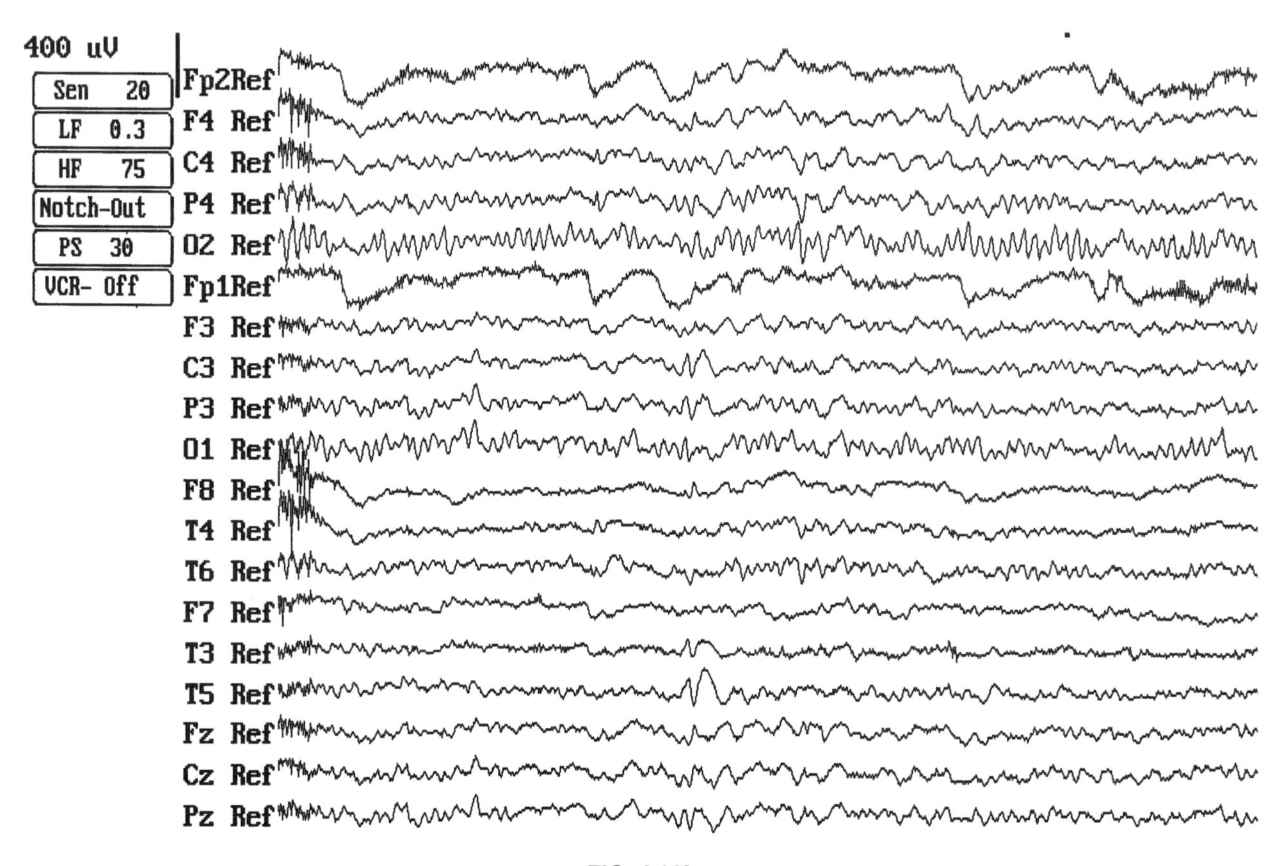
400 uV
Sen 20
LF 0.3
HF 75
Notch-Out
PS 30
VCR- Off
Fp2Ref
F4 Ref
C4 Ref
P4 Ref
O2 Ref
Fp1Ref
F3 Ref
C3 Ref
P3 Ref
O1 Ref
F8 Ref
T4 Ref
T6 Ref
F7 Ref
T3 Ref
T5 Ref
Fz Ref
Cz Ref
Pz Ref

FIG. 4-80b

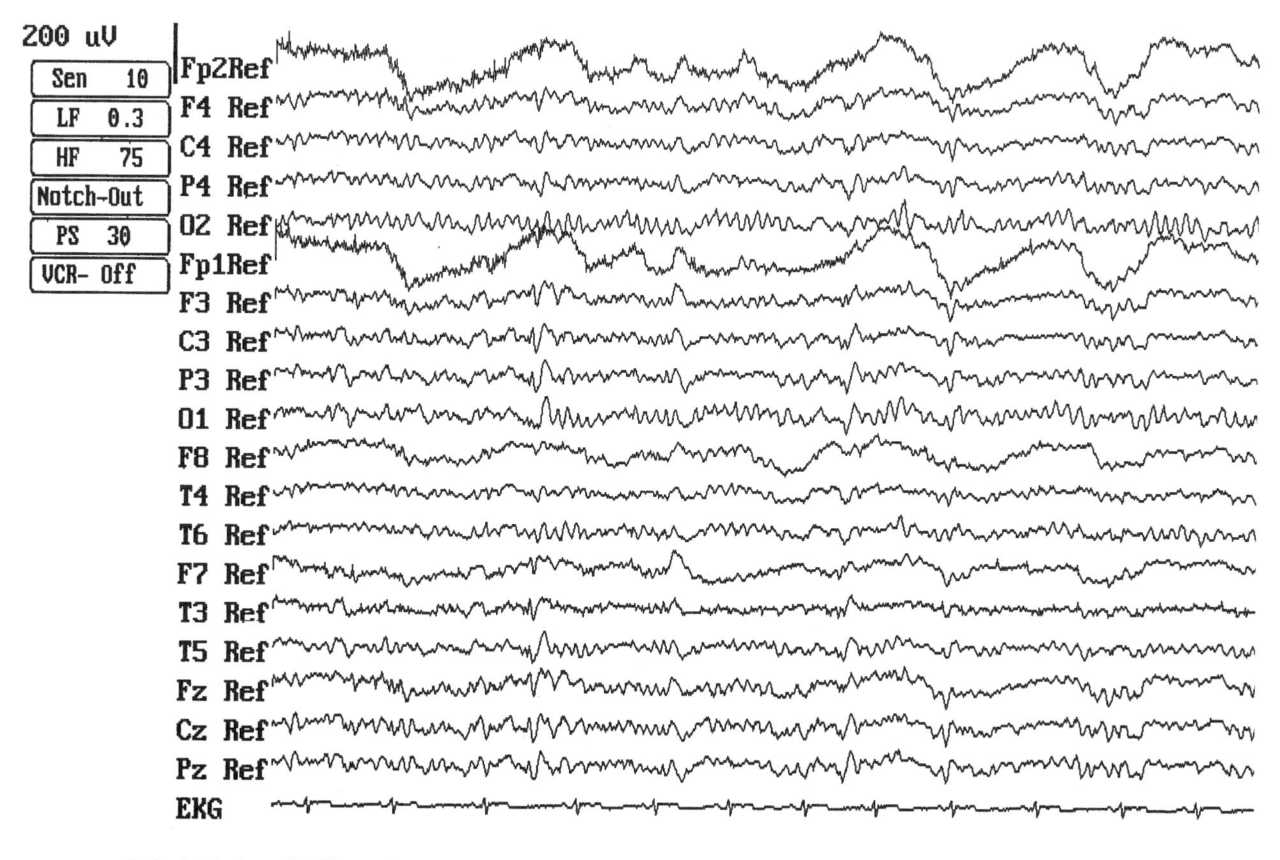

FIG. 4-81a,b,c A diffuse sharp wave maximal over the left hemisphere is seen on run 1. Run 3 shows it only at the end of chain channels, while run 2 does not show any hint of it. Here another reference might be helpful.

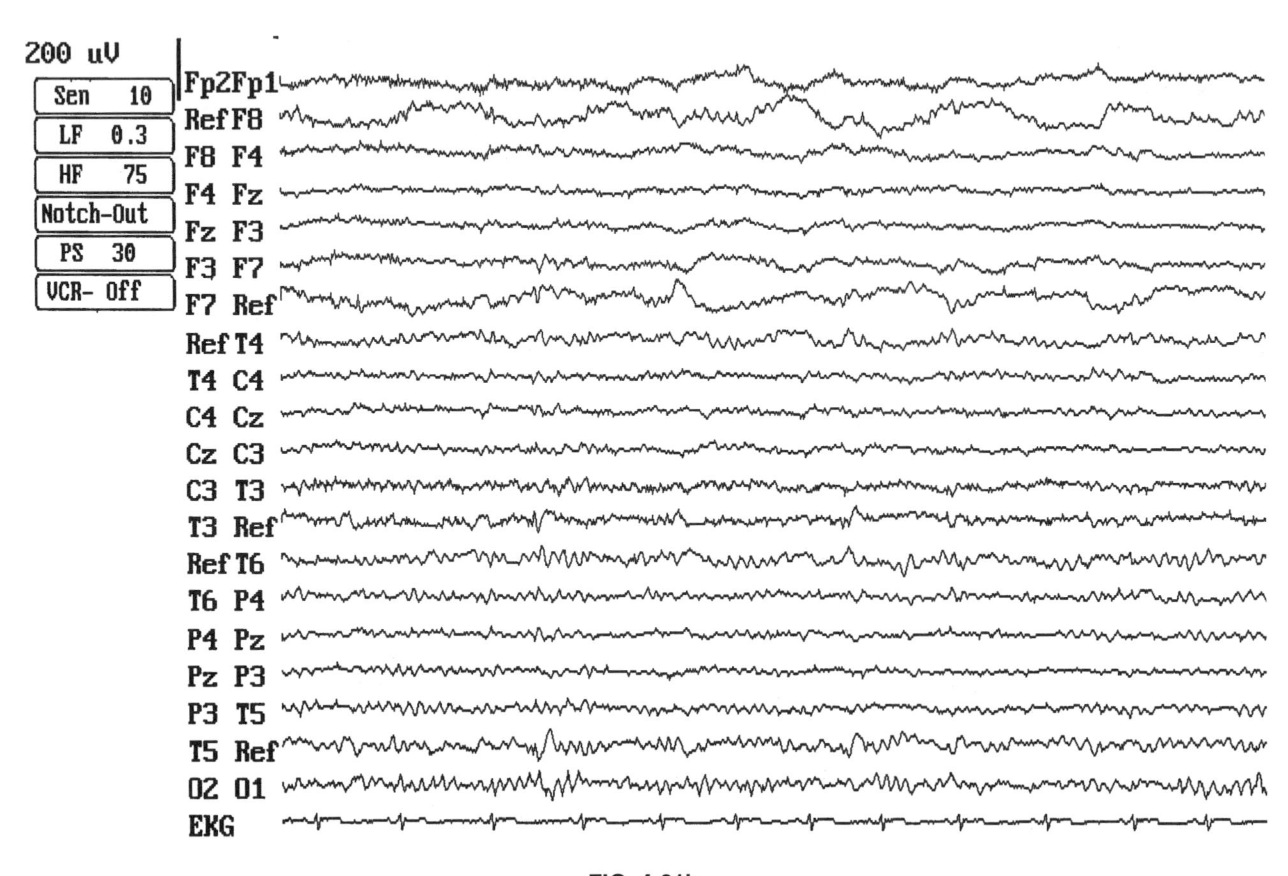
200 uV
Sen 10
LF 0.3
HF 75
Notch-Out
PS 30
VCR- Off
Fp2Fp1
Ref F8
F8 F4
F4 Fz
Fz F3
F3 F7
F7 Ref
Ref T4
T4 C4
C4 Cz
Cz C3
C3 T3
T3 Ref
Ref T6
T6 P4
P4 Pz
Pz P3
P3 T5
T5 Ref
O2 O1
EKG

FIG. 4-81b

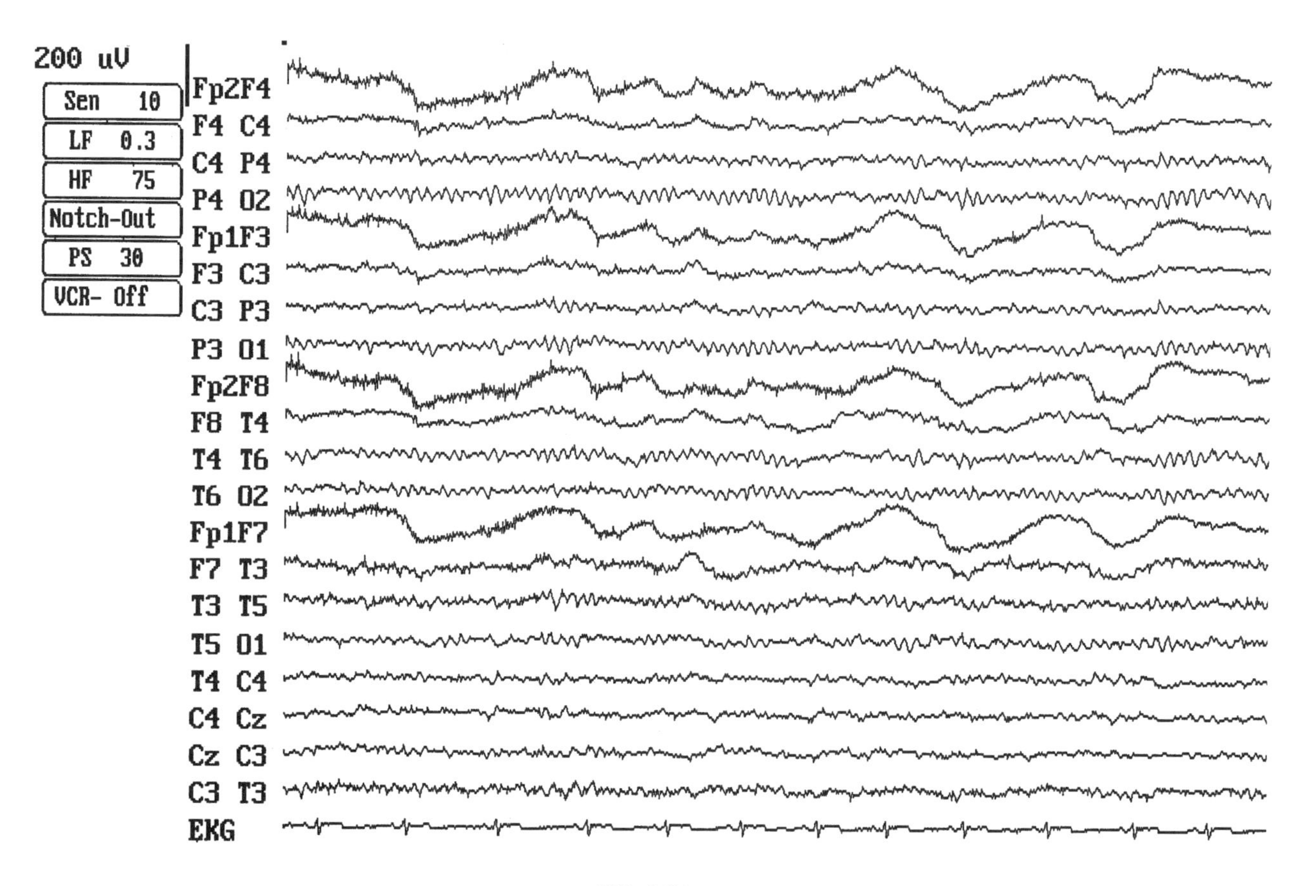
200 uV
Sen 10
LF 0.3
HF 75
Notch-Out
PS 30
VCR- Off
Fp2F4
F4 C4
C4 P4
P4 O2
Fp1F3
F3 C3
C3 P3
P3 O1
Fp2F8
F8 T4
T4 T6
T6 O2
Fp1F7
F7 T3
T3 T5
T5 O1
T4 C4
C4 Cz
Cz C3
C3 T3
EKG

FIG. 4-81c

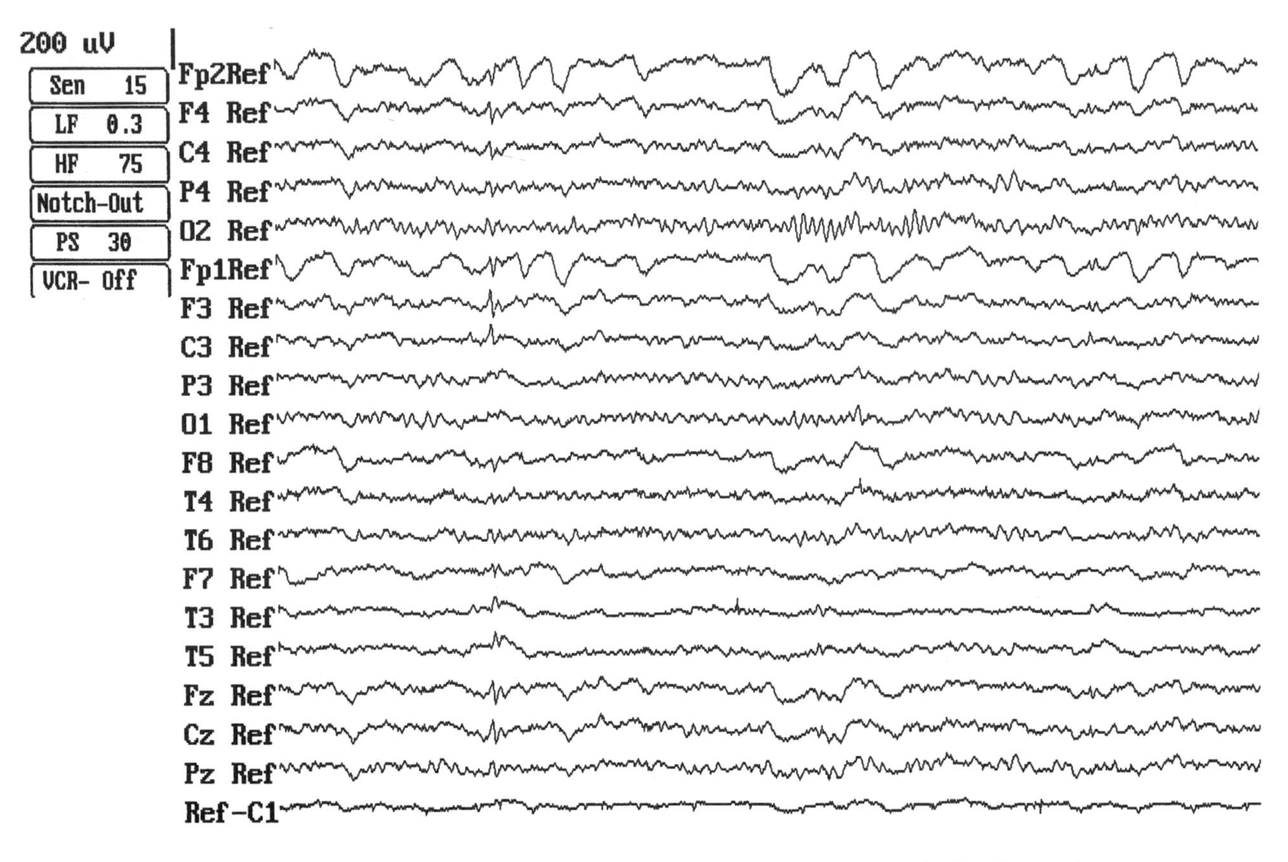

FIG. 4-82a,b,c,d,e Run 2 shows a left central-temporal spike, maximal over C3/T3. Run 1 shows a complex field, with simultaneous positivities and negativities overlapping at various electrode positions. This is best displayed using the 8 channel, 60 mm/s (e) page.

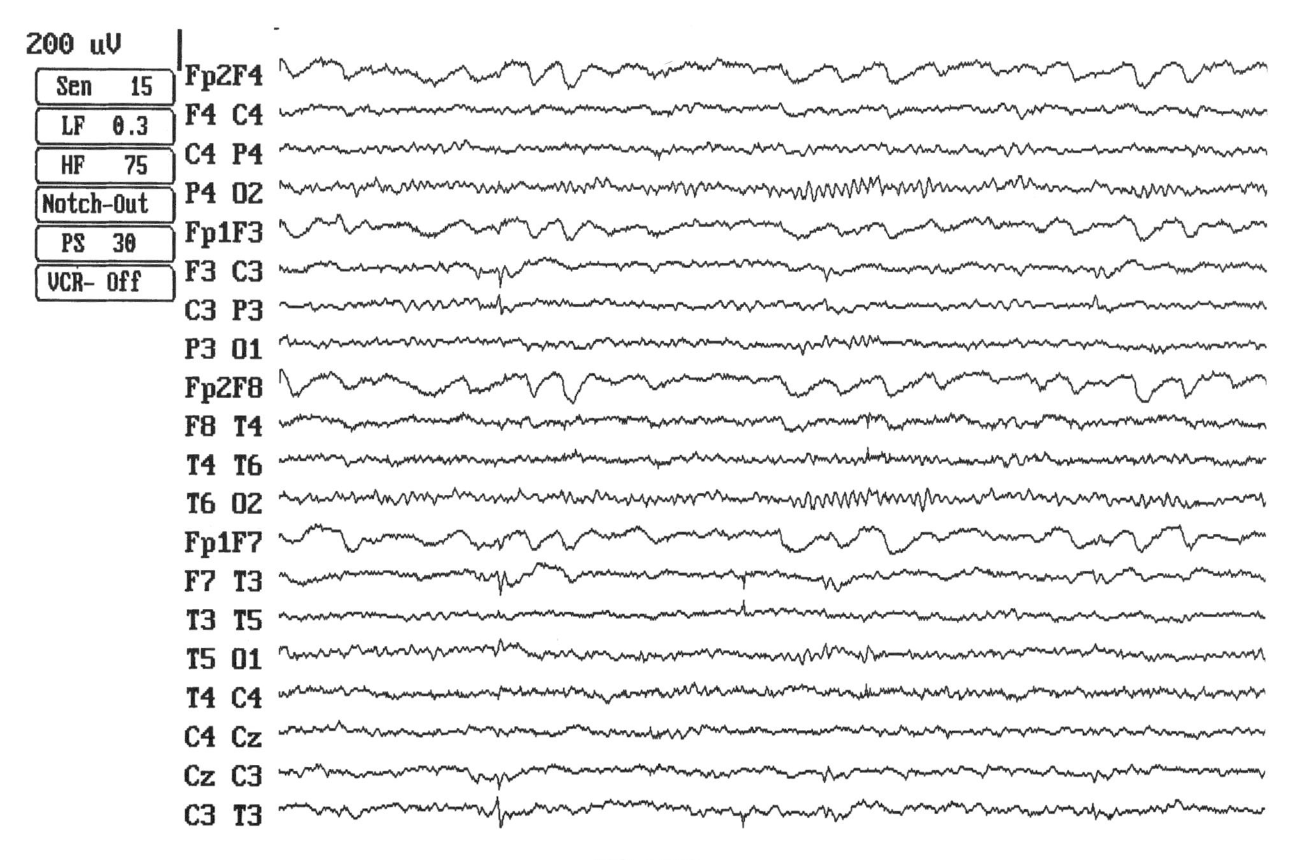
200 uV
Sen 15
LF 0.3
HF 75
Notch-Out
PS 30
VCR- Off
Fp2F4
F4 C4
C4 P4
P4 O2
Fp1F3
F3 C3
C3 P3
P3 O1
Fp2F8
F8 T4
T4 T6
T6 O2
Fp1F7
F7 T3
T3 T5
T5 O1
T4 C4
C4 Cz
Cz C3
C3 T3

FIG. 4-82b

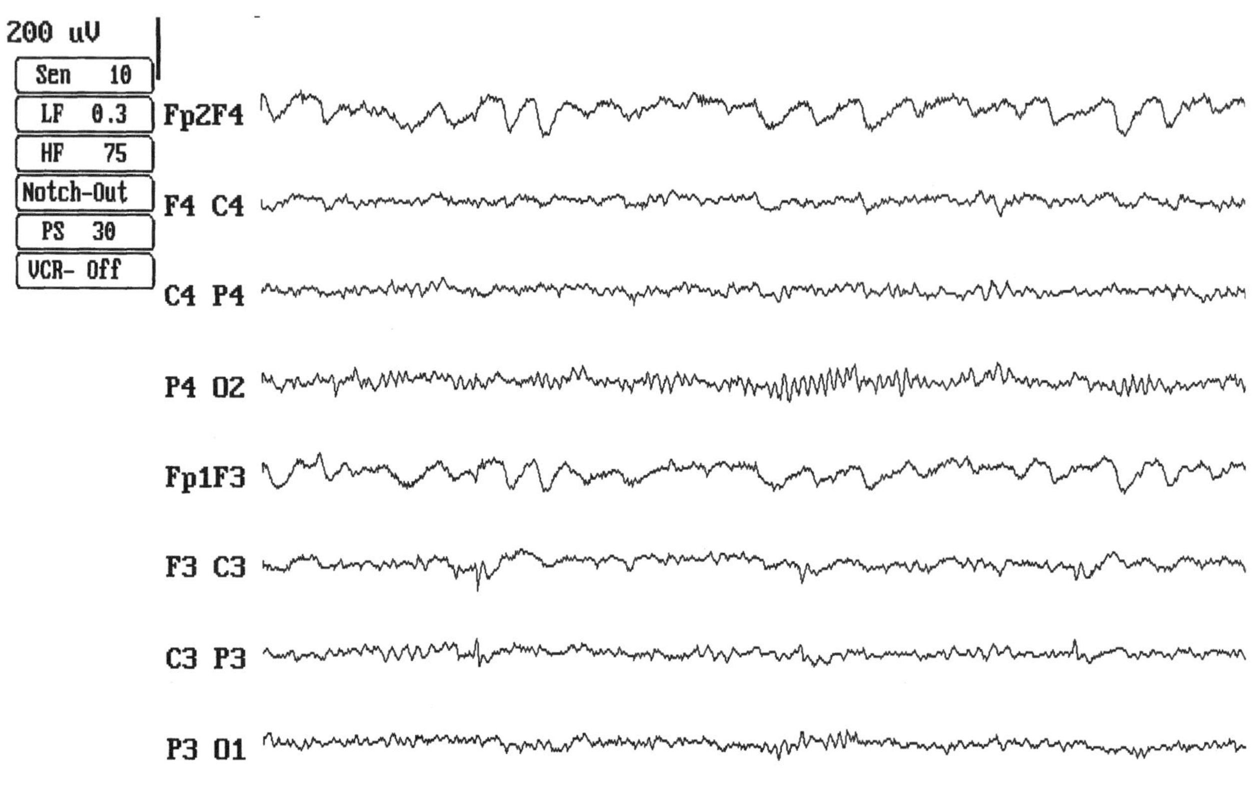
200 uV
Sen 10
LF 0.3
HF 75
Notch-Out
PS 30
VCR- Off
Fp2F4
F4 C4
C4 P4
P4 O2
Fp1F3
F3 C3
C3 P3
P3 O1

FIG. 4-82c

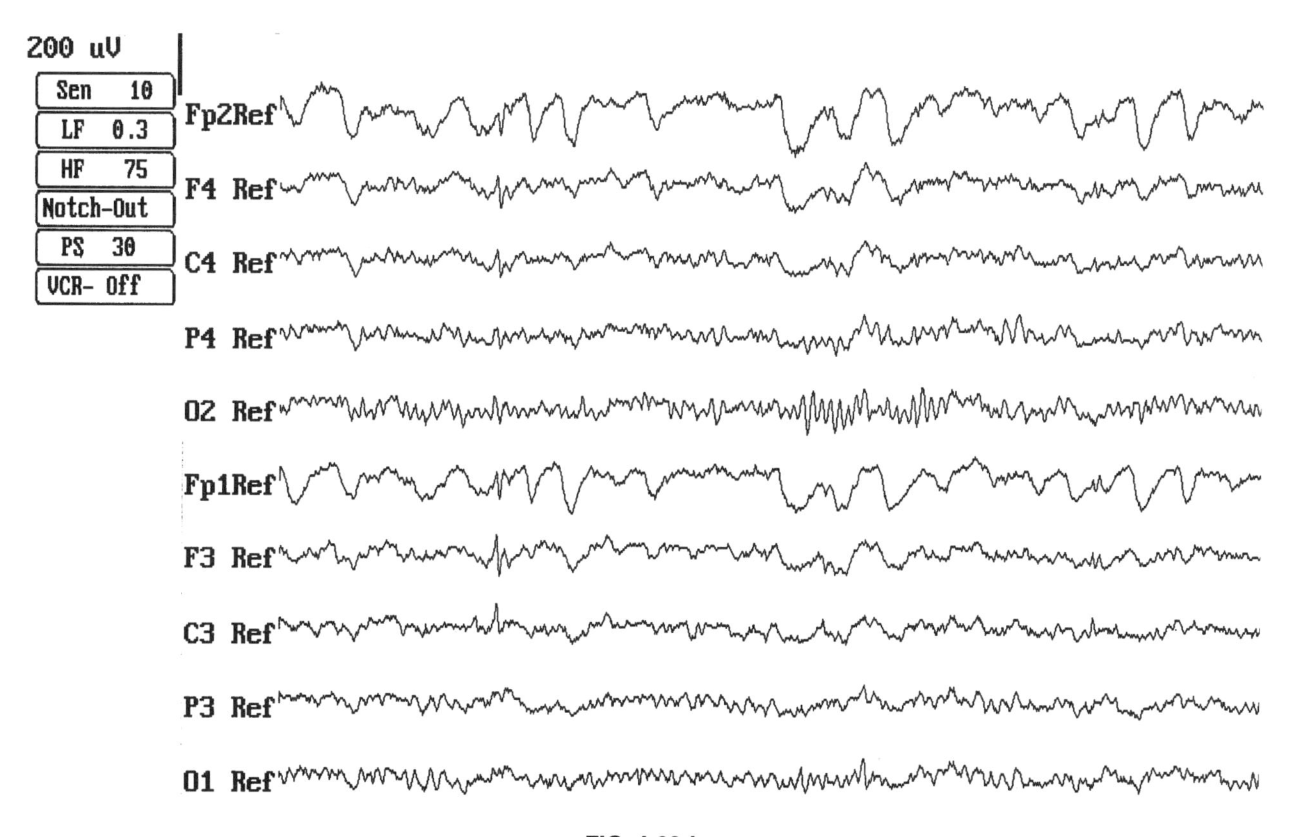
200 uV
Sen 10
LF 0.3
HF 75
Notch-Out
PS 30
VCR- Off
Fp2Ref
F4 Ref
C4 Ref
P4 Ref
O2 Ref
Fp1Ref
F3 Ref
C3 Ref
P3 Ref
O1 Ref

FIG. 4-82d

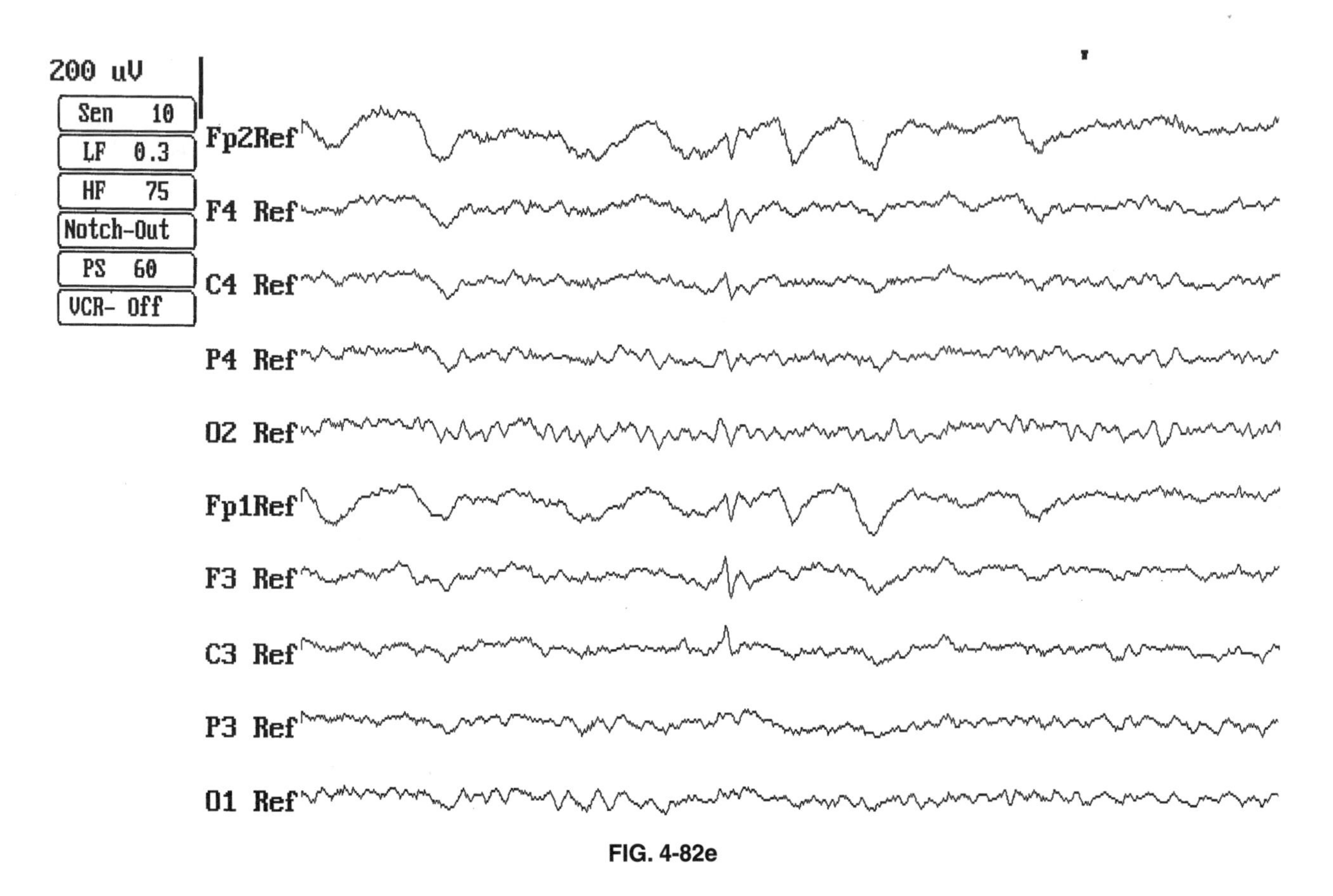
200 uV
Sen 10
LF 0.3
HF 75
Notch-Out
PS 60
VCR- Off
Fp2Ref
F4 Ref
C4 Ref
P4 Ref
O2 Ref
Fp1Ref
F3 Ref
C3 Ref
P3 Ref
O1 Ref

FIG. 4-82e

5
Quantitative Analyses

As well as visual interpretation, the recorded EEG can be subjected to post-processing using a variety of computation methods. The following are several examples that have been demonstrated to be useful because they assist the clinician in discriminating between clinical groups (i.e., a limited diagnostic capability) or have research purposes.

SPECTRAL ANALYSIS

One important characteristic of the EEG background is the frequency content of the underlying activity. A quantitative breakdown of EEG segments can be done using a computer, and this breakdown expressed in numeric or graphical format. Numeric output usually tabulates the average amplitude in each frequency band (delta, theta, alpha, and beta) (1). In an EEG fast Fourier transform (FFT) spectrum, the most prominent peak is usually the alpha peak. It is at once clear should there be an asymmetry in the occipital areas, and the degree of asymmetry is easily quantified from the FFT tracings. This can be done by the maximum alpha peak value, which can be simply read off the graph, or by the ratio of the alpha bands of O2 to O1, represented by the area under the FFT tracing from 8 to 13 Hz, which includes the alpha peak. The latter is the more accurate measure of alpha amplitude (referring to the spectral alpha content, in units of μV, rather than the alpha power, in units of μV^2).

The FFT is the most common computation technique, although many other faster algorithms exist. However, other algorithms tend to have unacceptable qualities, e.g., instability, spurious errors, inaccuracy, etc. FFT results are usually expressed as the square root of the spectral power, i.e., in microvolts. The appearance of the frequency graphs is markedly different if the results are expressed in powers, i.e., in microvolts squared.

MAPPING OF BACKGROUND AND SPIKE TRANSIENTS

In order to convey the topographic information contained in the set of EEG tracings from the multiple scalp leads, the simplest way is to use map displays. Depending on the objective, and what specific topographic feature is desired, the variable to be mapped can be chosen. The following maps can be created from digital EEG data:

Voltage Map

This is the simplest map, and displays the instantaneous voltage distribution (i.e., field) of the set of scalp voltages at a given instant. By "cartooning" (displaying successive maps in rapid sequence) a selected segment (typically 1 s of data), a good visual understanding can be obtained. Areas of high voltage can be differentiated from areas of low voltage, and areas of rapid change differentiated from areas of no change. This method is best suited to following fast events, such as interictal spikes, where the timing relationships between channels are important. But this is a tedious way to analyze large amounts of data (2).

Summated Map

The summated voltage over a given segment can be displayed, either as the mathematical average (which is not very meaningful except for the important case of averaging several identified events), or as the sum of the absolute voltages (i.e. the rectified voltage). The latter shows the relative amount of "activity" at different scalp sites, and is useful as a screening display. Comparisons can easily be made of different patients, or of data from the same patient but under different conditions, or of different trials of a test. Even for the simple interictal spike this display is useful.

Averaging

Averaging events that can be clearly identified is a particularly useful technique in studying interictal spikes and other transients. A single transient may be very small in amplitude, just barely distinguishable from the background activity. By carefully time-locking several segments each containing a spike onto a logical point of the event (e.g., the peak negativity of the same channel), the mathematical procedure of averaging several EEG segments together then produces the EEG equivalent of the averaged evoked potential (EP), which is based on the same principle. In this case, the "trigger" is the internal event which caused the spike to be generated (3).

Other derived measures are described below, including statistics, probabilities, current flow, source locations etc., and these also can be mapped.

CURRENT SOURCE DENSITY (LAPLACIAN, HJORTH METHODS)

The voltage map can be transformed into one of current flow by taking the mathematical second derivative of the voltage distribution. Usually, the voltage map is known from the scalp measurements at each electrode, in the form of a set of numbers for each time point. This is then numerically transformed into the so-called current source density (CSD). The convention is that current flows from the positive to the negative: the location of the former is called a "source" as electric current seems to emerge from the skull there, whereas the location of the latter is called the "sink" as current seems to disappear into the skull there. If the density of the electrode array is increased, by increasing the number of electrodes on the same scalp area, then the resultant CSD estimation is improved. The practical limit for the number of electrodes appears to be around 128 (4).

In another approach, the voltage map is represented by an equation for a two-dimensional mathematical function that approximates the voltage surface. By calculating the Laplacian value of this function, the CSD is obtained. The accuracy depends on how well the voltage function models the actual data. Again, high electrode density is helpful. Examples can be found in Gevins et al (4) and Perrin et al (5).

In a similar vein, Dr. Bo Hjorth derived a method to estimate the true contribution from local sources. His "Hjorth derivation" technique works by removing the contribution of volume conduction from distant sources, while emphasizing the contribution from local source(s). This method does not differentiate between contributions from one or more sources, as long as the sources are in the same location. It is capable, however, of separating the contributions of individual local sources by focusing on the electrodes where the individual sources are reflected. In this way a good estimate of the underlying generators (i.e., sources) can be obtained. For examples illustrating the use of Hjorth derivation, see Wong (6).

SOURCE MODELLING (DIPOLE LOCALIZATION METHOD)

A more precise approach (mathematically speaking) of source localization is the dipole localization method (DLM) in which an exhaustive (some may say brute force) search is carried out for a voltage map (the model) that is mathematically closest to the raw data. The current sources that make up that model and their locations and directions are then taken to be the best estimate of the source configuration. Such an approach does not guarantee the accuracy of the model: rather, it is entirely a mathematical exercise, once the decision is made as to how many sources are represented in the model.

If used with a clear understanding of its limitations and assumptions, DLM based on one source (so-called single dipole model) can lead to a greater understanding of the data, and can ultimately generate ideas and observations that shed light on the clinical problem. An example is the use of DLM in studying the interictal spike activity from children with benign rolandic epilepsy, or benign childhood epilepsy with central temporal spikes (6–13).

Single source DLM requires a minimum of approximately 20 electrodes for satisfactory results. Otherwise, the localization error can be unacceptably high and render the results meaningless.

FOCUS (EEG SOURCE ACTIVITIES ANALYSIS)

By making use of DLM and the placement of stationary sources in certain locations in the hemispheres (e.g., one source in each lobe), it is possible to take the raw EEG data and estimate the contribution to it from each of these fixed sources. If there is a large temporal activity for instance, then the temporal source will show high activity and all other sources will show low activity. Theoretically, such an approach [the FOCUS method(12,14)] behaves like the CSD or Hjorth derivation, and can be used as another electrode derivation for purposes of localization. In practice, at least 28 electrodes are required in order for FOCUS to work properly, as fewer electrodes gives too sparse an electrode array.

Fig. 5a,b illustrate data from a patient, consisting of two separate interictal spikes analyzed by FOCUS. The top left panel is the original 24 electrode referential montage, to its right is the common average reference montage, with cursor. The top right is the scalp potential topography of the cursor time point; the bottom left is the source montage, using 19 source locations; the bottom right is the diagrammatic representation of the proportional amount of activity at the cursor point of the source montage. The two spikes have almost identical scalp appearance and topography; the source montage and diagram show the subtle difference: (a) is more anterior temporal, while (b) has an inferior temporal component.

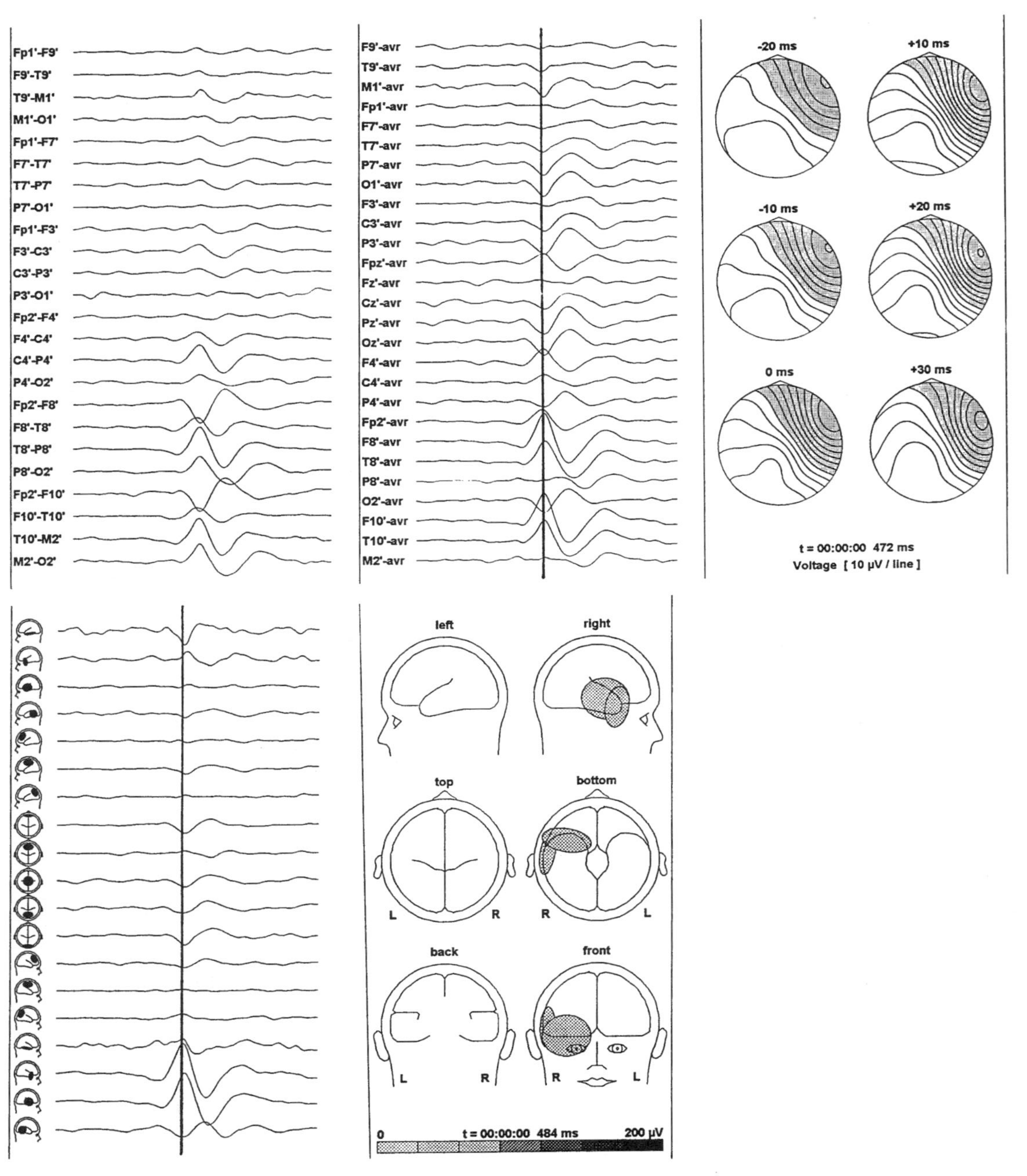

FIG. 5a,b FOCUS analysis. Two interictal spikes analyzed by FOCUS. Top left = original referential montage. Top right = common average reference montage, with cursor and topography to the right. Bottom left = source montage with 19 source locations. Bottom right = diagrammatic representation of the proportional amount of source activity at the cursor point. The spikes have almost identical scalp appearance; the source montage and diagram show the subtle difference: (a) is more anterior temporal, while (b) has an inferior temporal component not obvious from the tracings (Data courtesy of Dr. John Ebersole).

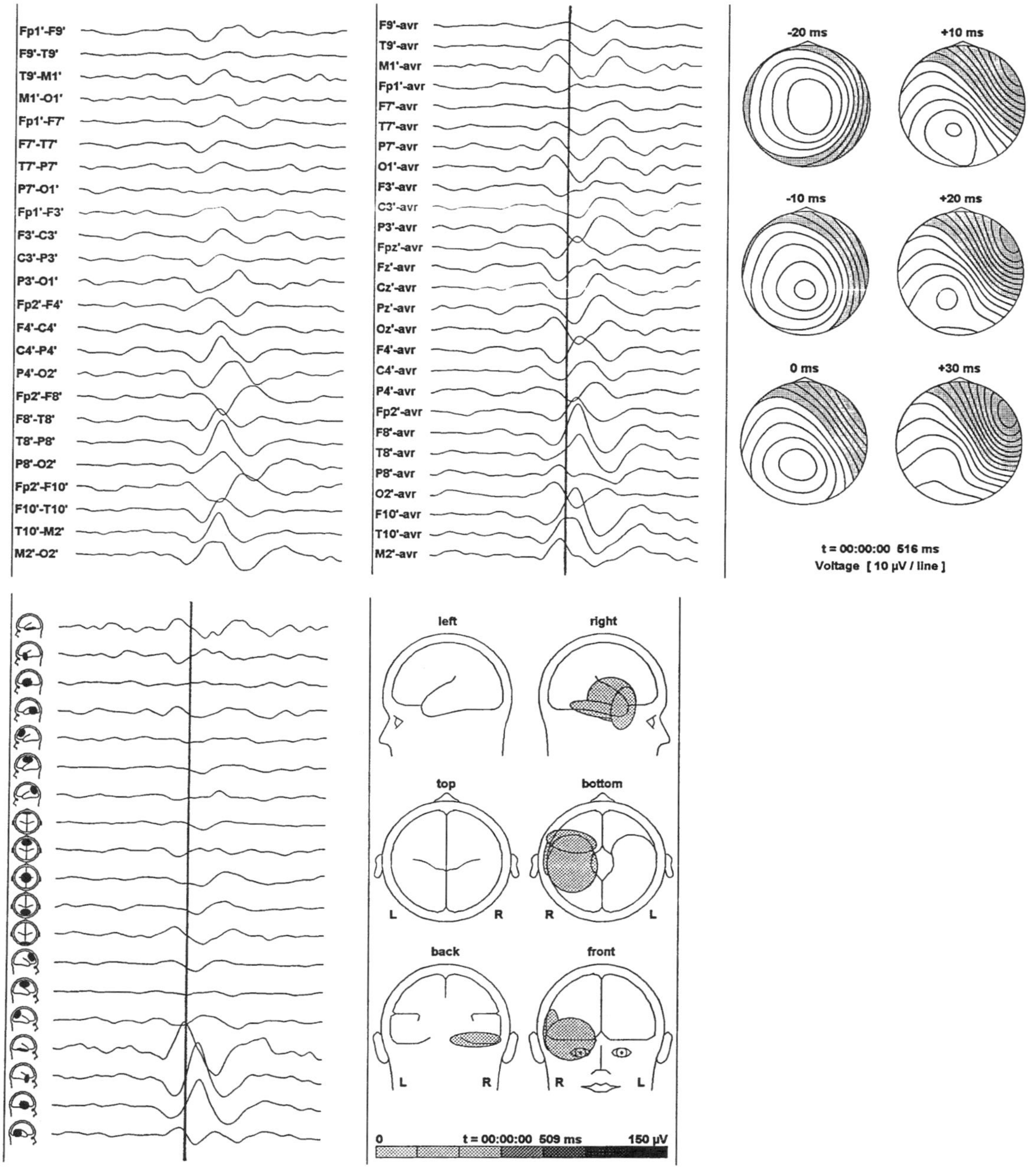

Fp1'-F9'
F9'-T9'
T9'-M1'
M1'-O1'
Fp1'-F7'
F7'-T7'
T7'-P7'
P7'-O1'
Fp1'-F3'
F3'-C3'
C3'-P3'
P3'-O1'
Fp2'-F4'
F4'-C4'
C4'-P4'
P4'-O2'
Fp2'-F8'
F8'-T8'
T8'-P8'
P8'-O2'
Fp2'-F10'
F10'-T10'
T10'-M2'
M2'-O2'
F9'-avr
T9'-avr
M1'-avr
Fp1'-avr
F7'-avr
T7'-avr
P7'-avr
O1'-avr
F3'-avr
C3'-avr
P3'-avr
Fpz'-avr
Fz'-avr
Cz'-avr
Pz'-avr
Oz'-avr
F4'-avr
C4'-avr
P4'-avr
Fp2'-avr
F8'-avr
T8'-avr
P8'-avr
O2'-avr
F10'-avr
T10'-avr
M2'-avr
-20 ms
+10 ms
-10 ms
+20 ms
0 ms
+30 ms
t = 00:00:00 516 ms
Voltage [10 µV / line]
left
right
top
bottom
L
R
R
L
back
front
L
R
R
L
0
t = 00:00:00 509 ms
150 µV

FIG. 5b.

SPIKE/SEIZURE DETECTION

Another value-added post-processing method is the detection of electrically significant events, like seizures or interictal spikes. There are many techniques that have been described to achieve rapid and accurate detection. All work by taking the incoming EEG (in real-time or off-line) from the multiple scalp leads and passing the values through a mathematical filter. When the filter detects an event, it sends an output signal to alert the technologist or the interpreter. Such a filter does not have to be perfect, as it can mark all suspicious segments for visual confirmation: indeed, visual confirmation is always the final step in this detection process as no filter is 100% accurate. The downside is that sometimes a lot of probable detections need to be screened, and this increases the chance of false positive results through carelessness.

These filter techniques include template matching, statistical analysis, rise/fall time profile and other morphological characteristics, slope and rate of change of slope measures (15), and neural net (16). All these methods have been shown to perform well under limited circumstances (e.g., small data sets), but when applied to the clinical arena where a diagnostic decision is required from 24 h seizure monitoring, the results of which will influence seizure surgery, no single method has been proven to be accurate enough as to render visual review redundant (17,18). Most centers at present appear to be using automated detection systems as the screening "front end," and relying on visual review to discard the false positive detections. This is done with full awareness that well over half, and sometimes close to 90%, of detected events will not be genuine seizures (or spikes), being usually due to artifacts (muscle, movement, electrode pop, static electricity, eye blink, tongue movement, etc.) or physiologic transients (e.g., v-wave).

Despite the best intentions, sometimes the visual review portion of the above procedure may suffer due to time pressure, so that not all the falsely detected events are recognized as such and discarded. This results in the reporting that ictal (or interictal) events were detected, thus confirming the clinical suspicion of epilepsy. For this reason, the choice of the detection system should be done with care, and each center should test it against a set of clinically-diagnosed cases covering the entire age range of potential patients. The objective is to acquire full awareness of its detection characteristics and idiosyncrasies. Many commercially available systems tend to work well for certain EEG characteristics (i.e., waking-only recordings) and perform poorly for other cases (e.g. pediatric or neonatal seizures).

6
Possible or Desirable Improvements

HEAD SHAPE SENSING

A very time consuming chore in a routine EEG (apart from the recording itself) is measuring the head for electrode positioning. With the help of commercially available three-dimensional location measuring devices, it is possible to construct a computer outline of the skull surface. Next the 10 and 20% points are computed and used for guiding the actual placement of electrodes. Such a computer-aided system has the added advantage of being able to measure the precise location of additional electrodes that may be required in the course of the recording. It can be estimated that such a procedure may take approximately 10 min, thus resulting in significant time savings. Errors in measurements are small, usually much less than those incurred routinely using a tape measure.

In the case of digital EEG units, the computer is already available, so that the only additional hardware is the three-dimensional sensor, and software. The skull outline and actual electrode positions can be saved in the data file, and thus are available for display alongside information from MRI and other modalities. The software can easily provide for the ability to rotate the head outline, so that the angle at which it is viewed can be varied at will.

The resultant system should be able to display EEG, as well as all computed results (spectrum, CSD, source models, etc.), superimposed onto an accurate skull outline of the patient, on which the three-dimensional MRI can be added. Depth electrode information can be introduced as easily as scalp EEG data. This system can be further adapted to show brain slices at any angle and depth, from any skull window (as might be contemplated for a craniotomy and grid ECoG recording prior to biopsy or resection).

ASSISTED ELECTRODE APPLICATION DEVICES

For electrode application, the fundamental requirements are precise locations, good electrical contact, and recording stability. Other desirable features include non-irritation of the skin, easy application/removal, standardization for different head sizes, etc. For purposes of facilitating this, a device called the Electro-Cap (Electro-Cap International Inc., Eaton, Ohio, USA) has been available for several years. It is based on a stretchable fabric mesh to which gel-filled electrodes are sewn. When the cap is worn, these electrodes are pressed against the scalp by an elastic strap passed under the arms or the chin for good electrical contact. Various sizes are available. The advantages of such a system are its availability and its relatively low cost. The problems include somewhat imprecise electrode locations, with little ability to adjust for asymmetrical heads (anatomic or iatrogenic, e.g., head dressings, etc.). Laboratories that demand precision over a wide range of head sizes and shapes usually find these restrictions unacceptable.

It should be possible to construct a device that is similar in principle to the cap, but with superior electrode contacts, both in terms of placement flexibility and low electrical impedance. Coupled with an automated measurement system for head shape, a very efficient system for electrode application can be made (19).

DISPLAY DEVELOPMENTS

As computer hardware and software achieve faster computing speeds and greater capabilities, graphical displays of larger size and higher resolution will become available, thus allowing more channels to be displayed, with equivalent or greater detail. Currently, special 21″ video monitors can display 32 simultaneous EEG channels with excellent clarity, although the tracings are packed closely together. With larger screen size, this problem will be alleviated.

Projection display technology that currently allows computer graphics to be projected onto a large wall screen can provide an alternative to small display size, provided that resolution is high enough to maintain the clarity of details. Current projection panels use liquid crystal display (LCD) technology. These will be replaced by an active matrix (using phototransistors etched into the glass panel) with color capability. Such large displays are suitable for review purposes only, and not for data collection, if size and portability are important considerations for bedside use.

In a different vein, digital video will revolutionize the routine EEG. Providing it is convenient and inexpensive, it will be very desirable to have both the EEG and the simultaneous video image of the patient for comparison: if a suspicious EEG segment is encountered, the patient's behavior will verify whether it was a seizure or not. Currently, video is stored in VCR cassettes that are inexpensive but slow: a search for particular point usually requires agonizingly laborious shuttling back and forth. If the video information was digitized similarly to the EEG, then it could be stored onto digital media (diskette or cartridges). The problem is that video signals require large amounts of storage, and without some form of data compression it is simply not economically feasible. Commercial data compression protocols being developed include the JPEG (Joint Photographic Experts Group) and MPEG (Motion Picture Experts Group) video standards. Hardware compression solutions are also being developed, consisting of special purpose electronic chips that can achieve quite impressive results.

SPECIALIZED COMPUTER DEVELOPMENTS

New computer central processor unit (CPU) chips are continually being announced: these have higher clock rates (a measure of the basic computing speed), greater amount of integral chip ("cache") memory, higher density of packaging (i.e., the number of transistors per square inch), faster input-output channels (for communicating with other chips), and smarter execution instruction sets. The current leaders are the 486 family (486, 586 or Pentium) made by Intel Corporation (and other look-alike clone chips), and the 68000 family used in the Apple Computer Company computers. New greatly enhanced hardware is usually followed within a few months by similar advances in software performance. At this point the end user gets the benefit in the form of enhanced performance. Features that in the past took too long to carry out (e.g., spike/seizure detection) and thus could not be done in "real time" now can be carried out "live," at the same time the data is being collected. Thus any significant event is detected immediately, an alarm activated, and appropriate action taken.

Newer software capabilities are also reflected in operating systems (the executive program that starts the computer) that allow several operations or tasks to be carried out concurrently (i.e., multitasking). This means that while one procedure is being done (e.g., calibration or data print out onto paper), other tasks can be performed (e.g., reviewing data while yet another task, such as seizure detection, is going on). Such multitasking ability is desirable, but is only efficient if the individual tasks can be done without being slowed down: a slow computer will only be able to multitask by running all the concurrent tasks at a proportionately slower speed.

Indeed, it is conceivable that hardware and software improvement will produce integrated circuits (IC) that have both analog amplifiers and digital filters on a single chip. Specialized ICs then will perform the functions that currently are done by an entire computer system. At that point the digital electroencephalograph will be embodied within a tiny package placed at the electrode grid. The operator will view the EEG at a distant facility, perhaps monitoring the collection of EEG from several patients in different locations. This implies a semiautomated recording environment with minimal human input. Certainly raw EEG must be intelligently collected, with human intervention should problems occur (annotations, artifacts), or if significant events occur (spikes, seizures). This may be possible due to refinements in computer artificial intelligence that can be embedded into modules that effectively monitor the ongoing EEG. Of course, it would be necessary for high quality simultaneous video information to be displayed along with the EEG.

PORTABILITY/CONNECTIVITY ENHANCEMENTS

The digital instrument can be miniaturized so that it can be used anywhere. Battery power means true freedom from the electrical mains. Connectivity with networks means sharing data with other centers. Artificial intelligence means competent and complete recordings with minimal supervision.

The EEG laboratory of the future may be a specialized center monitoring satellite laboratories that are all under its control. EEG interpretation would no longer be limited to the laboratory: the interpreter could use a portable computer to access the EEG/video information via the network by telephone.

INCREASED NUMBER OF CHANNELS

One of the reasons that routine EEG suffers from poor spatial localization precision when compared to other imaging modalities is due to the relatively few number of electrodes used, thus resulting in a low spatial sampling density. For the 10-20 system, the interelectrode distance is approximately 5 cm. For this to drop to 2.5 cm, the number of electrodes rises from 21 to approximately 69. If the more inferior locations are also sampled (e.g., the subtemporal chain) then even more electrodes are needed. The practical limit appears to be 128 (19).

With this maximum number of electrodes, there is an increased amount of information available, which allows more analytical computations like DLM and FOCUS, particularly the latter which performs poorly with only 20 electrodes.

QUANTITATIVE PROCEDURES

Deblurring

Gevins et al (19) and Le et al (20) described the estimation of cortical surface activity derived from a large scalp electrode array. Their procedure is based on the CSD approach, with correction for skull defects from high resolution MRI images. Such a procedure allows a greater resolution by decreasing the uncertainty from bone attenuation, particularly as bone thickness varies over the skull. This in essence allows ECoG with noninvasive means. The accuracy, of course, is inferior to direct ECoG, but as a noninvasive technique it has much attraction.

Dipole Localization (Realistic Heads/Sources)

By using realistic head shapes instead of the usual spherical head, and by correcting for bone thickness variations (including the various foramina), DLM models can be successful under certain circumstances in localizing cortical sources accurately.

PHYSIOLOGIC INTEGRATION AND MULTIMODAL INFORMATION DISPLAY

Combination of physiological information from various sources allow a more comprehensive assessment of the brain. Anatomic information from high resolution MRI, electrical information from EEG, magnetic information from magnetoencephalography (MEG), metabolic information from positron emission tomography (PET), SPECT, or functional MRI, etc. can be made available to the interpreter during review (21). The outcome can be a much better understanding of brain function, thus facilitating more accurate diagnosis. These disparate images need not be superimposed together, as this is not always logical: the EEG reflects cortical activity, while the others have three-dimensional characteristics. Just having convenient access to all these kinds of information for cross-reference purposes will be advantageous.

The integration of digital video into digital EEG machinery will alleviate the labor intensive aspect of video monitoring. No longer will it be necessary to catalog and maintain a large library of VCR cassettes. All the episodes of interest can be stored together in a multimedia digital file, instantly available for review or conference presentation. The addition of neuroimaging data (from the radiology department via the hospital network) will add another dimension of information. In fact, the MRI scan images can be in the form of a multimedia presentation of selected slices, with voice and cursor illustration of the important points for consideration, much like a slide-tape show. In this manner, the MRI files need never leave the radiology library. It is even conceivable that epilepsy surgery conferences might be carried out on-line, with no requirement for attendees to be in the same room.

Appendix A
Forms Used in CMS

1. INTERPRETATION WORKSHEET

1. Classification code:
   Waking: Drowsiness: Sleep: Meds:
2. Seizure occurred (dUring / Immed before / few (Min/Hr/Day) before) this EEG.
3. Patient was [Uncooperative / Moving with artifacts / not Asleep] {Good backgd unobtainable}.
4. (Alert / Drowsy / stUpor / Coma) bkgd {R/L} was (Well / mOd / Min / Poor) organized {α ( ) – ( ) Hz}
   and {Was / Not/ Mild/ mOd/Invariant} reactive. Hyperventilation {Hv normal}.
5. {Rare/ Occ/ Freq/ Pers/ Cont/ pErio} [Indepen/Synchr/ Gen/ Vert/Mltif/miX]
   [bUrst of/Spike/sHarp wave/spike-Wave n/Fragmentary s-w n/Atypical s-w/Polyspike/sLow wave/paroXysmal/Delta/Theta/Beta/Complexes] {[R/L/Bilat/mId] – [Anter/poSt/Hem/Quad/F/C/T/P/O]} area(s) in {[Wake/ Drowsy/ Sleep/ Arousal/ Hv/ Ps]} states. *This sentence can be repeated as necessary.*
6. Noxious stimulation produced (No / Minimal/ mOderate/ marKed change/ Suppression) in the EEG background.
7. [Spindles/ V waves/ K complexes] were {[Normal/ Seen/ aBsent/ Poorly seen/ asYnchronous/ Asymmetric]}. {Disorganized sleep background.}
8. Photic stimulation: (Good/ Moderate/ Little/ No/ High amplitude) driving.
9. No [Lateraliz / Focal/ Abnormal/ Epileptiform/ electrical Seizure] activity noted.

! IMPRESSION: [Wake/ Drowsy/ Sleep/Brief sleep/ stUpor/ Coma/ Quiet-Active] is (Normal/Essen. norm/Abnor/Mildly abnor/mOderately abnor/Severe abnor).

$ Background is [Normal/Essen. norm/Slow/dysRhyth/suPpressed/Asymmet].

& This EEG is (Suggestive / Compatible / Diagnostic) of [Non-specific changes / sEizure disorder / Structural lesion].

+ It would be (Useful / Desirable / Important) to repeat (Routine / Waking/ Sleep deprived / sEdated) EEG. {This may be (/Few) (Days/Weeks/Months)}.

*= Compare last EEG {(/Few) (Days/ Weeks/ Months/ Years) ago} is (Similar/ Deterior/ imProve) {Min/ mOd/ Greatly} {Incomparable to previous}.

2. EXAMPLE OF EEG REPORT GENERATION

Keyboard Entry

4AW9-10WH 5FSRTS 7S+V+KN 8G !W+SA "There was evidence for focal epileptiform activity in the left temporal region."

Individual Translation of the 5 Coded Sentences

4 The **A**lert background shows **W**ell organized posterior dominant activity (alpha rhythm **9–10** Hz), which **W**as reactive to eyes open/closing. **H**yperventilation was normal.
5 **F**requent **S**pike activity was seen in the **R**ight **T**emporal area in **S**leep.
7 **S**leep potentials, **V**-waves, and **K**-complexes were **N**ormal.
8 Photic stimulation showed **G**ood driving response.
! Impression: This EEG, obtained in **W**aking and **S**leep, is **A**bnormal.

Final Wording of Report

Findings:

The alert background shows well organized posterior dominant activity (alpha rhythm 9 to 10 Hz), which was reactive to eyes open/closing. Hyperventilation was normal.

Frequent spike activity was seen in the right temporal area in sleep. Sleep potentials, V-waves, and K-complexes were normal. Photic stimulation showed good driving response.

Impression:

This EEG, obtained in waking and sleep, is abnormal. There was evidence for focal epileptiform activity in the left temporal region.

3. HISTORY FORM (ABBREVIATED)

HOSP#:_______ FIRSTNAME:________ SURNAME: _________

DOB: ________ VISIT DATE: ________ NO History AVAIL:____

GA:__________ wks BW: ___lb ____oz ____g

Pregnancy/Delivery Complications:

NIL ABruptio Placenta AspHyxia low APGars BREech C/S DRugs Fetal Distress FoRceps InFection INDuced MEconium Pregnancy Comp PRolonged ResUscitation SPoTting ToXemia TWin Other_______________________

Neonatal Complications:

NIL APnea BRAdycardia CArdiac Failure to Thrive JAundice IVH NEC PDA PVL ReSp distress SeiZures SEpsis VEntilated VP Shunt Other: ______________________

Past History

NIL ASthma FAints FC Physical ABuse Renal Transplant SeiZures TRauma Other:__________________

Family History

/? NIL CaNcer CArdiac DM FAints FC LA MiGraine MR PsYch SZ Other: ____________

EEG #: __________ Disk #: __________

Doctor: __________ Copies To: __________ Tech: __________

4. PATIENT VISIT FORM (ABBREVIATED)

Development

N/A N Slow Motor slow SPeech Devel Delay MR Severe mR REgression Other: __________

School

N/A INTegrated Appropriate Grade Learning Assistance Below Grade Special Class/or ScHooL Other: __________

Intelligence

N/A Above Average AVerage Low AVerage BorDerline miLd mR Mod MR Severe mR Other: __________

Sz Type(s)

NIL /Seizure? 1=gen 2=2° gen Partial ComPLex partial Unclass PseUdo sz BreathHolding NEOnatal APnea ALternating Hemiplegia CYcling ELectrographic MIgratory MOuthing POsturing SUbclinical UNilateral ABsence ADversive APHasia ATonic ATypical Absence Atypical FC Always with Fever Sometimes with Fever Benign Rolandic Ep CLonic Febrile Convulsions Frontal ESES Tonic Clonic INfantile spasms JME Staring Spells Motor Sz L side Motor Sz R side MYoclonic NOCturnal NiGht Terrors Occipital PhotoSensitive Post Traumatic SENsory STatus Temporal TOnic VAsovagal Eye Deviation Other: __________

Sz Freq: __________ Total # of Seizures: __________
Onset Date: __________ Date of Last Attack: __________

N.Exam

N /N? ABsent DTRs ATaXia Cranial NErve palsy DIplegia DYsarthria DySmorphic GAit HypeRtonic HypOtonic L Hemi R Hemi R or L Motor Fine Motor/Gross Motor MicroCephalic NYstagmus Optic Atrophy Optic Neuritis PAPilloedema Spastic Quad TREmor visual Field Defect R L BrainStem dysfunction Min Brainstem Reflexes fixed Dilated Pupils no WIthdrawal Withdrawal to deep pain Minimal Gag No Gag VEntilator Stupor Vegetative State Other: __________

Other

NIL ANoxia ATTention deficit BEhaviour CNS Tumour Congen.Malformation ENcephalitis DegeNerative disease DiZziness HeadAche HYdrocephalus InFection Lennox-Gastaut MENingitis METabolic MiGraine MS MYOpathy VERtigo Near Drowning NEurofibromatosis PaChygyria PsYchiatric ReTTs RETinopathy RUEbella SHUnt STructural Lesion ScHool problems TRauma Tuberous Sclerosis VAsovagal VAScular VP Shunt

CT: ______________________ MRI: ____________________
Teaching File: ______________Tech Comment: _____________

Appendix B
EEG Classification System

1. GENERAL RULES

1. Classify background abnormalities first then other abnormalities in order of severity starting with the most severe.
2. Waking is always the first state classified. If an acceptable sufficient waking recording was not obtained, then the drowsiness or sleep recording only should be classified.
3. All abnormalities classified as above must be definite findings. If there is suspicion of an abnormality that is assumed genuine but not persistent enough to warrant an abnormal classification, it can be classified as a "questionable" abnormality by placing a question mark before the classification.

2. RULES FOR CLASSIFYING WAKING AND SLEEP

1. If an abnormality occurs only in waking, it will be classified under waking accordingly, with drowsiness and sleep classified as normal (N).
2. If present, the waking recording is always classified first. If a new abnormality appears in drowsiness or sleep the appropriate classification is to be given in the state separately.
3. An abnormality present consistently through waking, drowsiness, and sleep is not rewritten beside each state. It will be classified in the waking state only, and no change (n) will appear under drowsiness and sleep.
4. If an abnormality is present in the resting waking record and enhanced during photic stimulation, hyperventilation, sleep, finger tapping, or auditory stimulation, a slash (/) is put after the waking classification followed by the mode of enhanced activation, e.g., hyperventilation, photic, sleep, tactile stimulation, or auditory stimulation. If there is a right occipital spike focus present while awake that is enhanced by photic stimulation and sleep it would be classified as a waking dysRhythmia grade 4 Right Occipital Spike, enhanced by Photic and Sleep (W: R4RO-S/P/S). When used in this way the slash follows only those classifications that are enhanced by an activator. If there were more than one abnormality in waking but only the right occipital spikes were activated by photic and sleep,

it would appear as a dysRhythmia grade 4 Right Occipital Spikes activated by Photic and Sleep, and a Delta 1 Right Occipital (W: R4RO-S/P/S D1RO S: /). Note that when using a slash to denote enhancement in sleep a corresponding slash is put at the sleep classification as a reminder. Any new abnormality appearing in sleep that was not classified in waking would then follow the slash.

5. If all findings listed during waking are activated by sleep, one double slash (//) can be placed at the end of the waking classification and a double slash under sleep, e.g., R1G, R4LO-S + RC-P//S, S: //

3. CLASSIFICATION PROCEDURE

Normal (N)

Within normal limits for age.

Essentially Normal (E)

Minor variations that are at the borderline limits of normal.

Dysrhythmia (R)

Grades 0 to 3 are general categories containing waves that are usually slow, rhythmic, repetitive, and tend to be inhibited by eye opening and accentuated by hyperventilation. This classification must always be accompanied by a grade and a qualifier. Grade 4 is for specific epileptiform activity. Grade 5 is for specific nonepileptiform activity.

Grade 0: Minimal abnormalities slightly worse than essentially normal.
Grade 1: Minimal abnormalities, continuous or paroxysmal, amplitude up to 30 μV above that of normal activity.
Grade 2: Moderate abnormalities, continuous or paroxysmal, amplitude up to 100 μV above that of normal activity.
Grade 3: Severe abnormalities, continuous or paroxysmal, amplitude exceeding 100 μV above that of normal activity.
Grade 4: Specific epileptiform waveforms, i.e., Spikes, sHarp waves, spike and Wave, Multifocal spikes, recorded seiZures, dipoles, Recruiting rhythms, Photic Sensitivity, Electrodecremental or Incremental events, Fragmentary spike and wave, etc.
Grade 5: Specific nonepileptic waveforms, i.e., ctenoids, small sharp spikes, 6/s spike and wave, Extreme spindles, Beta, FIRDA, hYpsarrythmia, Alpha coma, theta coma, and Triphasic waves.

Grades 0 to 3 must be accompanied by the location. If a mild diffuse dysrhythmia is present it is a dysRhythmia grade 1 Generalized (R1G). If there is a moderate focal abnormality in the left frontal region, it is classified as a dysRhythmia grade 1 Left Frontal (R1LF). If more than one location is involved they appear in order of severity, e.g., dysRhythmia grade 1 Left Frontal Central Temporal (R1LFCT).

Grades 0 to 3 on their own imply a continuous dysrhythmia. Placing an exclamation mark after the grade will denote a paroxysmal dysrhythmia, e.g., occasional bursts of generalized high amplitude theta would be classified as a paroxysmal dysRhythmia grade 2 Generalized (R2!G).

Grade 4 must be accompanied by the location, as above, and by a description of the specific waveform, e.g., dysRhythmia grade 4 Left Frontal Central Spikes (R4LFC-S). The waveform is always separated from the classification by a hyphen. If there are three independent noncontiguous foci between the two hemispheres, they are classified as dysRhythmia grade 4 Multiple independent spikes (R4M-S). If the multiple independent spikes are clearly maximum in one area the focality would appear after the descriptor, e.g., a dysRhythmia grade 4 Multiple independent spikes maximum Right Frontal (R4M-S/RF). The slash denotes maximum in that area.

Grade 5 lateralized waveforms must have a location following the classification grade as for grade 4, e.g., dysRhythmia grade 5 Left Temporal small sharp spikes (R5LT-s) or focal Right Frontal Beta (R5RF-B). The other specific but unlateralized waveforms do not require location, e.g., ctenoids, hYpsarythmia, Alpha coma, Theta coma, 6/s Spike and Wave, Triphasic waves, etc.

Delta (D)

Random slow (0 to 3.9 Hz) waves. Arrhythmic and nonrepetitive. Usually unaffected by eye opening and hyperventilation.

Grade 1: Amplitude up to 30 μV, 2 to 3 Hz.
Grade 2: Amplitude up to 100 μV or 1 Hz or less.
Grade 3: Amplitude above 100 μV.

Delta abnormalities are classified along the same lines as dysrhythmias. Each grade must be accompanied by the location. If there is a low amplitude delta diffusely it is classified as a Delta grade 1 Generalized (D1G). If there is a focal left central delta it is classified as a Delta grade 1 Left Central (D1LC). Delta can also be categorized as generalized and maximal in one area, e.g., Delta grade 1 Generalized maximum Left Central (D1G/LC).

Asymmetry (A)

Represents an amplitude asymmetry of normal components (background rhythms) between homologous regions of the two hemispheres. The severity of the asymmetry may be graded with increasing degree.

Grade 1: Consistent and 25 to 50%.
Grade 2: Consistent and 50 to 75%.
Grade 3: Consistent and greater than 75%.

An adjective (less “<” or greater “>”) and the location follows the grade, e.g., if the activity from the left frontal region is 30% lower in amplitude than the right frontal region it is classified as an Asymmetry grade 1 lower Left Frontal (A1<LF). The classification of an asymmetry denotes an amplitude asymmetry only. It does not indicate which area is abnormal. It does not describe a frequency asymmetry.

Suppression (S)

Indicates an abnormal decrease in physiologic cerebral electrical activity.

Grade 1: Mild suppression.
Grade 2: Moderate suppression.
Grade 3: Electrocerebral silence (ECS).

Each grade must be accompanied by a location, e.g., if there is mildly less than expected activity for age diffusely it is classified as a Suppression grade 1 Generalized (S1G). If there is a marked suppression of activity over the right central region, it is classified as a Suppression grade 2 Right Central (S2RC).

Technically Unsatisfactory (U)

For technical reasons the record cannot be interpreted. Can be used in the classification of one state only or all states, e.g., if only the waking recording had a pulse artifact at C3 that interfered with an interpretation of a delta in that region, it would be classified as Technically Unsatisfactory in waking and sleep would be normal (W: U S:N).

Sleep (Z) Potentials

Asymmetric Sleep Potentials (ZA)

Used when there is a persistent asymmetry of V-waves, sleep spindles, or K-complexes.

Abnormal Sleep Potentials (ZB)

Used when there are abnormal sleep potentials for age, e.g., absence of spindles and V-waves at 8 months of age.

Asynchronous Sleep Potentials (Za)

Used when sleep potentials are consistently asynchronous.

These adjectives are used in the sleep classification only, either alone or with another abnormality, e.g., if an entire waking and sleep EEG was normal except that the sleep spindles were present only on the left, it would be classified as: Waking: normal, Sleep: Asymmetric sleep potentials (W: N, S: ZA<R).

If there is a normal background and a right central spike focus in waking that then spread to also involve the temporal frontal regions in sleep, and the V-waves and spindles are absent on the right, it would be classified as: Waking: dysRhythmia grade 4 Right Central Spikes; Sleep: dysRhythmia grade 4 Right Central Temporal Frontal, Asymmetric Zsleep potentials <lower on the Right (W: R4RC-S S: R4RCFT-S, ZA<R).

Dipole and Tripole Topography Spikes

Describe dipoles by negative pole first then positive pole. Separate opposite poles with periods. Describe tripoles as negative pole, positive pole, negative pole, starting anteriorly and moving posteriorly.

E.g., R4LT.F - Sd or R4LaF.T.O – St

Variable finding indicated by an inverted comma after dipole, i.e. R4LT.F – Sd'

4. CLASSIFICATION SYMBOLS

States

W = waking
D = drowsiness
S = sleep
A = arousal
C = coma
T = stupor
P = pavulonized

Locations

G = generalized
M = multifocal
b = bilateral
H = hemisphere
Q = quadrant
i = independent
I = mid
F = frontal
C = central
P = parietal
O = occipital
T = temporal
a = anterior
s = posterior

Classifications

N = normal
E = essentially normal
R = dysrhythmia (grade 0 to 5)

R4 Qualifiers

S = spike
R = recruiting rhythm
B = PBDA (paroxysmal posterior delta activity)
H = sharp
S = photic sensitivity
X = periodic epileptiform discharges (PLEDs)
W = spike and wave
d = dipole
t = tripole
W3 = 3/s spike and wave
A = atypical spike-wave
L = slow wave
F = fragmentary spike and wave
P = polyspikes
SBS = 2° bilateral synchrony
O = positive spike/sharp wave
I = electroincremental event
E = electrodecremental event
z = electrographic seizure only
Z = clinical and electrographic seizure
M = multifocal

R5 Qualifiers

C = ctenoids
Y = hypsarrhythmia
H = theta coma
6 = 6/s spike and wave
s = small sharp spikes
F = FIRDA (frontal intermittent rhythmic delta activity)
E = extreme spindles
B = beta
A = alpha coma
T = triphasic waves

U = burst suppression
x = bilateral periodic epileptiform discharges (biPLEDs)
P = psychomotor variant
V = alpha variant SSP
SSPE = subacute sclerosing pan-encephalitis
O = OIRDA (occipital intermittent rhythmic delta activity)

General Qualifiers

! = paroxysmal finding
/ = maximum (area or condition)
? = questionable finding
= tech's classification
' = variable
^ = rare finding
~ = rhythmic, repetitive
// = whole of preceding class max in

Delta (D)

Grades 1 to 3

Asymmetry (A)

Grades 1 to 3
< = lower amplitude, > = greater amplitude

Suppression (S)

Grades 1 to 3

Reactivity (X)

1 = definite
2 = some
3 = none

Technically Unsatisfactory (U)

Conditions

N = noise–auditory stimulation
EO = max. with eyes open
o = only with eyes open
EC = max. with eyes closed
ec = only with EC
H = maximum in hyperventilation
h = only in hyperventilation
P = maximum in photic stimulation
p = only in photic stimulation
A = maximum on arousal
a = only on arousal
tn = no response with tapping
T = tactile evoked

Sleep

N = normal
E = essentially normal
n = no change
ZB = abnormal sleep potentials
ZA = asymmetric sleep potentials
Za = asynchronous sleep potentials
Zt = paroxysmal theta bursts
ZP = sleep potentials seen in coma
ZF = FAR (frontal arousal response)

References

1. Dummermuth G, Molinari L. In: Gevins AS, Remond A, eds. *Handbook of EEG and clinical neurophysiology, volume 1*. Amsterdam: Elsevier; 1987:85–125.
2. Gregory DL, Wong PKH. Clinical relevance of a dipole field in rolandic spikes. *Epilepsia* 1992;33(1):36–44.
3. Gregory DL, Wong PKH. Topographical analysis of the centrotemporal discharges in benign rolandic epilepsy of childhood. *Epilepsia* 1984;25(6):705–711.
4. Gevins A, Le J, Martin N, Brickett P, Desmond J, Reutter B. High resolution EEG: 124 channel recording, spatial deblurring and MRI integration. *Electroencephalogr Clin Neurophysiol* 1994;90:337–358.
5. Perrin F, Pernier J, Betrand O, Giard MH, Echallier JF. Mapping of scalp potentials by surface spline interpolation. *Electroencephalogr Clin Neurophysiol* 1987;66:75–81.
6. Wong PKH. Source modelling of the rolandic focus. *Brain Topogr* 1991;4(2): 105–112.
7. Wong PKH. Topographic EEG analysis. In: Wada JA, Ellingson RJ, eds. *Handbook of EEG and clinical neurophysiology, volume 4*. Amsterdam: Elsevier; 1990:389–405.
8. Wong PKH. The importance of source behaviour in distinguishing populations of epileptic foci. *J Clin Neurophys* 1993;10(3):314–322.
9. Ebersole JS, Wade PB. Intracranial EEG validation of spike topography and dipole modelling in the presurgical localization of epileptic foci. *Epilepsia* 1989;30:696.
10. Ebersole JS, Wade PB. Temporal spikes are not all the same—a topographic EEG analysis in surgical candidates. *Neurology* 1989;39(Suppl 1):299 (abstract).
11. Ebersole JS, Wade PB. Spike voltage topography identifies two types of fronto-temporal epileptic foci. *Neurology* 1991;41:1425–1433.
12. Ebersole JS. EEG dipole modelling in complex partial epilepsy. *Brain Topogr* 1991;4:113–123.
13. Aktari M, McNay D, Mandelkern M, Teeter B, Cline HE, Mallick J, Clark G, Tatar R, Lifkin R, Chan R, Rogers RL, Sutherling WW. Somatosensory evoked response source localization using actual cortical surface as the spatial constraint. *Brain Topogr* 1994;7:63–69.
14. Scherg M, Ebersole JS. Models of brain sources. *Brain Topogr* 1993;5(4):419–423.
15. Panych LP, Wada JA. Computer applications in data analysis. In: Wada JA, Ellingson RJ, eds. *Handbook of EEG and clinical neurophysiology, volume 4*. Amsterdam: Elsevier; 1990:361–385.
16. Webber WR, Litt B, Wilson K, Lesser RP. Practical detection of epileptiform discharges in the EEG using an artificial neural network. *Electroencephalogr Clin Neurophysiol* 1994;91(3):194–204.
17. Pauri F, Pierelli F, Chatrian GE, Erdly WW. Long-term EEG-video-audio monitoring, computer detection of focal EEG seizure patterns. *Electroencephalogr Clin Neurophysiol* 1992;82(1):1–9.
18. Gotman J, Burgess R, Darcey T, Hasner R, Ives J, Lesser R, Pijn JP, Velis DN. Computer applications. In: Engel J Jr, ed. *Surgical treatment of the epilepsies, 2nd ed.* New York: Raven Press; 1993:429–444.
19. Gevins A, Brickett P, Costales B, Le J, Reutter B. Beyond topographic mapping: towards functional-anatomical imaging with 124-channel and 3-D MRIs. *Brain Topogr* 1990;3(1):53–64.
20. Le J, Gevins AS. Method to reduce blur distortion from EEGs using a realistic head model. *IEEE Trans Biomed Eng* 1993;40:517–528.
21. Stefan H, Schneider S, Feistel H, Pawlik G, Schuler P, Abrahams-Fuchs K, Schlegel T, Neubauer U, Huk WJ. Ictal and interictal activity in partial epilepsy recorded with multichannel MEG: correlation of EEG/ECoG, MRI, SPECT and PET findings. *Epilepsia* 1992;33(5):874–887.

Index

T

ISBN 0-397-51635-5
9 780397 516353

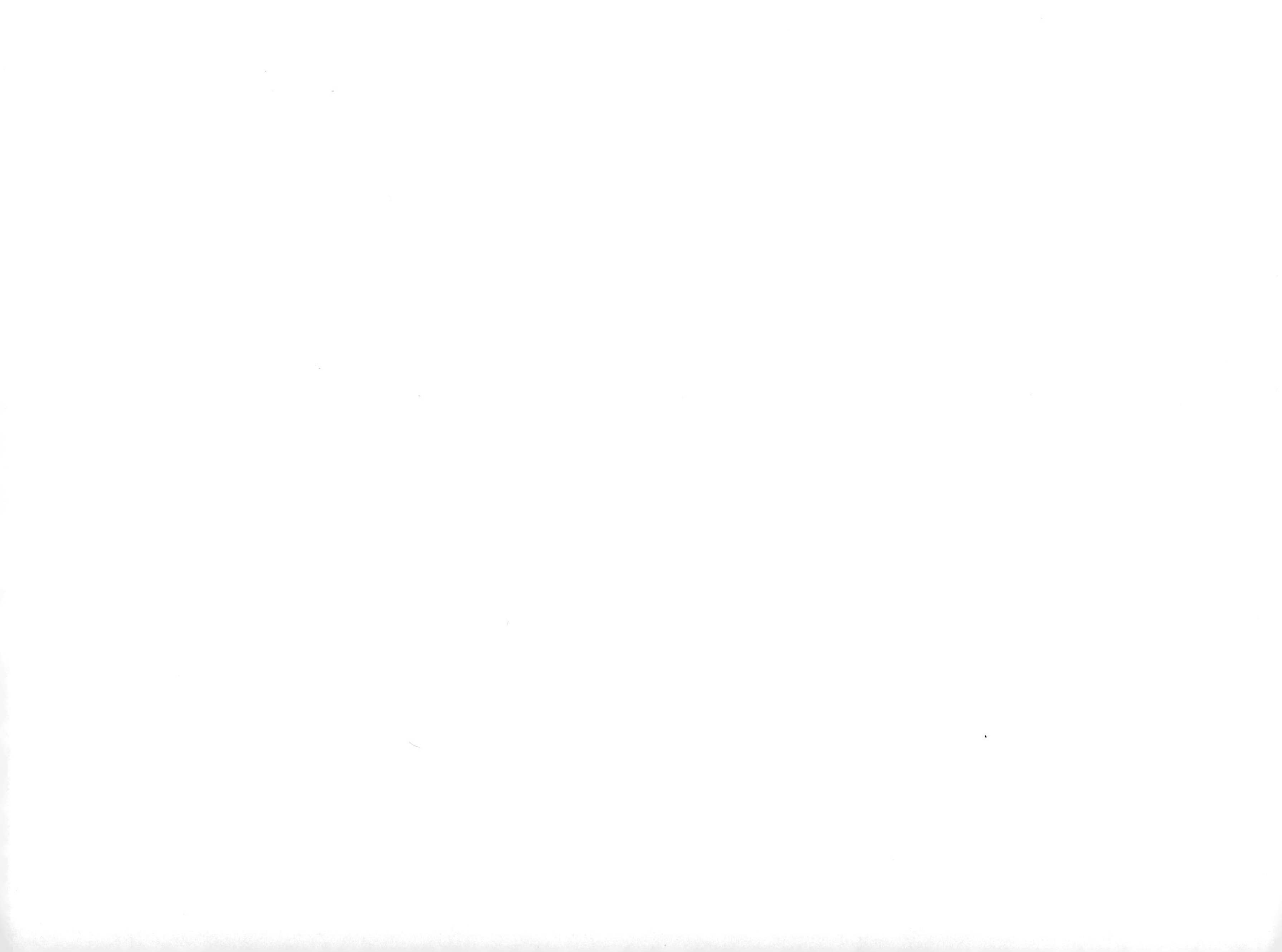